Critical Perspectives on Technological Innovations in Healthcare

Andreas Charalambous
Editor

Critical Perspectives on Technological Innovations in Healthcare

Building the Future

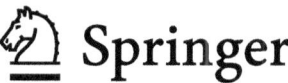 Springer

Editor
Andreas Charalambous
Faculty of Health Science
Department of Nursing Science
Cyprus University of Technology
Limassol, Cyprus

ISBN 978-3-031-87157-3   ISBN 978-3-031-87158-0   (eBook)
https://doi.org/10.1007/978-3-031-87158-0

This Springer imprint is published by the registered company Springer Nature Switzerland AG
The registered company address is: Gewerbestrasse 11, 6330 Cham, Switzerland

If disposing of this product, please recycle the paper.

Foreword

A new healthcare landscape is emerging, shaped by unprecedented technological advancement, accelerated by global challenges like the SARS-CoV-2 pandemic, that enabled the rapid adoption of technologies that would have taken years otherwise. That experience teaches us about the possibilities and limitations of digital health solutions—many of which are analysed in *Critical Perspectives on Technological Innovations in Healthcare*. This is a timely and comprehensive review of technological innovations in healthcare—an issue very relevant to our current healthcare landscape in early 2025. All who wish to keep up with the latest developments in healthcare should read this book, particularly its impact on cancer care and treatment.

We are positioned at the interface between traditional healthcare delivery and newer technological possibilities that promise to reshape how we prevent, diagnose, treat, and manage diseases. This moment is urgent, and the innovations discussed herein are paradigm shifts in healthcare delivery.

Its scope reflects the broad nature of technological integration in healthcare. With their unparalleled experience, the authors navigate the maze of telemonitoring, digital literacy for healthcare professionals, cultural competence in healthcare AI, and robotics in twenty-first century cancer care. Especially noteworthy is the consideration of health inequalities and how technological innovations might reduce these gaps.

The work is especially balanced. The authors celebrate the potential of technological innovations while also being critical of obstacles to implementation. Discussing the training requirements for professionals and patients and the cultural competence of healthcare technologies shows an appreciation of what it takes to integrate these innovations into clinical practice.

Looking forward, technological innovation will undoubtedly become increasingly central to healthcare. However, our ultimate viability will depend not so much on the sophistication of our technologies as much as on how we apply them—fairly, justly, and ethically. This book gives valuable suggestions about how to reach those ends—providing practical strategies and solutions for healthcare professionals, technology developers, policymakers, and anyone interested in the future of healthcare delivery.

It is an indispensable guide for the practical application of these innovations—an indispensable guide for all those working towards better healthcare through technological innovation.

The authors created a helpful guide that will undoubtedly influence how we think about and implement technological advances in healthcare. Their work informs and encourages us to see the thoughtful application of such tools in the context of patient care as the ultimate success of healthcare innovation.

While we face complex healthcare challenges like the fight against cancer, the perspectives and insights in this volume will be a useful road map through the technological transformation of healthcare. The authors of this critical dialogue deserve my highest recommendation. They have dedicated their expertise to those working to improve healthcare through technological innovation.

European Cancer Organisation   Dégi László Csaba
Brussels, Belgium

Preface

In recent years, there has been an unprecedented infiltration of technological solutions in healthcare. I have, as a healthcare professional but mostly as a researcher, contributed to the introduction of technological solutions in various fields of healthcare. Caught up in an overwhelming feeling that technology can possibly solve most problems in healthcare, I have begun a journey with the aim to improve cancer care through the inception, designing, and testing various technological solutions. Solutions that are being utilised across the disease continuum can facilitate the provision of care that ranges from simple tasks to more complex ones. The evidence show clearly that technology has become a valuable tool in the hands of healthcare professionals in an effort to provide comprehensive and quality care focusing on addressing complex and/or unmet needs. Equally, in the hands of patients and caregivers, technology has been viewed as the means for a smooth continuation of care to the home setting, a tool to increase their self-management (i.e. symptom and adverse event management) and achieve empowerment by increasing their ability to participate in health-related decision-making.

Looking at the past, the way cancer was treated and the way patients perceived and received care has changed drastically. Technological breakthroughs have allowed us to better understand how cancer develops and to find new ways and improve existing ones to better treat the disease. It has improved our chances of early and more accurate diagnosis (e.g. artificial intelligence-enhanced imaging and AI-powered pathology) and enhanced our knowledge of how to best treat patients through precision medicine. This was achieved by improving the process of tailoring treatment to an individual patient's genetics and lifestyle as well as the cellular and molecular features of the tumour and its microenvironment (e.g. personalised medicine, AI-enhanced integration of genetic and medical imaging data). Now more than ever, technology has allowed a more person-centred approach to care, offering the ability to constantly adapt to the needs of the person. As the landscape of cancer changes, there is also a shifting of traditional systems of providing care within the hospital to providing care closer to home. The evolution of treatments, the desire of the patient to receive care in a familiar environment, and the fiscal pressures on health systems together with the development and availability of the appropriate technology (e.g. wearables for monitoring) have led to an increase in the services that are provided at home and the community.

Despite the fact that scepticism still remains, technology in healthcare has been widely embraced; however, it cannot be seen as a panacea. The new technologies have the potential to radically transform healthcare; however, they still pose significant challenges, including regulatory barriers, difficulties in retrieving quality data, and effectively digitising patient data. Furthermore, global trends such as an ageing population and general constraints on government spending are factors that make effective digital transformation of the healthcare industry imperative, with digital technologies playing a central role in this change. Just as any digital solution introduced in a different context can suffer from personalisation issues during its development phase, the same goes for healthcare. Hence, possible poor personalisation practices can result in technologies that do not meet the needs of the users or might be too disruptive. Technological solutions have diverse learning curves, but almost in every case, a necessary level of digital skills background is necessary to support the effective and efficient utilisation of the technology and ensure its sustainability over time. There are however concerns whether, for example, the healthcare professionals have the necessary knowledge and skills and therefore the appropriate readiness to take advantage of these opportunities to their full potential.

This book was therefore conceived to provide critical perspectives on the issues that surround the introduction of technological innovations in healthcare.

This book has been prepared by specialists from diverse disciplines and professions in an attempt to provide critical perspectives on technological innovations in healthcare, highlighting discussions on contemporary issues in the sphere of technology in healthcare. The SARS-CoV-2 beyond the shockwaves that it sent across healthcare (and beyond), it has contributed to the fast track introduction of numerous technological innovations mediating this way the change in the landscape of technological innovation in healthcare. As the introduction of any technological innovation largely relies on the capacity and preparedness of the healthcare professionals, this book records the experiences of researchers leading the TRANSiTION project, which has been specifically designed to address these challenges across Europe. The challenges faced by any innovative, interdisciplinary research project aiming to develop socially assistive robots that are culturally aware is discussed thoroughly, drawing on projects such as the CARESSES. This book brings the collective experience of researchers developing solutions such as telemonitoring, teleconsultation, rehabilitation, and virtual environments (AI powered) that primarily aim at providing supportive care to different groups of patients (e.g. AYAs) and informal caregivers. Furthermore, covering another part of the disease continuum, this book highlights recent research evidence on the use of AI in screening (i.e. AI-powered medical imaging). Healthcare being governed by a significant number of inequalities across the disease continuum, the ways, and the potential of technological innovation to help address these inequalities is discussed. The central role that data generated within healthcare define the way care is being planned and delivered is thoroughly discussed, drawing also on their influential role on techno-logical innovations. The use of innovative technology solutions in healthcare, as mentioned above, is not without challenges. This book provides an insight into these challenges that developers and users of such technologies might face and how these can be changed into opportunities.

"Supportive Care should be Context-Free, as such it can thrive through the appropriate Technological Solutions and the necessary human oversight".

Limassol, Cyprus   Andreas Charalambous

Contents

How SARS-CoV-2 Changed the Landscape of Healthcare: Opportunities for Technological Innovation

Andreas Charalambous

1   Introduction

An extensive body of evidence demonstrates the significant impact of the COVID-19 pandemic on health systems on a global scale [1, 2] but also on the continued impact to this day that threatens the efficiency of systems [3, 4]. Such crises/emergencies have an impact on the primary goal of public healthcare which is to make healthcare resources more efficient and accessible. The unpredictability of diseases or pandemics and other emergencies, may cause problems for health systems to deliver suitable and timely resource allocation.

Although the full grasp of the impact is difficult to be estimated, it is widely accepted that the pandemic has affected health systems in their totality. Aspects such as the provision as well as the utilization of healthcare services because of such measures as lockdowns and stay-at-home orders were consider to have suffered a major impact. The healthcare workforce as the main driver of these health systems has also experienced a heavy impact as a result of the direct and indirect implications of the pandemic. Although the disruptions in the health service delivery have been recorded on a global scale, evidence indicate that the COVID-19 pandemic has made more significant disruption in health service delivery particularly in resource-limited countries potentially due to their reduced ability to absorb the increased demands placed by the disease [5].

The COVID-19 crisis had and is still having a huge impact on individuals, organizations, and society. Despite all the tragedy it caused, it also created room for learning and change. It is evident that the COVID-19 pandemic acted as a transformation catalyst, accelerating the implementation and adoption of changes in healthcare interventions across the disease continuum [5, 6]. These changes can be viewed

A. Charalambous (✉)
Faculty of Health Science, Department of Nursing Science, Cyprus University of Technology, Limassol, Cyprus
e-mail: Andreas.charalambous@cut.ac.cy

© The Author(s), under exclusive license to Springer Nature
Switzerland AG 2025
A. Charalambous (ed.), *Critical Perspectives on Technological Innovations in Healthcare*, https://doi.org/10.1007/978-3-031-87158-0_1

as a new model of healthcare delivery that places emphasis on care closer to home (e.g., telemonitoring and teleconsultation) and substantial technological dependence (e.g., Digital Care Pathways). However, these are contrasted against ongoing technical challenges to meet the surge capacity in remote care which is furthered complicated by the complexity of the care required (e.g., patients with cancer), the fast-tracked implementation of new technologies, the allocation of financial resources concerns, the inappropriate preparedness of the healthcare workforce (Please also refer to chapter "Digital Literacy and Preparedness of Healthcare Professionals: The TRANSiTION Project") to uptake and integrate the technological solutions, and the protection of privacy and personal data that the new model of healthcare delivery entails.

1.1 Health Systems

The disruptions in the provision as well as the utilization of healthcare services was not merely attributed to the direct effects of the COVID-19 pandemic but also it pressurized the health systems and stretched others beyond their capability indirectly. The COVID-19 pandemic presented itself at a point in time where health systems have already been facing existing gaps and challenges resulting in their exacerbation and maximizing their impact [7]. While many sectors of public structures were impacted by the pandemic, it particularly highlighted shortcomings in medical care infrastructures as well technology-based infrastructure's around the world that highlighted the need to restructure medical systems, as they were vastly unprepared and ill-equipped to manage a pandemic and simultaneously provide general and specialized medical care [8]. The COVID-19 pandemic has disrupted both preventive and curative services for communicable and noncommunicable diseases [9]. Many of essential services have been delayed by the healthcare facilities, patients were also unable to attend follow-ups and acute care visits due to the fear and anxiety they experienced during the pandemic waves [10]. It has been challenging to estimate the number of individuals who could not access screening programs, faced delays in diagnosis, and encountered barriers to appropriate care within the EU. However, within the cancer context, the European Cancer Organization [11] as part of the Time to Act Campaign reported that due to the pandemic nearly one million cancer cases in Europe are being missed. As part of the same study, it has been estimated that doctors saw 1.5 million fewer people with cancer in the first year of the pandemic, and approximately 100 million cancer screening tests were not performed [12].

1.2 The Physical Environment of Healthcare Delivery

A major component of modern healthcare systems that witnessed transformation during COVID-19 was the physical context in which care was delivered. The creation of new conditions as a result of the pandemic highlighted the importance of team-based medicine and infrastructural flexibility in medical systems in order to safely and efficiently correspond to the increased and diverse demand. From the safety perspective of both patients and healthcare professionals and organizational perspective, hospitals across the globe adopted several cross-cutting strategies in response to the surge in COVID-19 cases, such as creating buffer areas between wards, and placing dividers between contaminated and non-contaminated areas [13]. However, such strategies inevitably had a cumulative impact on the healthcare professionals' working conditions creating an unprecedented working context. For example, hospitals began allowing employees to work from home to minimize the number of people on site, and retraining staff for areas of need. Staff had to adapt to the new work environments and were only allowed to have limited interactions with colleagues owing to social distancing, which resulted in psychological stress and burnout [14].

As health systems around the world were struggling to respond to the realities imposed by the pandemic, many examples were recorded in successfully modifying facility features to be more appropriate to the pandemic conditions. For example, to modify facility features in response to the pandemic, the Mt. Sinai Hospital in New York City drew on the experience of a non-profit architecture organization with extensive experience in regions of the globe where infectious disease poses major design threats. As part of the modification strategy cameras were fitted on the bodies of healthcare staff as a means to provide detailed visualizations of the hospital layout and outline recommendations for redesign. Based on the retrieved data, the hospital's facilities were modified to meet the new needs posed as a result of the pandemic. Modifications included the introduction of transparent plastic sheeting as see-through walls that allowed staff to monitor COVID-19 patients without endangering themselves from contracting the disease. Other restructuring of the physical environment included patient rooms, floors, and doorways being painted or taped in a color-coded fashion to provide quick visual cues to healthcare professionals about risk zones and sterile zones [1].

1.3 Delivery Models Shifting to Care Closer to Home

During the first COVID-19 wave which developed further during the following waves, many healthcare organizations restructured patient care accommodating for emergent and urgent care that were mostly needed at the time of the health emergency. In addition, the limited knowledge of this novel virus deterred patients from receiving the needed care therefore, elective cases were postponed. People in the communities were scared to enter a hospital for fear of contracting COVID-19 therefore directing many aspects of the care at the home setting. The World Health Organization (WHO) defines home-based care as "any form of care given to ill people in their homes, including physical, psychosocial and palliative activities" [15].

The trend of moving care from the hospital to the patient's home is not a new one, but one that began in the 1990s and has been gathering steam ever since.

A combination of factors has contributed to the onset and development of this trend, however, demographic impetus, increased cost and health care delivery system reform hold a prominent place [15, 16].

Growing costs across the board—from national economic hardship to increased regular care costs—are driving care from hospitals to alternative locations, including skilled nursing facilities and patients' homes. Misuse and overuse of acute care resources and unavailable space will drive increases in home care utilization as providers and patients seek out alternatives to hospital stays.

Traditionally, home care has primary focused on the elderly and people living with chronic disease. Projections show that the percentage of people aged 60 years and older will increase by 34%, from 1 billion in 2020 to 1.4 billion by 2030 [17]. With an increasingly ageing population, there is a significant rise in the demand for long-term care. Certain conditions are more prevalent among the elderly, such as chronic diseases including cancer, frailty, mental disorders, and physical disability; these conditions impose a substantial care burden on hospitals and primary care centers, as they require complex disease-specific management [18, 19].

During the pandemic, with hospitals at or near capacity due to COVID-19 and other factors straining hospital resources, home care was expanded to include the younger populations and those without chronic conditions. As the healthcare landscape continues to evolve, healthcare professionals should prepare to provide home care for a population that would prefer receiving care at home and payors are willing to reimburse the costs in an effort to potentially decrease hospitalization and readmissions.

1.4   Healthcare Workforce

Another aspect of medical systems that the pandemic significantly altered was staffing frameworks. This had a two-fold perspective: one in relation to the increased demands on healthcare professionals needed and the other one in terms of managing the infected professionals. With respect to the latter, the management of COVID-19 infected healthcare personnel became a priority: as a possible carrier of contagion (e.g., risk of overexposure of already hospitalized patients with serious diseases), healthcare staff are suspended from work, causing also serious consequences on the operational capabilities of the treatment centers [20]. However, in this process, the management of infected healthcare personnel was supported by very heterogeneous and not integrated digital tools such as text documents and spreadsheets resulting in poor outcomes that weakened the ability of the hospitals to effectively respond to the increased demand and reduce infection rate and deaths [21]. The development of digital tools for the management of infected healthcare personnel became an urgent necessity to foster more organized and integrated solutions, able to process huge amount of heterogeneous information, which later proved to be more effective in this respect [22]. These digital health tools facilitate efficiencies and enable rapid scale-up, near-instantaneous data sharing, and quick data aggregation and analysis. The challenge that remains is to sustain and replicate lessons learned from implementing digital tools during the pandemic, toward leveraging their potential to ensure healthy lives and promote well-being for all [22]

Hospitals were forced to significantly increase their patient-to-nurse ratios due to hospital crowding and lack of resources. Increased reliance on contingent staffing arose out of necessity to help overwhelmed healthcare systems meet the increased demand for intensive critical care during the pandemic. The increasingly prominent role of traveling nurses and critical care physicians highlighted the value of a flexible workforce in a time of global health crisis [23].

Shifting workforce dynamics reflect other ways in which healthcare facilities adapted to personnel shortages during the pandemic. During the pandemic, one strategy to manage the increasing medical staff shortage included the medical schools providing the opportunity for an earlier graduation to fourth year students so that they could assist hospitals in patient care during the pandemic [1].

There is an increased attrition of health workers that is due to: an aging workforce; increased absenteeism and resignations (62% increase during the COVID-19 pandemic); increased number of deaths during the COVID-19 pandemic (50,000 health workers in Europe are estimated to have died); and increased migration of health and care workers in certain countries (27% and 79% increase in the global migration to OECD countries after the COVID-19 pandemic) [20, 23]. These challenges additionally to drops in long-term employment, inadequate relief resources, and declines in treatment success rates have led to a massive change in the healthcare workforce and will continue to exacerbate the care accessibility challenges on a global scale.

1.5   The Transformed Landscape of Technological Innovation in Healthcare

Worldwide healthcare systems face significant challenges, including rising healthcare costs [24], outcome problems, aging populations with a high prevalence of multimorbidities [25], shrinking healthcare workforce [20], and continuing (post-) pandemic management [26]. These challenges have highlighted the poor design of systems and processes, the system's inability to respond to changing patient demographics and related requirements, a failure to assimilate the rapidly growing and increasingly complex science and technology base (e.g , telemonitoring and teleconsultation) and slow adoption of information technology innovations. To face these challenges, innovative healthcare solutions as part of an overall digital transformation strategy present as a key social and economic priority and are crucial for achieving high-quality healthcare and increased access to healthcare services [27, 28].

Digital health care refers primarily to the utilization of technology to improve patient care. Digital transformation represents "a process that aims to improve an entity by triggering significant changes to its properties through combinations of information, computing, communication, and connectivity technologies" [29, p. 118]. The topic of digital transformation in healthcare has received increased attention in recent years from scholars, practitioners to policy makers. Marques & Ferreira [30] in a systematic literature review on digital transformation within the healthcare context demonstrated the increased attention in research in this field over the last 20 years and highlighted integrated management, medical images and electronic medical records as the most common technology-related research themes within this domain. From a policy perspective, the European Commission for example has placed emphasis on the digital transformation across business and services, and hence it incorporated a corresponding regulation namely Regulation (EU) 2021/694 of the European Parliament and of the Council of 29 April 2021, 21 establishing the Digital Europe Program and repealing Decision (EU) 2015/2240 [31].

Digital innovations and digital transformation, however, are perceived as an opportunity to improve the quality of and access to care while at the same time containing costs [32]. Yet, despite this potential, healthcare providers were quite hesitant in adopting and using digital innovations in the past. According to Charalambous [31], the main reasons for the slow adoption of digital technologies in health can be attributed to performance expectancy, effort expectancy, and facilitating conditions, which act as significant determinants to users' behavioral intention. Others have drawn on regulatory, compliance, and legal challenges that the digital health revolution is creating for the healthcare sector. Thus, until recently digitalization in healthcare progressed only slowly.

After years of slow movement advancing telehealth, remote patient monitoring and other digital health technologies, the landscape changed rapidly during the COVID-19 pandemic. In the realm of healthcare, technological innovation stands as a beacon of hope, continually transforming the landscape of medical practices and patient outcomes. From cutting-edge treatments to advanced diagnostic tools, the fusion of technology and healthcare has ushered in an era of unprecedented possibilities. In the following section, we draw on the horizons that technologies such as virtual reality (VR), artificial intelligence (AI), machine learning (ML), and telehealth offer within the healthcare context.

Virtual reality interventions have been implemented at various conditions within the healthcare realm making it one of the biggest adopters of VR. Evidence from a systematic review showed that VR intervention is more effective compared with the control (i.e., standard care) for anxiety, depression, fatigue, and pain. VR can reduce effectively these symptoms in different contexts and diseases, including cancer [33]. In a randomized crossover trial with 50 cancer patients on active chemotherapy treatment, VR interventions based on mood induction strategies were shown to be a feasible and effective procedure for promoting positive mood in cancer patients during chemotherapy [34]. Other applications of VR encompass robotic surgery, phobia treatment, surgery simulation, medical diagnostics, and skills training to name a few.

Within the medical fields of radiology and pathology, for example, the application of AI is particularly popular in the analysis of imaging data toward disease classification, detection, segmentation, characterization, and monitoring [35]. Nowadays AI is applied in cancer imaging including digital pathology (low- and high-level image processing and clarification tasks), radiographic imaging (differentiation between high- and low-risk lesions) and clinical photographs [36]. The capability of AI to analyze massive data retrieved through electronic health records (EHRs) enabled pattern recognition of clinically relevant parameters using individual and historical data as aggregated data. This has allowed for more precise risk stratification that takes into consideration genomics, advanced imaging, and serum markers in addition to data streaming from the TNM staging [35].

Machine learning-based applications within healthcare assumed a prominent role as a result of greater data availability and computing capabilities [37]. Machine learning has been deployed in healthcare primarily as a supportive tool to a physician or analyst's ability to fulfill their roles, identify healthcare trends, and develop disease prediction models to help health care systems improve the quality of care and use resources more accurately and efficiently. Machine learning-based approaches have also been implemented to achieve increased efficiency in the organization of electronic health records, identification of irregularities in the blood samples, organs, and bones using medical imaging and monitoring, as well as in robot-assisted surgeries [38]. Machine learning algorithms have been particularly effective to extract insights from large data sets, helping researchers to uncover new connections and relationships that would be difficult to detect using traditional methods [39]. The use of ML in clinical environments has hitherto experienced diverse adoption patterns, with the field of radiology raising considerable attention due to the notable capability of ML (in particular, deep learning [DL]) models to extract valuable information from medical images [40, 41].

The need and implementation of telehealth services escalated with the COVID-19 pandemic as a response tool to meet the altered patients' needs for remote access. Telehealth is a broad term that includes Telemedicine and a variety of non-physician services (e.g., telenursing, telepharmacy, and linguistic interpretation) and can be discussed synonymously with integrated remote care modalities, such as mobile health and E-health platforms [42]. Telehealth presents with many strategic advantages as it can improve healthcare access including those who live in remote and hard to reach areas [43]. Moreover, telehealth can improve healthcare access options for people with disabilities by reducing travel for medical visits whist the telehealth video conferencing may mask in-person characteristics that invoke provider bias [42].

2   Conclusion

The pandemic has caught healthcare systems around the world by surprise, exposing systemic weaknesses in infrastructures, supply chains, government preparedness and actions, human resources, and public health systems. Moreover, the pandemic presented challenges for government health officials and administrative managers of health care systems to maintain a consistent narrative on technological innovation as a means to better respond to the conditions created by the COVID-19. As part of the challenges that have been recorded during the virus outbreak, it became clear that many health care facilities were ill-equipped and unprepared from a technological point of view to remotely manage the care needs of patients due to the forced change of the physical environment of healthcare delivery.

The COVID-19 experience conveyed a clear message to the healthcare community on the need of building resilient and sustainable health systems that are digitally prepared for future challenges. In doing so, strong investment to strengthen the health systems including the health workforce development with emphasis on digital solutions, creating attracting working conditions, providing continues training and equipment (e.g., AI, machine learning, virtual reality), especially in the areas of remote monitoring and teleconsultation (i.e., telehealth) is required. Such an investment can make the difference in terms of personalizing the care but also sustaining the care when challenges threaten its physical provision. Digital preparedness and digital health literacy are tools that can also facilitate the current reshaping of healthcare delivery systems that promote the care closer to home approach. Despite the COVID-19 pandemic has catalyzed innovations in digital health, but scaling and sustaining the innovations remains a challenge. Social dialogue is essential to building resilient health systems, and therefore has a critical role both in crisis response and in building a future that is prepared for health.

References

1. Davis B, Bankhead-Kendall BK, Dumas RP. A review of COVID-19's impact on modern medical systems from a health organization management perspective. Health Technol (Berl). 2022;12(4):815–24. https://doi.org/10.1007/s12553-022-00660-z. Epub 2022 Mar 25.
2. Moynihan R, Sanders S, Michaleff ZA, Scott AM, Clark J, To EJ, Jones M, Kitchener E, Fox M, Johansson M, Lang E, Duggan A, Scott I, Albarqouni L. Impact of COVID-19 pandemic on utilisation of healthcare services: a systematic review. BMJ Open. 2021;11(3):e045343. https://doi.org/10.1136/bmjopen-2020-045343.
3. Jazieh AR, Kozlakidis Z. Healthcare transformation in the post-coronavirus pandemic era. Front Med. 2020;7:429. https://doi.org/10.3389/fmed.2020.00429.
4. Manavgat G, Audibert M. Healthcare system efficiency and drivers: re-evaluation of OECD countries for COVID-19. SSM—Health Syst. 2024;2:100003. https://doi.org/10.1016/j.ssmhs.2023.100003.
5. Menendez C, Gonzalez R, Donnay F, Leke RGF. Avoiding indirect effects of COVID-19 on maternal and child health. Lancet Glob Health. 2020;8:e863–4.
6. Steinhauser S. COVID-19 as a driver for digital transformation in healthcare. In: Glauner P, Plugmann P, Lerzynski G, editors. Digitalizatiphon in healthcare. Future of business and finance. Cham: Springer; 2021. https://doi.org/10.1007/978-3-030-65896-0_8.
7. WHO. Attacks on health care in the context of COVID-19. Geneva: WHO. [Sep 20, 2021]. https://www.who.int/newsroom/feature-stories/detail/attacks-on-healthcare-in-the-context-of-covid-19.
8. Filip R, Gheorghita Puscaselu R, Anchidin-Norocel L, Dimian M, Savage WK. Global challenges to public health care systems during the COVID-19 pandemic: a review of pandemic measures and problems. J Pers Med. 2022;12(8):1295. https://doi.org/10.3390/jpm12081295.
9. Haileamlak A. The impact of COVID-19 on health and health systems. Ethiop J Health Sci. 2021;31(6):1073–4. https://doi.org/10.4314/ejhs.v31i6.1.
10. Papautsky EL, Hamlish T. Patient-reported treatment delays in breast cancer care during the COVID-19 pandemic. Breast Cancer Res Trea. 2020;184(1):249–54.

11. European Cancer Organisation. 2021. https://www.europeancancer.org/resources/news/time-to-act.html.
12. Baird AM. Re-engaging EU citizens with national screening programmes and cancer diagnosis post-pandemic. Lancet Oncol. 2022;23(5):566–7. https://doi.org/10.1016/S1470-2045(22)00090-0.
13. Capolongo S, Gola M, Brambilla A, Morganti A, Mosca EI, Barach P. COVID-19 and healthcare facilities: a decalogue of design strategies for resilient hospitals. Acta Bio Med Atenei Parm. 2020;91:50.
14. Bae S. A qualitative study of hospital interior environments during the COVID-19 pandemic. Int J Environ Res Public Health. 2023;20(4):3271. https://doi.org/10.3390/ijerph20043271.
15. Lizano-Díez I, Amaral-Rohter S, Pérez-Carbonell L, Aceituro S. Impact of home care services on patient and economic outcomes: a targeted review. Home Health Care Manag Pract. 2022;34(2):148–62. https://doi.org/10.1177/10848223211038305.
16. Landers S, Madigan E, Leff B, Rosati RJ, McCann BA, Hornbake R, MacMillan R, Jones K, Bowles K, Dowding D, Lee T, Moorhead T, Rodriguez S, Breese E. The future of home health care: a strategic framework for optimizing value. Home Health Care Manag Pract. 2016;28(4):262–78. https://doi.org/10.1177/1084822316666368. Epub 2016 Oct 5.
17. World Health Organization. Decade of healthy aging 2020–2030. Published 2020. https://www.who.int/docs/default-source/decade-of-healthy-ageing/full-decade-proposal/decade-proposal-fulldraft-en.pdf?sfvrsn=8ad3385d_6. Accessed 6 May 2020.
18. Che RP, Cheung MC. Factors associated with the utilization of Home and Community-Based Services (HCBS) among older adults: a systematic review of the last decade. J Gerontol Soc Work. 2024;67(6):776–802. https://doi.org/10.1080/01634372.2024.2342455.
19. Mah JC, Stevens SJ, Keefe JM, et al. Social factors influencing utilization of home care in community-dwelling older adults: a scoping review. BMC Geriatr. 2021;21:145. https://doi.org/10.1186/s12877-021-02069-1.
20. Smallwood N, Harrex W, Rees M, Willis K, Bennett CM. COVID-19 infection and the broader impacts of the pandemic on healthcare workers. Respirology. 2022;27(6):411–26. https://doi.org/10.1111/resp.14208. Epub 2022 Jan 19.
21. Raimo N, De Turi I. Albergo F, Vitolla F. The drivers of the digital transformation in the healthcare industry: an empirical analysis in Italian hospitals. Technovation. 2023;121:102558. https://doi.org/10.1016/j.technovation.2022.102558. Epub 2022 May 27. PMCID: PMC9135505.
22. Mason C, Lazenby S, Stuhldreher R, Kimball M, Bartlein R. Lessons learned from implementing digital health tools to address COVID-19 in LMICs. Front Public Health. 2022;10:859941. https://doi.org/10.3389/fpubh.2022.859941.
23. Azzopardi-Muscat N, Zapata T, Kluge H. Moving from health workforce crisis to health workforce success: the time to act is now. Lancet Reg Health Eur. 2023;26(35):100765. https://doi.org/10.1016/j.lanepe.2023.100765. PMID: 38115956; PMCID: PMC10730309.
24. Wulfovich S. Digital health entrepreneurship. Cham: Springer International Publishing AG; 2020.
25. Chowdhury SR, Chandra Das D, Sunna TC, Beyene J, Hossain A. Global and regional prevalence of multimorbidity in the adult population in community settings: a systematic review and meta-analysis. EClinicalMedicine. 2023;57:101860. https://doi.org/10.1016/j.eclinm.2023.101860. PMID: 36864977; PMCID: PMC9971315.
26. Oleksa-Marewska K, Tokar J. Facing the post-pandemic challenges: the role of leadership effectiveness in shaping the affective Well-being of healthcare providers working in a hybrid work mode. Int J Environ Res Public Health. 2022;19(21):14388. https://doi.org/10.3390/ijerph192114388. PMID: 36361264; PMCID: PMC9655828.
27. Weimar SN, Martjan RS, Terzidis O. Conceptualizing the landscape of digital health entrepreneurship: a systematic review and research agenda. Manag Rev Q. 2024; https://doi.org/10.1007/s11301-024-00417-0.
28. Bratan T, Schneider D, Heyen N, Pullmann L, Friedewald M, Kuhlmann D, Brkic N, Hüsing B. E-health in Deutschland: entwicklungsperspektiven und internationaler vergleich. Studien zum deutschen Innovations system. 2022; https://doi.org/10.24406/publica-fhg-416796.

29. Vial G. Understanding digital transformation: a review and a research agenda. J Strateg Inf Syst. 2019;28(2):118–44.
30. Marques IC, Ferreira JJ. Digital transformation in the area of health: systematic review of 45 years of evolution. Heal Technol. 2020;10:575–86.
31. Charalambous A. Digital transformation in healthcare: have we gone off the rails? Asia Pac J Oncol Nurs. 2024;11(5):100481. https://doi.org/10.1016/j.apjon.2024.100481. PMID: 38774536; PMCID: PMC11107189.
32. Agarwal RG, DesRoches GC. The digital transformation of healthcare: current status and the road ahead. Inf Syst Res. 2010;21(5):796–809.
33. Ioannou A, Papastavrou E, Avraamides MN, Charalambous A. Virtual reality and symptoms management of anxiety, depression, fatigue, and pain: a systematic review. SAGE Open Nurs. 2020;6:2377960820936163. https://doi.org/10.1177/2377960820936163. PMID: 33415290; PMCID: PMC7774450.
34. Ioannou A, Paikousis L, Papastavrou E, Avraamides MN, Astras G, Charalambous A. Effectiveness of virtual reality vs guided imagery on mood changes in cancer patients receiving chemotherapy treatment: a crossover trial. Eur J Oncol Nurs. 2022;61:102188. https://doi.org/10.1016/j.ejon.2022.102188. Epub 2022 Aug 13.
35. Charalambous A, Dodlek N. Big data, machine learning, and artificial intelligence to advance cancer care: opportunities and challenges. Semin Oncol Nurs. 2023;39(3):151429. https://doi.org/10.1016/j.soncn.2023.151429. Epub 2023 Apr 20.
36. Hesso I, Kayyali R, Charalambous A, Lavdaniti M, Stalika E, Lelegianni M, Nabhani-Gebara S. Experiences of cancer survivors in Europe: has anything changed? Can artificial intelligence offer a solution? Front Oncol. 2022;12:888938. https://doi.org/10.3389/fonc.2022.888938. PMID: 36185207; PMCID: PMC9515410.
37. Gama F, Tyskbo D, Nygren J, Barlow J, Reed J, Svedberg P. Implementation frameworks for artificial intelligence translation into health care practice: scoping review. J Med Internet Res. 2022;24(1):e32215.
38. Habehh H, Gohel S. Machine learning in healthcare. Curr Genomics. 2021;22(4):291–300. https://doi.org/10.2174/1389202922666210705124359. PMID: 35273459; PMCID: PMC8822225.
39. Coelho L, Glotsos D, Reis S. The COVID-19 pandemic: how technology is reshaping public health and medicine. Bioengineering. 2023;10:611. https://doi.org/10.3390/bioengineering10050611.
40. Ardito V, Cappellaro G, Compagni A, Petracca F, Preti LM. Implementation of machine learning applications in health care organizations: protocol for a systematic review of empirical studies. JMIR Res Protoc. 2023;12:e47971.
41. Lazic I, Agullo F, Ausso S, Alves B, Barelle C, Berral JL, Bizopoulos P, Bunduc O, Chouvarda I, Dominguez D, et al. The holistic perspective of the INCISIVE project—artificial intelligence in screening mammography. Appl Sci. 2022;12(17):8755. https://doi.org/10.3390/app12178755.
42. Phuong J, Ordóñez P, Cao J, Moukheiber M, Moukheiber L, Caspi A, Swenor BK, DKN N, Mankoff J. Telehealth and digital health innovations: a mixed landscape of access. PLOS Digit Health. 2023;2(12):e0000401. https://doi.org/10.1371/journal.pdig.0000401.
43. Alhussein MS, Liu XM. Patient perspectives on telehealth during the pandemic in the United States. Int J Med Eng Inform. 2022;16(5):70–6.

Digital Literacy and Preparedness of Healthcare Professionals: The TRANSiTION Project

Iolie Nicolaidou
and On behalf of the TRANSiTION Consortium

1 Introduction: The Importance of Developing Healthcare Professionals' Digital Literacy

The digital transformation of health and care has the capacity to act as a key enabler to enhance health and care. The potential of digital solutions to improve the quality and safety of healthcare has been recognized decades ago [1] and as a result, the landscape of healthcare is becoming increasingly more technology-dominated.

Previous research in the area of digital transformation in healthcare has focused on different areas, one of which is improving patient-centered approaches [2]. Digital health approaches are particularly relevant to cancer care, given the growing numbers of cancer survivors and their complex long-term healthcare needs, which include the need for them to manage their health [3]. One of the major barriers to the uptake of digital health solutions across the cancer continuum is the lack of continuous training for the cancer healthcare workforce.

Despite their promises, digital innovations have scarcely translated to technologies used in routine clinical practice [4] and a potential barrier to this inconsistency may be healthcare professionals' digital literacy. Previous studies within the context of healthcare that focused on clinical staff found a discrepancy between healthcare professionals' scores in healthcare literacy and digital literacy [4]. Specifically, healthcare professionals scored high with respect to healthcare literacy, which is their area of expertise, but the same finding was not observed for their digital literacy. Another study found that the majority of clinical staff reported high digital literacy levels, expressing confidence in using technology. However, one-fifth

On behalf of the TRANSiTION Consortium

I. Nicolaidou (✉)
Department of Communication and Internet Studies, Cyprus University of Technology,
Limassol, Cyprus
e-mail: iolie.nicolaidou@cut.ac.cy

A. Charalambous (ed.), *Critical Perspectives on Technological Innovations in Healthcare*, https://doi.org/10.1007/978-3-031-87158-0_2

of respondents reported anxiety and reduced levels of confidence when using information systems [5].

Healthcare professionals (HCPs) need to acquire digital health literacy or improve their digital health literacy to assess the impact of eHealth solutions and use them consciously on a systematic basis. Digital literacy for healthcare professionals and cancer patients is of paramount importance for the successful, effective, and ethical implementation of digital solutions in healthcare. Therefore, education and training relating to digital health have been recognized as a priority for empowering the future healthcare workforce and benefiting cancer patients.

Kuek and Hakkennes recognized the need for health services to provide targeted education and training to address staff with low digital literacy levels and/or confidence with using information systems [5] especially given poor staff engagement with information systems, which adversely affects the safety and quality of patient care. Pfob et al. demonstrated the need to develop transdisciplinary curricula to bridge skill gaps and to drive the implementation of digital health initiatives [4]. Kraus et al. stressed the importance of needs assessment and curricula updates which would provide a sufficient scale for linking traditional clinical practice and medicine in the digital age and support the training and upskill of healthcare professionals and nursing staff [2].

Recognizing the need to support HCPs digital literacy and focusing on professionals fighting cancer, the EU Funded TRANSiTION project (https://www.europeancancer.org/eu-projects/impact/resource/transition.html), designed training on digital skills for the health workforce focusing on the needs of clinical professionals, non-clinical professionals, patients and their informal carers for cancer prevention, diagnosis, treatment and survivorship.

Furthermore, TRANSiTION aims to improve HCPs' digital skills, support the safe and effective use of existing digital tools and at the same time increase their preparedness and readiness for the adoption of new ones. This chapter will describe the methodology of how TRANSiTION designed engaging and effective learning experiences, focusing on HCPs in particular.

2   Methodology

The first step was conducting a systematic literature review that identified the content and utilization of digital solutions in the field of Oncology for HCPs and explored the landscape of mobile applications (apps) for cancer care for HCPs. Next came a needs analysis, whose aim was twofold, to define HCPs' learning needs and identify areas where they needed training the most and to describe their current level of knowledge of digital skills. The third step was the curriculum development of 11 modules with their respective learning activities and tasks. Principles of Learning eXperience Design (LXD) were applied for curriculum development. This chapter describes these steps and demonstrates how theory was introduced into practice to design learner-centered, goal-oriented modules that create cognitive dissonance, use the right technology to create an appropriately supported learning environment, constitute a creative solution to an important learning challenge, and engage learners through gamification and virtual reality.

2.1 Systematic Literature Review on Digital Solutions in Oncology for Healthcare Professionals

A systematic literature review conducted in the early stages of the project identified the content and utilization of digital solutions in the field of oncology for HCPs and non-clinical professionals—NCPs (i.e., health managers) and explored the landscape of apps for cancer care for these two target groups of professionals. The systematic review followed the guidelines provided by PRISMA 2020 and covered the databases PubMed, EMBASE, and CINAHL (EBSCO). The review included studies conducted between the years 2018–2023 and involved HCPs and NCPs in the field of oncology engaged across the care continuum from prevention to survivorship, palliative care and end-of-life care. The review used the following keywords: oncology OR cancer prevention OR cancer treatment OR cancer therapy OR cancer support, healthcare professional* or doctor* or nurse, nursing*, health manager*. Studies included any type of digital tools applied in cancer care such as mHealth apps, eHealth platforms, telemedicine, and other digital solutions. To complement the results of the systematic review and to explore the landscape of apps for cancer prevention, treatment, therapy or support for healthcare professionals, doctors, nurses and health managers, a review of apps in Google Play and AppStore has also been conducted.

Following the screening phase of the initial 26,596 studies that were retrieved, the final number of studies for the systematic review was 30. The majority of the studies followed a randomized control trial (RCT) design and included interventions such as mobile applications (mHealth), web-based interventions (eHealth), virtual reality, and /or text messages. Some of these digital tools aimed to support the decision-making process and improve the quality of treatment decisions of HCPS, and to support remote monitoring of chemotherapy-related side effects such as burden, quality of life, and anxiety. The review showed the wide range of areas where digital health technologies are being utilized in healthcare as well as their importance in improving the quality of cancer care. The findings of the review also supported the cost-effectiveness of digital technologies compared to the standard of care, and decision-making enhancement of digital technologies for HCPs in clinical practice.

For the app review, through the search strategy, 221 apps were identified (77 in Google Play, 144 in the App Store). After applying exclusion criteria, 27 apps were included (20 in Google Play, 7 in the App Store). Most apps were either medical or educational, focused on HCPs, doctors, nurses or students (none was found for health managers) and very few were empirically validated.

The systematic review showed the benefits of integrating digital health technologies to improve the quality of cancer care across the cancer continuum and across different cancer diagnoses and identified a few mobile apps that could be included in the training modules as decision-support tools.

2.2   Needs Analysis: Defining Learning Needs

As part of identifying user requirements, the current needs and knowledge of clinical and non-clinical professionals involved in cancer care were analyzed.

The Digital Competence Framework for Citizens (DigComp) [6], which provides a common understanding of digital competence, was used as a basis to identify basic areas to be included in the curriculum. The EU digital framework was used as a model to inform the process of identifying even more specific contents to address the specific needs of HCPs. The training needs for clinical professionals and non-clinical professionals were identified, and they focus on the following areas: digital information, communication, content creation, security, problem-solving, ethics, and patient empowerment skills.

Furthermore, their educational preferences, Internet usage habits and access to available online resources were explored. This was achieved using two rounds of an eDelphi questionnaire and a user experience (UX) design workshop. The clinical professionals who participated in both rounds of the eDelphi survey represented ten countries within the consortium: Belgium, Bulgaria, Croatia, Cyprus, Greece, Italy, Lithuania, Portugal, Slovenia, and Spain. Regarding their profession, 42.4% were physicians specializing in cancer care, 30.3% were oncology nurses, 15.1% were researchers working on cancer, and 12.2% were working in other clinical professions related to cancer care.

Clinical professionals have reached a consensus that all proposed digital skills are necessary for cancer care. Given that almost half of clinical professionals reported they have never received any training in digital skills and considered their co-workers as basic digital users (i.e., low proficiency in digital skills), the results of the needs analysis supported the implementation of a comprehensive training program covering all the digital skills analyzed and highlighted the need for comprehensive training and broad rather than specialized knowledge.

The user experience design workshop showed that clinical professionals were mainly concerned with two aspects. The first was how to adapt the digital environment to the needs of patients/caregivers. According to clinical professionals, patients and caregivers need to accept digital cancer care. This implies the development of specific communication and patient empowerment skills for clinical professionals, to increase patient acceptability of digital cancer care. Secondly, they were concerned with keeping patients' medical information confidential and proceeding in a safe and ethical manner. Therefore, the development of a module for clinical professionals on data security and ethics was also identified as necessary.

With respect to their training preferences, the majority of HCPs expressed a preference for a training program in a hybrid format, with a long duration (≥ 9 contacts) and a limited amount of written content. A formal course in an oncology platform, which could be followed asynchronously allowing for flexibility to accommodate the HCPs' busy schedules, was therefore decided as ideal for the online component of the training.

2.3   Curriculum Development. Defining Learning Activities and Tasks

The systematic, scientific perspective of instructional design was used for curriculum development, and, as shown previously, the starting point was a needs assessment to identify the learners' needs and preferences. The traditional instructional design model was enhanced with a learning experience design approach, using a more creative perspective to focus on the learners, their goals, and their tasks.

The project involved the creation of 11 modules in total, one of which is shared between clinical and non-clinical professionals (Fig. 1). Participants follow different learning pathways depending on their clinical profile. This chapter focuses on clinical professionals, specifically oncology nurses, for showcasing purposes. It showcases the design and development of one module (Module 11), which focuses on problem-solving digital skills for oncology nurses. All modules followed a similar pedagogical approach.

The module has a challenge as a starting point: How can we address the need for working oncology nurses and nursing students to enhance their digital literacy skills and their problem-solving critical thinking skills? An example of a digital literacy skill in this context is for them to identify mobile apps that address their needs and to use them in their daily professional life in a critical way to solve a problem.

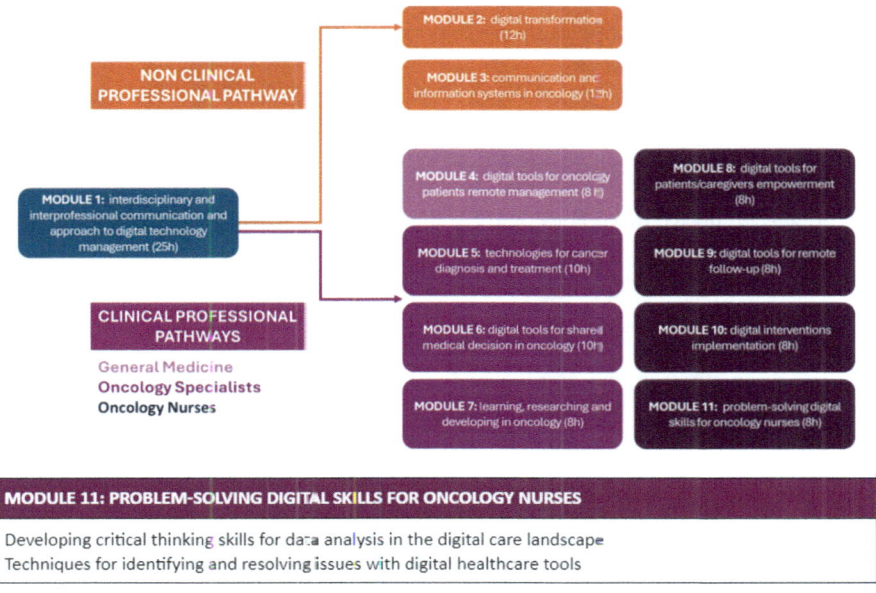

Fig. 1 Learning pathways in the TRANSiTION training program showing the clinical and non-clinical professionals' pathways

The module "Problem Solving Digital Skills for Oncology Nurses" consists of two submodules: "Developing Critical Thinking Skills for Data Analysis in the Digital Care Landscape" and "Techniques for Identifying and Resolving Issues with Digital Healthcare Tools" (Fig. 1). The submodule "Developing critical thinking skills for data analysis in the digital care landscape," which has an approximate duration of 8 hours for completion, is shown as an example in this chapter and its main contents are the following:

1. *Critical thinking skills*
   - *What are critical thinking skills?*
   - *Why are critical thinking skills important for oncology nurses?*
2. *Applying critical thinking in data analysis*
   - *to provide patient support*
   - *to select digital care tools for patients, and*
   - *to select apps that can be used as decision-support tools*

2.4   Applying Principles of Learning eXperience Design (LXD)

The Learning Experience Design (LXD) was used for curriculum development. Learning Experience Design (LXD) is "a human-centric, theoretically-grounded, and socio-culturally sensitive approach to learning design, intended to propel learners towards identified learning goals, and informed by user experience design methods" [7]. From a theoretical perspective, according to Reigeluth [8], the literature has shown that an effective learning experience has specific characteristics. "An effective learning experience:

(a) is learner-centered (focused on the learner, including the learner's needs and interests, and on the process that the learner goes through

(b) is goal-oriented (oriented toward a desired learning outcome that is valuable and meaningful)

(c) creates cognitive dissonance and epiphany that has a lasting positive impact on the learner

(d) uses the right technology to create an appropriately supported learning environment

(e) is usually a creative solution to an important learning challenge

(f) harnesses emotion and enjoyment but does not focus too much on entertainment" [8]

These six theoretical characteristics were implemented into practice in curriculum design and the next sections explain how this was done. The module was framed using a Performance Learning Activity as follows:

> In their shifts, nurses act effectively without using critical thinking as many decisions are mainly based on habit and have a minimum reflection. Thus, higher critical thinking skills are put into operation when some new ideas or needs are displayed to take a decision beyond routine. As an oncology nurse, you make decisions related to clinical practice on a daily basis. Patients need personalized support to address their needs. How do you apply critical thinking in data analysis to provide patient support, select digital care tools for patients, and select apps that can be used as decision-support tools in your professional life?

As can be seen from the Performance Learning Activity used above, oncology nurses who are our learners in this case, are placed in the center.

To explain what the general goal is, they are presented with the main competency they will develop through this submodule, as follows:

Upon completion you will be able to: critically analyze outcomes from digital processes and technologies and select the most fitting digital tools for each situation, through critical thinking approaches, to optimize the implementation of digital technologies in healthcare settings.

To explain the goal of the module and why the desired learning outcome is valuable and meaningful, the learners are first prompted to think about how they apply their critical thinking in data analysis in their everyday practice for three different cases, to: (1) provide patient support, (2) select digital care tools for patients, and (3) select apps that can be used as decision-support tools in their professional life. Applying critical thinking skills in these three cases also acts as a precursor, or advance organizer, for the hands-on practical activities that will follow in respective scenarios.

Prerequisite knowledge in this module refers to defining "critical thinking skills in general" and "critical thinking skills in nursing" in particular, which represent the theoretical part of the module (Fig. 2). These are explained using limited text, with the use of informative graphics and short videos, that direct the learners' attention to a specific element, for example, the importance of critical thinking skills for oncology nurses.

The learning material was based on scientific references, which are provided at the end of the module, while, in some cases, they are also integrated into the learning activities (Fig. 3). To create cognitive dissonance, the learners' attention is directed to a specific task, in this instance to access and read the article which focuses on the importance of critical thinking skills in nursing, with the goal to reflect on their own professional experience about their cancer patients'

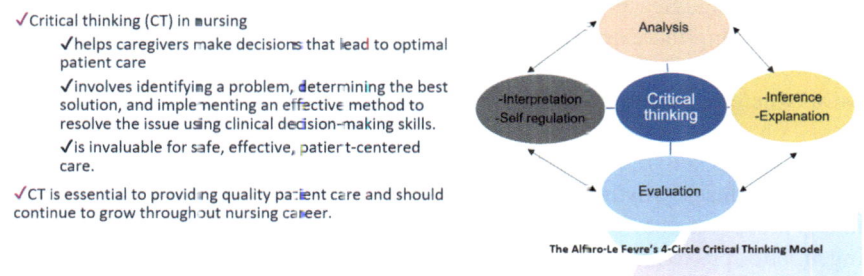

Fig. 2 The theoretical part of the module, explaining critical thinking skills using graphics and limited text. (© American Nursing Association [9]; Reji and Sushma [10]. With permission)

Why are critical thinking skills important for oncology nurses?

✓ Scan the QR code to access the article

✓ Papathanasiou, I. V., Kleisiaris, C. F., Fradelos, E. C., Kakou, K., & Kourkouta, L.
   (2014). Critical thinking: the development of an essential skill for nursing
   students. Acta Informatica Medica, 22(4), 283. Source:
   https://www.ncbi.nlm.nih.gov/pmc/articles/PMC4216424/

✓ Read this article

Reflect in the (Moodle) forum:

✓ In your daily professional life, what do your cancer patients expect from you
   when they reach out for your support?

Fig. 3 The theoretical part of the module, explaining the importance of critical thinking skills in nursing using a scientific article. (© Papathanasiou et al. [11]. With permission)

expectations as a way for them to identify any dissonance between theory (the scientific article) and practice (their professional clinical practice experiences).

In this module, as well as in all other modules of the curriculum the right technology to create an appropriately supported learning environment was used. Fully aligned with the learners' training preferences as identified in the needs assessment, the training program has a hybrid format, a long duration ($\geq$9 contacts), and a limited amount of written content as much as possible, presented as a formal course in an oncology platform using Moodle for the online component. Articles that can be accessed either using a QR code or a link, graphics, tables, figures, short videos and forums all represent technologically supported learning material that provide easy access for participants using either a computer or a mobile device (tablet or smartphone).

The practical, hands-on part of the module focuses on applying newly acquired skills in three scenarios, two of which are shown in (Figs. 4 and 5). An important learning challenge for healthcare professionals focusing on cancer care is that they often face difficulties in identifying the most appropriate apps for their needs as well as in evaluating the extent to which scientific evidence supports their use [12]. A creative solution to this challenge was to ask learners to simulate a task in the real world where they were asked to conduct searches for mobile apps using given keywords, on their own and report on their results (Figs. 4 and 5).

These activities require learners to analyze data in a structured context, with specific feedback provided to them after each step (Fig. 6). Learners are scaffolded in this process as they are provided with some criteria that can be used for evaluating mobile apps to practice in evaluating retrieved results (Fig. 6), while at the same time, they are directed to relevant resources that guide them to already evaluated mobile apps that address their needs to simplify their professional life (Fig. 7).

Applying critical thinking to select digital care for patients (Scenario 2)

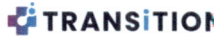

✓ Seeing how Phil uses technology a lot in his daily life and spends a lot of time online on his smartphone, you can a so suggest that Phil use a mobile app that provides support.

✓ Try a search on Google Play or App Store with these keywords: **"cancer patient support"**

Fig. 4 Scenario 2 applying critical thinking skills to select digital care for patients

Applying critical thinking to select apps that can be used as decision-support tools (Scenario 3)

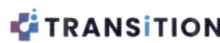

✓ Digital decision support tools can often assist oncology nurses.

✓ You decided to integrate a decision support tool in your work. Try a search on Google Play or App Store with these keywords: **"cancer decision support tool"**

✓ Approximately 30 results are retrieved.

✓ What are some criteria you would use to select the most appropriate app for your work?

Fig. 5 Scenario 3 applying critical thinking skills to select apps that can be used as decision-support tools

Applying critical thinking to select apps that can be used as decision-support tools

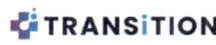

Criteria you can consider are the following:

✓ a)   apps that target health care professionals or nurses

✓ b)   apps that focus on oncology, cancer prevention, treatment, therapy or support

✓ c)   apps available at east in the English language

✓ d)   apps that have a high evaluation score

An app that satisfies all criteria, ONCOASSIST, appears as a top choice in your search.

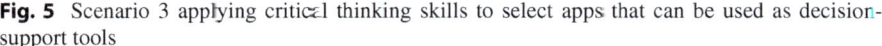

Fig. 6 Some evaluation criteria for mobile app evaluation

Applying critical thinking to select apps that can be used as decision-support tools

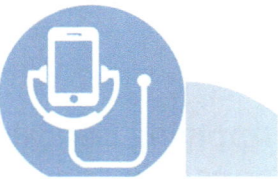

✓ Deciding on criteria to select digital resources and evaluating retrieved results takes a lot of time. As a busy professional you cannot evaluate all retrieved results. The TRANSiTION project developed a **Digital Health Tools Guide** for oncology professionals after systematically searching for apps that are available at the moment.

✓ The Digital Health Tools guide is available in English and 12 additional languages here.

Fig. 7 Healthcare professionals are directed to relevant resources to guide them to already evaluated mobile apps that address their needs

2.5   Embedding Immersive Virtual Reality in the Curriculum for Inexperienced Learners

To help us envision future learners, two personas were developed during the design phase of the curriculum. The primary persona for this module is a young nursing student and the secondary persona is an experienced nursing professional.

The primary persona, Artemis, "is an 18-year old undergraduate student at the Cyprus University of Technology, in her second year of studies. As a typical digital native, she's an excellent user of social media and she holds positive attitudes to using emerging technologies for learning. As a typical undergraduate student, she has a rather short attention span, she's easily distracted and she's reluctant to speak up in class. Her motivation for attending training may be grade-oriented, and she faces some challenges, including the need to be taught in her native language (Greek) and the fact that she lacks professional experience as she's a novice who has not yet done her practicum in a hospital or health center."

To address the undergraduate nursing students' lack of professional experience and advance their critical thinking skills, the enhancement of the module with an immersive virtual reality (VR) component was suggested. The VR component will provide a simulated environment in a face-to-face setting that will make it easy for nursing students to practice specific protocols in assessing, monitoring or treating a patient without the risk of hurting actual patients, to increase their skills, internalize protocols until they become an automatic process for them, and become more efficient in their future work.

2.6   Gamification to Increase Engagement

Gamification refers to using game attributes in a non-gaming context [13]. A systematic review that focused on empirical evidence for the effectiveness of gamification approaches in health showed only positive outcomes for using gamification and improved learning outcomes for all studies that met inclusion criteria ($n = 44$). Almost all studies used gamification for assessment purposes ($n = 40$), and several studies ($n = 27$) used it in combination with a conflict or challenge [14]. A meta-review on serious games and gamification in healthcare found that serious games and gamification techniques are increasingly being used for a wide range of health conditions, including cancer, while the research focus is shifting toward the use of mobile and digital platforms and virtual reality to personalize and adapt interventions [15].

With respect to using gamification in the context of training in healthcare in particular, previous studies assessed healthcare workers' experiences, attitudes, and knowledge regarding serious games in training and found that the majority of healthcare workers were not familiar with serious games or gamification but reported positive attitudes toward the use of serious games for training. Mainly by Younger people working in healthcare were significantly more motivated than older generations to use serious games for training in the future [16].

The training modules that were designed in the TRANSiTION project embed gamification techniques involving challenges to be solved as part of the assessment of each module, in an effort to increase learners' engagement.

3   Conclusion

This chapter explained the TRANSiTION approach for designing a curriculum to develop and support oncology healthcare professionals' digital literacy. The prototype of the curriculum was rigorously developed in a multidisciplinary context and through several stages that incorporated the perspectives of end-users (i.e., HCPs and NCPs) and recipients of digital health technology interventions (i.e., patients and caregivers). Future steps involve piloting the curriculum in small-scale studies to make adjustments based on participants' feedback. The curriculum will then be available to an extensive pool of users (with the goal to reach more than 9000 healthcare professionals beyond the lifespan of the project). Moreover, small-scale studies will embed immersive VR in the training curriculum and evaluate its effectiveness on young oncology nursing students' digital literacy and problem-solving skills. Large-scale studies will evaluate the impact of the designed curriculum on healthcare professionals' digital literacy across Europe and beyond.

References

1. Marques ICP, Ferreira JJM. Digital transformation in the area of health: systematic review of 45 years of evolution. Health Technol. 2020;10(3):575–86.
2. Kraus S, Schiavone F, Pluzhnikova A, Invernizzi AC. Digital transformation in healthcare: analyzing the current state-of-research. J Bus Res. 2021;123:557–67.
3. Kemp E, Trigg J, Beatty L, Christensen C, Dhillon HM, Maeder A, et al. Health literacy, digital health literacy and the implementation of digital health technologies in cancer care: the need for a strategic approach. Health Promot J Austr. 2021;32(S1):104–14.
4. Pfob A, Sidey-Gibbons C, Schuessler M, Lu SC, Xu C, Dubsky P, et al. Contrast of digital and health literacy between IT and health care specialists highlights the importance of multidisciplinary teams for digital health—a pilot study. JCO Clin Cancer Inform. 2021;5:734–45.
5. Kuek A, Hakkennes S. Healthcare staff digital literacy levels and their attitudes towards information systems. Health Informatics J. 2020;26(1):592–612.
6. Vuorikari R, Kluzer S, Punie Y. JRC publications repository. 2022 [cited 2024 Jul 8]. DigComp 2.2: the digital competence framework for citizens—with new examples of knowledge, skills and attitudes. https://publications.jrc.ec.europa.eu/repository/handle/JRC128415.
7. Schmidt M, Huang R. Defining learning experience design: voices from the field of learning design & technology. TechTrends. 2022;66(2):141–58.
8. Reigeluth CM. What's the difference between learning experience design and instructional design? J Appl Instruct Design. 2023;12(3):237–53.
9. American Nursing Association. Critical thinking in nursing: Tips to develop the skill. 2024. Available from https://www.nursingworld.org/content-hub/resources/nursingleadership/critical-thinking-nursing/.
10. Reji RK, Saini SK. Critical thinking and decision making: Essential skills in nursing. Int J Pharm Sci Res. 2022;13(1):61–7. https://doi.org/10.26452/ijrps.v13i1.21.
11. Papathanasiou IV, Kleisiaris CF, Fradelos EC, Kakou K, Kourkouta L. Critical thinking: the development of an essential skill for nursing students. Acta Informatica Medica. 2014;22(4):283.
12. Ana FA, Loreto MS, José LMM, Pablo SM, María Pilar MJ, Myriam SLA. Mobile applications in oncology: a systematic review of health science databases. Int J Med Inform. 2020;133:104001.
13. Nicolaidou I, Tozzi F, Kindynis P, Panayiotou M, Antoniades A. Development and usability of a gamified app to help children manage stress: an evaluation study. Italian J Educ Technol. 2019;27(2):105–20.
14. van Gaalen AEJ, Brouwer J, Schönrock-Adema J, Bouwkamp-Timmer T, Jaarsma ADC, Georgiadis JR. Gamification of health professions education: a systematic review. Adv Health Sci Educ. 2021;26(2):683–711.
15. Damaševičius R, Maskeliūnas R, Blažauskas T. Serious games and gamification in healthcare: a meta-review. Information. 2023;14(2):105.
16. Katonai Z, Gupta R, Heuss S, Fehr T, Ebneter M, Maier T, et al. Serious games and gamification: health care workers' experience, attitudes, and knowledge. Acad Psychiatry. 2023;47(2):169–73.

Culturally Competent AI and Robotics in Healthcare

Irena Papadopoulos

1   Introduction

The notion of cultural competence has been around for almost 50 years. The term 'cultural competence' was first used in 1978, by Derald Wing Sue and colleagues in their book '*Counseling the Culturally Diverse: Theory and Practice*' [1]. However, it was Terry L. Cross and his colleagues who popularised cultural competence with their report titled '*Towards a culturally competent system of care: a monograph on effective services for minority children who are severely emotionally disturbed*' [2]. Despite its long existence, cultural competence only recently became mainstream, not only in health and social care, but in many other domains such as commerce, education, the justice system, environment, hospitality and more.

Closely linked to the notion of cultural competence are racism and inequalities worldwide, which have highlighted the suffering that can result from ignorance of cultural differences at personal, local, national and international levels. However, it is fair to say that many international organisations such as the United Nations (UN) [3], the UN Educational, Scientific and Cultural Organisation (UNESCO) [4–7], and the World Health Organisation (WHO) [8], have produced policies and strategies which promote cultural competence.

The Fourth Industrial Revolution (4IR) is now rapidly changing health and social care, with robots and other artificially intelligent (AI) devices being trialed or deployed within the health domains. The success of these devices will be dependent, to a large extend, on the adoption of a culturally competent approach.

I. Papadopoulos (✉)
Research Centre for Transcultural Studies in Health, Middlesex University, London, UK

A. Charalambous (ed.), *Critical Perspectives on Technological Innovations in Healthcare*, https://doi.org/10.1007/978-3-031-87158-0_3

This chapter explores the need for culturally competent (AI) devices and socially assistive robots (SARs) in healthcare, the challenges, strategies and ethical issues faced by the developers and users of these technologies, the benefits of using the new technologies, and the urgent need for training healthcare professionals to work with the new AI and robotics technologies. The CARESSES project [9] will be introduced and will be referred to in the sections of this chapter. A basic information about the CARESSES project is provided at the end of this chapter.

2   Definitions, and the Need and Benefits of Culturally Competent AI and Robotics

Papadopoulos [10] defined cultural competence as the capacity to provide effective and compassionate healthcare taking into consideration people's cultural beliefs, behaviourism, and needs. Cultural competence is not an end in itself, but a means to an end. The end is to improve health outcomes for patients and communities, reduce health inequalities and promote social justice. Cultural competence is an ongoing process of learning, reflection, and self-awareness. It requires nurses (and other health and care workers) to constantly examine their own cultural assumptions and biases and to engage in a process of lifelong learning and professional development [10, 11]. This definition and explanation were developed with humans in mind. The Papadopoulos model [10] of cultural competence includes four key constructs: cultural awareness, cultural knowledge, cultural sensitivity, and cultural competence in practice. However, during the CARESSES project (Culturally Aware Robots and Environmental Sensors Systems for Elderly Support), it was clear that a new definition of cultural competence was needed, one which, although based on my human definition, was now referring to a non-human entity. Therefore, a culturally competent socially assistive robot (CCSAR) was defined as a robot that has knowledge of the culture-generic characteristics of its user, whilst being able to adapt its behaviour to gain and use culture-specific knowledge in order to respond sensitively to the users' needs, preferences, and ways of living. To achieve this, the robot should be aware of factors such as the age, education, family structure, religion, and cultural heritage (cultural awareness). In addition to the robot's programmed culture-generic knowledge, the robot should be able to assess the needs of the user to obtain culture-specific information. This process is briefly described under the title 'ADORE' further down. If the user has a health problem the robot should take into consideration the user's cultural values, beliefs and attitudes about health and illness, as well as their self-care practices (cultural knowledge). The robot should be sensitive about the user's attributes like language, accent, interpersonal skills, communication skills, ability to trust others, and to be compassionate to others (cultural sensitivity). Finally, the robot should be able to put all the above into practice whilst promoting social justice by challenging discrimination, oppression, prejudice, and inequalities (cultural competence in practice).

3   Needs and Benefits for Culturally Competent AI and Robotics

As AI and robotics will become increasingly integrated into healthcare systems around the world, there is a growing recognition of the need to ensure these technologies are culturally competent and able to provide equitable, high-quality care to diverse patient populations. The development of culturally competent AI and robots in healthcare is not just a matter of improving patient experiences and outcomes, it is an ethical and practical necessity as healthcare systems strive to reduce inequalities and deliver more personalised, effective care. Figure 1 below provides the six interconnected factors influencing the needs and benefits of cultural competent AI and robotics in healthcare. These six factors are explained here.

Fig. 1 Factors influencing the needs and benefits of culturally competent AI and Robotics in healthcare

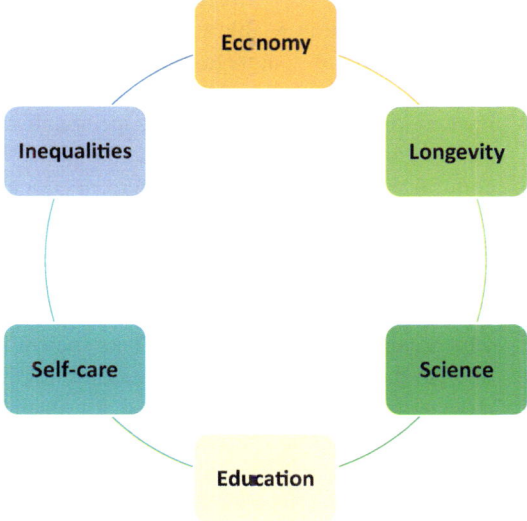

Economy: Globally, healthcare institutions are experiencing economic pressures due to all the factors shown in Fig. 1. AI and robotics are viewed as the tools which will enable policy makers and care providers to manage the economic challenges through new, faster, more sensitive, and accurate processes. However, these benefits will be achieved if, for example, cultural competence guides the development of the tools, the data collection and analysis.

Longevity: Research evidence and public consensus acknowledge the fact that humans are living longer and thus require healthcare for a longer period. This means that more resources are needed such as money and care staff. However, across the multicultural world there is a shortage of care workers. Research indicates that culturally competent AI and robotics will alleviate this challenge by taking over tasks currently performed by humans: a huge and positive benefit.

Science: One of the benefits coming from AI and robotics is their contribution in medical discoveries which enables humans to live longer and have better quality of life. On the one hand, these discoveries have the potential of saving monies due to healthier lifestyles and faster recoveries from illness and surgery, on the other hand, many diseases that had no cures or could not be diagnosed early, often resulting in premature death, are now cured or managed with expensive treatments. Scientists are gradually discovering that cultural factors can influence how patients describe symptoms or how diseases manifest. Culturally competent AI could improve much needed diagnostic accuracy and efficiency by accounting for these variations [12].

Education: This is a key influencing factor for the need of AI and robotics in healthcare. People are now able to access health and illness information anytime and anywhere, in any language, on their smart phones and other assistive devices. There is an explosion of AI platforms, models, devices, and many more, providing text, pictures, graphics, videos, personalised information, and so on, enabling them to take pro-active actions, and making informed decisions based on their cultural values and beliefs. The current educational tools are needed in order to nurture the many AI and robotics beneficial possibilities.

Self-care: Culturally competent care information and devices enable individuals to take control of their lives. Self-administered devices such as those measuring a number of blood elements and blood oxygen, robots, and assistive devices which can remind the person to take their medication or to do their exercises, or wear their smart prostheses are examples of benefits. However, as healthcare moves towards more personalised approaches, AI systems need to be able to account for the cultural factors that influence health behaviours, beliefs, and outcomes [13].

Inequalities: Ethnic minorities often experience worse health outcomes and quality of care, due in part to cultural and linguistic barriers [14]. There is a need for eradicating these inequalities. Culturally competent AI could help address these inequalities by providing AI-powered real-time translation services in healthcare settings, chatbots, and virtual assistants trained in multiple languages and cultural communication styles, AI-powered telehealth platforms designed to overcome cultural barriers to healthcare access, voice-activated systems that explain medical terms in culturally appropriate ways.

4   Challenges in Developing Culturally Competent Healthcare AI and Robotics

Whilst the previous section provided the examples of the need for culturally competent AI and robotics, there remain significant challenges in developing truly culturally competent AI and robotic systems for healthcare, some of which are summarised below:

Complexity of culture: Culture is multifaceted and dynamic, making it challenging to fully capture in AI systems. However, Kitsios et al. [15] discussing this matter in an article in the journal of Applied Sciences, emphasises the fact that the implementation of AI in healthcare is not only a technical challenge but also a socio-cultural one, as AI systems must navigate diverse cultural contexts and adapt to varying healthcare norms and practices. I will provide my solutions of this challenge within the CARESSES case study. A systematic literature review on ChatGPT's implementation in education, underscored the challenges AI faces in interpreting cultural heritage and values accurately. The study points out the potential for AI to misrepresent cultural nuances, stressing the importance of a critical approach when using AI in culturally sensitive fields [16].

Data bias and representation: One of the underpinning pillars of cultural competence is that of human rights. As stated above my cultural competence theory and model requires that health professionals challenge all behaviours that promote inequalities, including data bias. Many AI systems are trained on datasets that underrepresent minority populations, potentially leading to biased or less accurate results for these groups. In a recent article Agarwal et al. [17] state that whilst technological advances in data collection and processing as well as extraordinarily powerful machine learning methods have opened the door to a deeper understanding of patients, the social determinants of health continue to be important factors in achieving the goals of equity and fairness. They go on to state that the time has come to reimagine how AI/ML algorithms can better advocate for patients by finding more nuanced patterns rather than relying on group-level race corrections. Equitable AI will not happen without asking the hard questions to understand why we observe unequal outcomes. Simply relying on the current system will not fully address health inequities. Bias aware AI processes must be enforced so as not to exacerbate current inequities.

Ethical considerations: This challenge is connected to the previous one on data biases. Ethics is the fastest growing subfield of AI and almost all companies, governments and non-governmental international organisations involved in AI and robotics establish ethics teams to discuss the huge challenges faced by the sector. For example, the various UNESCO's reports [4–7], on AI ethics stress the need for AI to be developed and deployed in ways that respect human dignity, democracy, justice, privacy, diversity, and sustainable development. In a research study I conducted with colleagues exploring the views of care home workers regarding their acceptability of having socially assistive humanoid robots in their workplace, we discovered that their concerns were about the privacy, dignity and data collection about the residents [18]. This indicates that in order to gain the trust of the public culturally competent ethics must always be used. During the CARESSES project the research team, which included two ethicists, took great care to identify the ethical issues and apply culturally competent solutions [9].

Acceptability and technical limitations: The CARESSES study revealed that participants had a variety of opinions and views about the use of AI technology and robots. Several comments suggested that participants were generally accepting of robots and saw the potential benefits of using robots in society. Participants also recognised that technology was rapidly advancing within society, and although these innovations were welcomed, they were also the cause of fear, with some participants commmenting that they and their colleagues found robots frightening. Several participants were concerned that the older people in the care home, especially those with dementia, may also be fearful of robots. Another view was that humans should always be involved in the care of fellow humans. Participants expressed their awareness that care AI technology and robotics are work in progress and still have limitations such as lacking many human traits and qualities necessary for looking after older people.

All the challenges included in this section can be positively addressed if the AI and robotics developers engage with diverse communities and health professionals who can contribute in the creation of culturally competent designs, developments, and deployments of these technologies thus meeting real public needs and the health professionals' acceptance [12].

5   The Urgent Need for Training Healthcare Professionals to Work with the New AI and Robotics Technologies

The importance of training and education in relation to technological developments in health and social care was the focus of the UK Topol report which was published in 2019. Titled 'Preparing the healthcare workforce to deliver the digital future' the report suggested that the healthcare landscape in the UK is changing, as is the workforce. It recommends that National Health Service (NHS) staff will urgently need to have digital skills and digital literacy in order to be able to deal with new ways of working. Values of patient-centred care will need to be key to these efforts. Continuous investment in specialist skills as well as appropriate leadership and planning will be needed to achieve the outcomes required to deal with the changes brought about by the 4IR [19].

However, training efforts related to SARs have been limited, revealing inadequacies in the preparedness of health and social care professionals [20]. As mentioned in the previous section, healthcare staff desire to gain a range of skills, from basic operational skills to in-depth knowledge of ethical and legal aspects, data protection, and privacy [21].

One successful example of addressing the preparedness of multidisciplinary staff was the 2020 EU ERASMUS+ project titled 'Preparing health and social care workers to work with socially assistive artificially intelligent robots in health and social care environments'. Five European countries with six partner institutions participated in the project: UK (coordinator), Italy, Austria, Romania, and Cyprus. A massive online, open access course (MOOC) was developed, delivered, and evaluated. The quantitative analysis of the MOOC data on attendance, participation, assessments, and evaluation revealed improvements in participants' knowledge in relation to practical aspects, benefits and challenges of SARs implementation, relevant ethical issues and equality, diversity, and inclusion matters. Table 1 presents the four modules of the MOOC. Each module addresses one of the four constructs of the Papadopoulos model of cultural competence, which if you remember are 'cultural awareness', 'cultural knowledge', 'cultural sensitivity' and 'cultural competence in practice'. Each module includes four micro-learning units covering key content as they relate to each module.

Table 1 MOOC modules and learning units' topics

Modules	Learning unit 1	Learning unit 2	Learning unit 3	Learning unit 4
Module 1. Cultural awareness	Definitions, terminology, abbreviations and course orientation	The needs for SARs: the professional and the patient's perspective	Misconceptions and stereotypes about robots	Cultural values, attitudes, and views about SARs
Module 2. Cultural knowledge	Types and uses of SARs in different health and social care settings	Capabilities and the potential 'role' of SARs: imaginary vs existing robots	SARs' benefits and challenges in the context of health and social care	Cultural aspects in designing and interacting with SARs
Module 3. Cultural sensitivity	Human-robot interaction and communication of personnel, family, carers, and robots	Ethical and legal issues of SARs implementation	Working together: humans-robot collaboration	Culturally sensitive and compassionate human-robot companionship
Module 4. Cultural competence in practice	Practical skills and general abilities in the interface with robots and artificial agents	Safety in the use of robots for the care of the patient/client	Rights of patients/clients and inequalities in access to SARs	The ADORE approach/model

5.1   The ADORE Model and Approach

As mentioned in an earlier section of this chapter, the ADORE model and approach was developed by I. Papadopoulos during the CARESSES project (2017–2020). The ADORE acronym stands for Assess, Do, Observe, Revise, and Evaluate. The robot can use ADORE steps to obtain cultural-specific information by asking a question which will lead to an assessment (A), depending on the answer by the human in its care the robot proceeds to act on it (D), and observes the results (O), if the result is unsatisfactory the robot revises its actions (R) and then evaluates the outcome (E). This process is depicted as a spiral that goes on as long as it is needed [9].

6   The CARESSES Case Study

In 2017, the CARESSES European-Japanese multidisciplinary and multinational consortium commenced the process of developing the first culturally competent SAR (CCSAR). The team strongly believed that cultural competence would be as important to a robot carer/companion as it is to a human carer. Bruno et al. [22] stated that today, it is technically conceivable to build robots that reliably accomplish basic assistive services. However, the services provided by these robots are rigid and invariant with respect to the place, person, and culture. The consortium believed that if service robots are to be accepted in the real world by real people, they must take into account the cultural identity of their users. Therefore, cultural competence must be the approach in deciding how to provide their services.

The CARESSES team included robotics engineers, culturally competent nurse academics, ethicists, experts in health care trials, computer programmers, and psychologists. The key goals of the project can be summarised under two headings: (a) Innovation and (b) the development of Culturally competent robotic capabilities (see Table 2).

Table 2 Improving well-being, reducing loneliness of older people

Innovation/breakthrough	Culturally competent robotic capabilities
• Improving the acceptance of care robots • The development of the first ever culturally competent robot • No previous research or commercial enterprise has explored the possibility of culturally competent robot	AUTONOMOUS LEARNING: ability to collect, remember, and use person-specific information COMPANIONSHIP: communicating through speech and gestures; providing entertainment (e.g., reading aloud, playing music and games); connecting people; reminiscing HEALTH PROMOTION: providing health-related information; encouraging exercise, hydration, nutrition; reminders about health checks CARE: assisting the person in performing everyday tasks; reminding the person to take their medication; doctors/hospital appointments; working with SC team SAFETY and PREVENTION: alerting carers and emergency services about accidents such as falls, burns, cuts, acute pain, etc.

A conceptual framework for the development of culturally competent guidelines for the robotics engineers and software developers was produced as shown in detail in Fig. 2. The framework contained five domains and seven rules which were populated and informed by Hofstede's Cultural Dimensions Theory which is a framework used to understand the differences in culture across countries, and the principles of the Papadopoulos Transcultural Model and ADORE approach, to further develop the culturally competent guidelines [9].

Figure 3 provides the methodology used by the culturally competent experts in the development of the guidelines. For more information for every stage of the process included in the methodology please refer to the book 'Transcultural Artificial Intelligence and Robotics in Health and Social Care' [9]

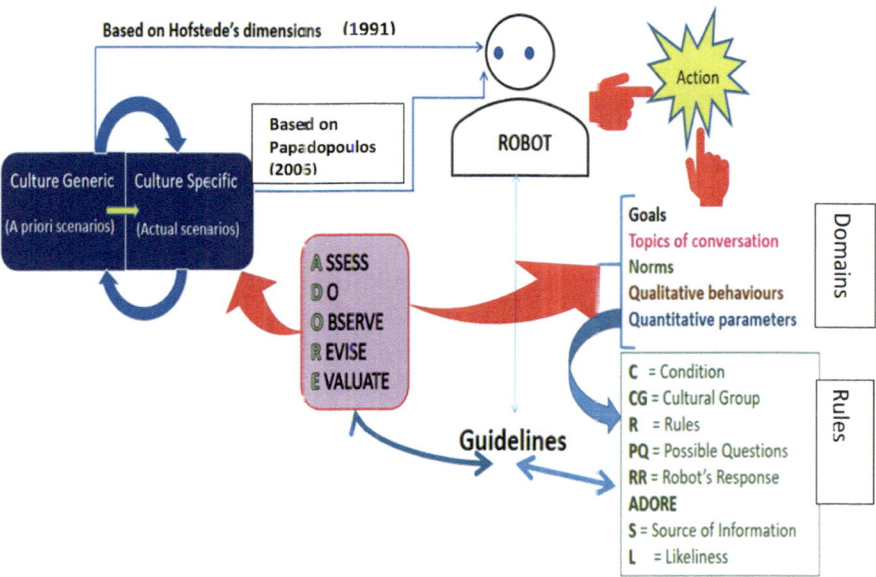

Fig. 2 Conceptual framework for the development of guidelines. (Reproduced with permission from Copyright Elsevier—This figure was published in the book 'Transcultural Artificial Intelligent and Robotics in Health and Social Care', authored by I. Papadopoulos, C. Koulouglioti, C. Papadopoulos, A. Sgorbissa, Chapter 7, page 136, Copyright Elsevier, 2022)

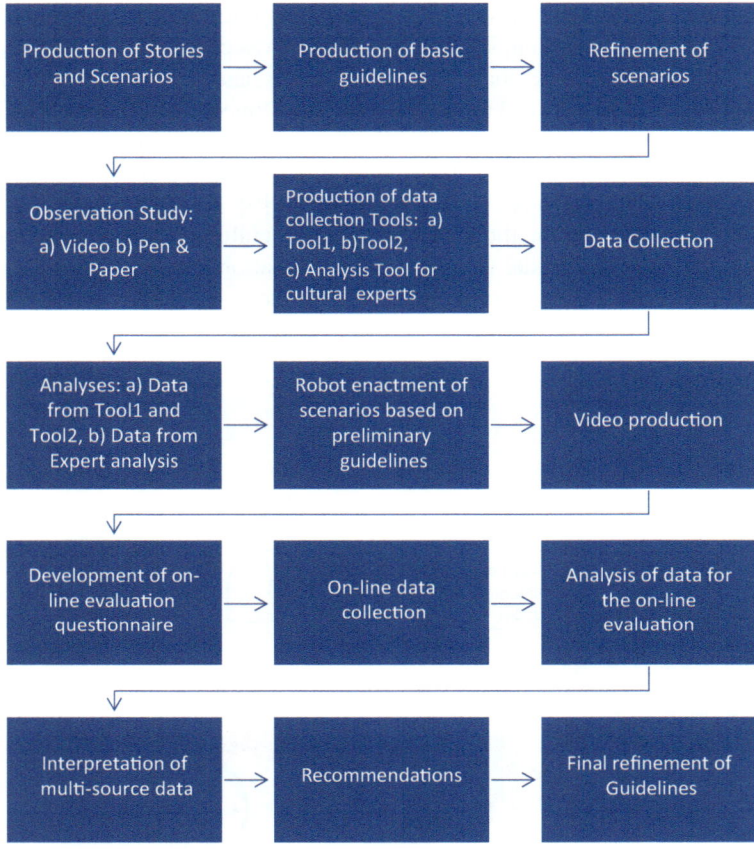

Fig. 3 Methodology. (This figure was published in the book 'Transcultural Artificial Intelligent and Robotics in Health and Social Care', authored by I. Papadopoulos, C. Koulouglioti, C. Papadopoulos, A. Sgorbissa, Chapter 7, page 135, Copyright Elsevier, 2022)

7 Conclusion

The development and deployment of culturally competent AI and robotic technologies in healthcare is not just a desirable goal; it is an urgent necessity as healthcare systems around the world strive to provide more equitable, effective, and personalised care. Whilst there are significant challenges to overcome, the potential benefits in terms of improved health outcomes, reduced disparities, and enhanced patient experiences are immense.

Moving forward, it will be crucial to prioritise cultural competence in the development of healthcare AI, adopt interdisciplinary collaboration, engage diverse communities, and establish robust frameworks for evaluation and continuous improvement. By doing so, we can harness the power of AI and robotics to create a healthcare future that truly serves all patients, regardless of their cultural background.

References

1. Sue DW, Sue D, Neville HA, Smith L. Counselling the culturally diverse: theory and practice. 9th ed. New Jersey: Wiley; 2022.
2. Cross TL, Bazron BJ, Dennis KW, Isaacs MR. Towards a culturally competent system of care: a monograph on effective services for minority children who are severely emotionally disturbed. Washington DC: Georgetown University Child Development Center, CASSP Technical Assistance Center; 1989.
3. United Nations Department of Economic and Social Affairs. Building an inclusive, sustainable and resilient future with indigenous peoples: a call to action. New York: United Nations; 2021.
4. UNESCO World Commission on the Ethics of Scientific Knowledge and Technology (COMEST). Preliminary study on the ethics of artificial intelligence. Paris: UNESCO; 2019.
5. UNESCO. UNESCO recommendation on the ethics of artificial intelligence (draft). Paris: UNESCO; 2020.
6. UNESCO. Recommendation on the ethics of artificial intelligence. Paris: UNESCO; 2021.
7. UNESCO. Reimagining our futures together: a new social contract for education. Paris: UNESCO Publishing; 2022.
8. World Health Organization. Global competency standards for refugee and migrant health services. Geneva: World Health Organization; 2022.
9. Papadopoulos I, Koulouglioti C, Papadopoulos C, Sgorbissa A. Transcultural artificial intelligence and robotics in health and social care. London: Elsevier; 2022.
10. Papadopoulos I. Transcultural health and social care: development of culturally competent practitioners. Edinburgh: Churchill Livingstone Elsevier; 2006.
11. Papadopoulos I. Culturally competent compassion. London: Routledge; 2018.
12. Gianfrancesco MA, Tamang S, Yazdany J, Schmajuk G. Potential biases in machine learning algorithms using electronic health record data. JAMA Intern Med. 2018;178(11):1544–7. https://doi.org/10.1001/jamainternmed.2018.3763.
13. Char DS, Shah NH, Magnus D. Implementing machine learning in health care—addressing ethical challenges. N Engl J Med. 2018;378(11):981–3. https://doi.org/10.1056/NEJMp1714229.
14. Hall WJ, Chapman MV, Lee KM, Merino YM, Thomas TW, Payne BK, et al. Implicit racial/ethnic bias among health care professionals and its influence on health care outcomes: a systematic review. Am J Public Health. 2015;105(12):e60–76. https://doi.org/10.2105/AJPH.2015.302903
15. Kitsios F, Kamariotou M, Syngelakis AI, Talias MA. Recent advances of artificial intelligence in healthcare: a systematic literature review. Appl Sci. 2023;13(13):7479. https://doi.org/10.3390/app13137479.
16. Mohebi L. Empowering learners with ChatGPT: insights from a systematic literature exploration. Discov Educ. 2024;3(1):1–13. https://doi.org/10.1007/s44217-024-00120-y.
17. Agarwal R, Bjarnadottir M, Rhue L, Dugas M, Crowley K, Clark J, et al. Addressing algorithmic bias and the perpetuation of health inequities: an AI bias aware framework. Health Policy Technol. 2023;12(1):100702. https://doi.org/10.1016/j.hlpt.2022.100702.
18. Papadopoulos I, Ali S, Papadopoulos C, Koulouglioti C. A qualitative exploration of care homes workers' views and training needs in relation to the use of socially assistive humanoid robots in their workplace Int J Older People Nursing. 2021;17(3):e12432. https://doi.org/10.1111/opn.12432.
19. NHS. The Topol review: preparing the healthcare workforce to deliver the digital future. An independent report on behalf of the secretary of state for health and social. London: NHS; 2019.

20. Papadopoulos I, Koulouglioti C, Lazzarino R, et al. Views about perceived training needs of health care professionals in relation to socially assistive robots: an international online survey. Contemp Nurse. 2023;59:344–61. https://doi.org/10.1080/10376178.2022.2162989.
21. Hung L, Mann J, Perry J, Berndt A, Wong J. Technological risks and ethical implications of using robots in long-term care. J Rehab Assist Technol Eng. 2022;9:20556683221106917. https://doi.org/10.1177/20556683221106917.
22. Bruno B, Chong NY, Kamide H, Kanoria S, Lee J, Lim Y, et al. The CARESSES EU-Japan project: making assistive robots culturally competent. arXiv:1708.06276v1 [cs.RO]. 2017 Aug 21.

Telemonitoring and Teleconsultation in Cancer Care

S. Mappouras, M. Gemenaris, and E. Kyriacou

1   Introduction

Cancer care involves complex and often prolonged, personalized treatment procedures that create the necessity for continuous monitoring and frequent consultations with specialized healthcare professionals that often lack time [1]. In the recent years, healthcare professionals are starting to identify the necessity of technology in their clinical workflows, that can enable and ease the provision of personalized healthcare and address the needs and modify their approaches tailored to the needs of each individual patient [2].

Telemonitoring and Teleconsultation in Cancer Care constitute 2 intertwined but also distinct pillars that aim on enhancing the effectiveness of monitoring and communication of Cancer patients during all Cancer phases.

Telemonitoring is an emerging technology that refers to the remote monitoring and assessment of patients' health status, which has a primary use of utilizing several digital tools and technologies to track the overall well-being of patients through continuous distant monitoring that includes, but is not limited to, vital signs, symptoms, treatment side effects, and other relevant health-related indicators [3]. The secondary use is to utilize the continuous streams of data generated from the telemonitoring activities, using real-time advanced data processing techniques to visualize the data in a readable and insightful form for the physicians, giving insights to drive personalized care, prevent bad situations, and make timely interventions by adjusting the treatment based on data-driven decisions.

S. Mappouras · M. Gemenaris · E. Kyriacou (✉)
Department of Electrical Engineering and Computer Engineering and Informatics,
Cyprus University of Technology, Limassol, Cyprus
e-mail: sm.mappouras@edu.cut.ac.cy; michalis.gemenaris@cut.ac.cy;
efthyvoulos.kyriacou@cut.ac.cy

© The Author(s), under exclusive license to Springer Nature   35
Switzerland AG 2025
A. Charalambous (ed.), *Critical Perspectives on Technological Innovations in
Healthcare*, https://doi.org/10.1007/978-3-031-87158-0_4

On the other hand, teleconsultation technology enables remote communication between the patient and the doctor, throughout the entire timeline of care, from the initial diagnosis and treatment planning to the follow-up care and palliative support [4]. Teleconsultation is keen to reduce hospital visits that sometimes exposes the patients to dangerous bacteria/environment, and at the same time, is keen to allow doctors to provide better support to their patients and enhance the ability of the doctors to monitor more patients within less time.

Digital tools have already demonstrated and evaluated the value of these technologies in cancer care through numerous research studies, research projects, and real-world use cases and applications [5, 6].

The remaining structure of this chapter is as follows: Sect. 2 explains the underlying technologies that enable telemonitoring and teleconsultation and facilitate data collection to be used for primary and secondary use. Section 3 describes the roles and benefits of telemonitoring and teleconsultation tools for Cancer Care. Section 4 presents the case studies that include eHealth, mHealth technological solutions. Finally, Sect. 5 concludes the chapter by identifying open research challenges and suggesting directions for future research in the field.

2 Underlying Technologies to Enable Telemonitoring and Teleconsultation

2.1 Metrics and Methodologies for Data Collection

To achieve the desired benefits from the utilization of Telemonitoring and Teleconsultation technologies in cancer care, it is essential to establish clear and well-structured methodologies for identifying and selecting the most relevant metrics and configure seamless and continuous streams for generation and collection of data. As a result of these technologies being inherently data-driven, meaning that in order to generate valuable insights and support effective decision-making, the collection of large volumes of high-quality data is a prerequisite [7].

One of the foundational elements for this data collection workflow is the monitoring of vital biosignals, which provide an easy way to forward physiological information about the patient's health status, through the use of IoT sensors that are embedded on smart devices such as smart watches and other types of wearable devices. Some types of biosignals might include, but are not limited to the heart rate, respiration, body temperature, and blood pressure that can be monitored in real time. This is significant for cancer patients regardless of stage and type of cancer, as biosignals constitute a vital way to facilitate early detection against infections, complications, or other medical issues that can be prevented [8]. In addition, questionnaires can play a key role in gathering subjective yet vital information directly from the patients regarding their symptoms, side effects, and overall Quality of Life (QoL). This might include questionnaires related to patient-reported outcomes (PROs), QoL, and others related to psychosocial and emotional health of the patient [9].

- PROs will give the patient the opportunity to self-report on specific symptoms such as pain, fatigue, nausea or cognitive difficulties, which are not always clearly visible through clinical trials.
- QoL will give a broader view on the effects of treatment on the patients physical, phycological, and social functioning, revealing how treatment affects not only the survival, but also the overall QoL of the patient.
- Psychosocial and emotional health questionnaires will assist the identification of stress, anxiety, depression and the overall emotional well-being, all of which play a significant role in the patient's ability to cope with the disease and adhere to the treatment protocols.

These types of questionnaires will provide an immediate, comprehensive view of how the disease and its treatment impact the patient's life and provide valuable insights toward more personalized care and timely interventions, enhancing both clinical procedures and patient's QoL. Some established examples include the EORTC QLQ-C30 [9] that assesses the PROs and QoL, and EQ-5D-5L [10] that is effectively used to evaluate QoL in terms of physical and emotional well-being for patients undergoing chemotherapy. Other types of useful data that could benefit the treatment process include the nutritional monitoring of the patient, the environmental data around the places that the patient spends his most time on. These constitute external factors that can affect the patient's QoL, distress that contribute positively or negatively to his treatment procedures. Furthermore, the collection of genomic and imaging data are a cornerstone in cancer care. Telemonitoring platforms can facilitate the remote sharing and analysis of image results such as CT scans and MRIs, allowing oncologists to assess tumor progression or regression over time. Similarly, genomic data allows for genetic mutations to be linked to cancer progression, and data-driven decisions can tailor treatments to target those mutations more effectively. All these could be enhanced using emerging technologies such as AI and image processing and analysis. Concluding, comparing the automatically monitored biosignals with information given directly from the patient (e.g., questionnaires), healthcare provides can adhere to data-driven decisions to prevent the progression of the disease and identify ways to improve the quality of care provided and the QoL of the patient [11].

2.2   Technologies and Tools for Telemonitoring

The successful implementation of telemonitoring in cancer care heavily relies on a range of technological tools that enable continuous streams of data collection, real-time monitoring, and seamless communication between the patients and healthcare providers. With nowadays technology, there is a wide range of available technological tools that can be used for telemonitoring, depending on each case, patient/physician preferences, or technological availability for specific regions, centers, or patients. This section distinguishes between the hardware and software that is utilized for telemonitoring for data collection. One of the most common hardware tools utilized for telemonitoring due to the ease of use, as well as the importance of the data recorded are wearable devices. Wearable devices usually include a number of IoT smart sensors for measuring vital biosignals such as the ones mentioned in Sect. 2.1, which are then recorded and transmitted seamlessly with minimal user intervention in a non-invasive manner, that are transmitted to a server and then to a platform/app accessible from the healthcare providers sometimes in even real time. Examples of the wearable devices include smart watches, fitness trackers and specialized medical wearables. Furthermore, smart patient ECG monitors and ultrasound devices are types of powerful hardware tools that can be used for telemonitoring, in collaboration with other doctors or nurses. However, especially for cancer care wearable devices remain the most widely used hardware tool [12]. In terms of software, solutions usually are comprised of multiple subsystems that are integrated together through a centralized database to exchange data. In this context, Mobile Health Applications (mHealth Apps) represent the software interface usually accessible through smart phones or tablets, that are used in conjunction with wearable devices to track symptoms, medications, biosignals, and more. In addition, in cancer care, mHealth apps enable patients to self-report on questionnaires, such as PROs or QoLs, or assist the patients to maintain their treatment schedule by providing medication reminders and tracking appointments. All the data recorded through the mHealth apps are analyzed and visualized through remote patient monitoring platforms (RPMs). These platforms act as the infrastructure for telemonitoring, allowing healthcare providers to monitor their patients' conditions remotely and make data-driver clinical decisions. Furthermore, in some cases, more advanced technologies are employed and integrated to the RPM such as machine learning algorithms to identify trends among disease evolution or make future projections and predictions for each patient individually [13–15].

2.3   Technologies and Tools for Teleconsultation

Teleconsultation tools are simpler in comparison to telemonitoring tools as the procedure is straight forward and does not require advanced and complex tools. To begin with, the foundational technology for teleconsultations is video conferencing, that allows patients and healthcare providers to have face-to-face consultations remotely. What is important here is the results of the teleconsultations to be recorded in a structured way in order to make it easier for further analysis. Thus, mHealth apps and RPMs can be utilized for documenting the results of teleconsultations, either in the form of standard forms such as questionnaires, or free text. Additionally, platforms that are used for teleconsultations must be compliant with specific regulations such as EU General Data Protection Regulation (GDPR) [16] to ensure that data that goes through the platform are private and secured. Also, the platforms should adhere to specific high-quality video and audio standards as well as screen sharing for viewing diagnostic results, analytics etc. Along with the video conferencing, secure messaging systems can be used for quick direct communication between the healthcare provider and the patient, for exchanging questions and answers, report symptoms, seek clarification on treatment instructions, or any other useful data exchange between the two parties without the need of a scheduled appointment [17–19].

2.4 Data Collection and Storage

As stated earlier, in order for telemonitoring and teleconsultation to be applied effectively there is a strong need for continuous and reliable collection of large volumes of data. Therefore, secure and efficient data collection and storage are critical to ensure that data are collected and stored in a secure manner, in a way that are easily accessible from authorized users. Modern storage solutions such as data lakes can be employed, to provide a flexible, quick, scalable, and efficient way to collect and store large volumes of data with different types (structured, semi-structured, and unstructured), that can be later utilized through machine learning models or undergo of statistical analysis either for individual patients or a group of aggregated patients to extract insights about cancer care in general. During large volumes of data collection, securing the transmission of data cannot be dismissed. Secure communication protocols such as SSL and TLS should be employed [20], to guarantee that all data that are exchanged between different devices, applications, and healthcare providers are encrypted and protected from unauthorized access or cyberattack attempts. The stored data must be stored taking into account the interoperability across different devices and platforms within healthcare systems. Interoperability standards such as HL7 FHIR [21] should be taken into consideration to accomplish smooth exchange of information between health-related software systems. This promotes collaborative care, enables external software systems to exchange data and maximize the impact of Telemonitoring and Teleconsultation. Lastly, the data collection and storage must comply with privacy regulations toward the sensitive data handling of the patients, such as the HIPAA [22] in the USA and GDPR in Europe [16, 23].

2.5 Primary and Secondary Use of Data

The collection of data serves multiple purposes, broadly categorized into primary and secondary uses that are both important for the efficient monitoring of the whole procedure (from diagnosis to treatment), to the future exploitation for improving healthcare protocols. Primary use of data refers to the direct utilization of data in patient care and clinical decision-making. More specifically, data such as biosignals, questionnaires, imaging and analysis results, are immediately made available to doctors for taking more informed decisions during the patient care procedures. This is with minimal analysis, in order to increase the speed that the data are provided to the doctor for quick results. For reference, continuously monitored vital signs recorded through smart watches are visualized in real time through an RPM, where the platform provides decision support to the doctor to detect early signs of infections [24]. The primary use of data may also encompass the integration proce-dures with electronic health records (EHRs), making sure that the health record of each patient remains up to date and the newly collected data are seamlessly inte-grated into the patient's comprehensive medical record [25]. This integration allows healthcare providers to have access to a complete, near real-time view of the patient's health, and also paves the way for cross-border transmission of health records. On the other hand, secondary use of data extends beyond the individual patient care where the data are aggregated and analyzed for purposes such as research, policymaking, machine learning and predictive analytics, and many more [26]. Lastly, this is also aligned with the European Health Data Space (EHDS) issued by the European Commission in 2022 that aims on providing to the citizens access, ownership and control of their health data across the whole European Union [27]. Figure 1 displays the ways in which eCAN project could manage the primary and secondary use of data collected from telemonitoring and teleconsultation activities.

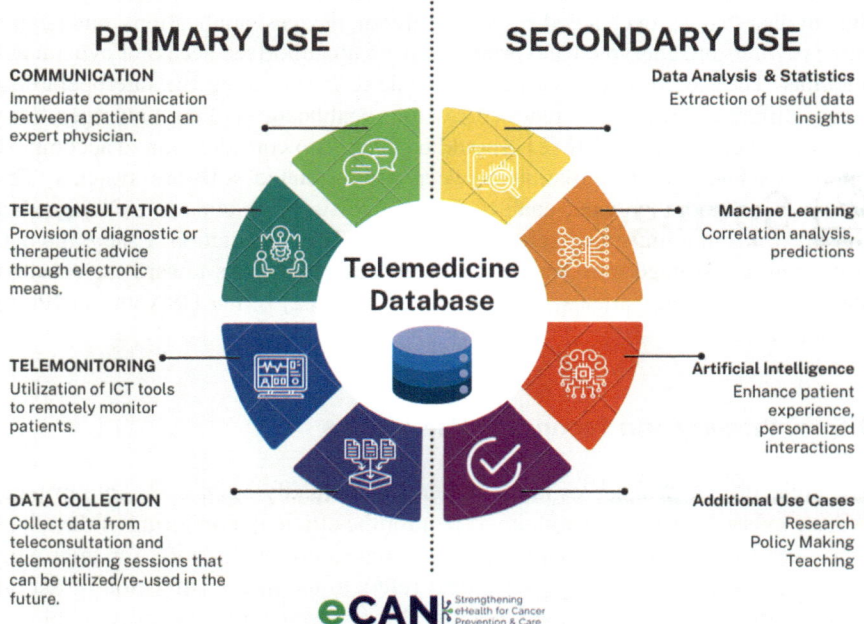

Fig. 1 Primary and secondary use of data in eCAN project. (Reproduced with permission from eCAN) (eCAN "Co-Funded by the European Union. Views and opinions expressed are however those of the author(s) only and do not necessarily reflect those of the European Union or HaDEA. Neither the European Union nor the granting authority can be held responsible for them")

3 Roles and Benefits of Telemonitoring and Teleconsultation in Cancer Care

3.1 Role of Telemonitoring in Cancer Care

From the previous sections, integrating telemonitoring practices in cancer care endorses numerous benefits that contribute both to the procedures of effective monitoring of patients and also the improvement of the healthcare practices. One of the primary roles is the ability to continuously track patient s health metrics remotely. Through the usage of smart devices, collection of vital biosignals can be established and provide the healthcare providers a real-time view of the patient's condition, reducing the need of frequent hospital visits, thereby decreasing the burden on both patients and healthcare system. This also supports the provision of personalized healthcare, meaning that doctor can support the patient based on data-driven decisions planning the treatment based on the needs of individual patients from information arising from the collected data acquired through the telemonitoring activities. The successful implementation and integration of telemonitoring in clinical practices could scale up to the integration into existing healthcare software systems. This can be facilitated through the creation of Application Programming Interfaces (APIs) that would enable secure data sharing of real-time data that can be integrated into the patient EHR. This would create an ecosystem and a workflow toward the management of the disease for each individual patient, tailored to his needs and specific challenges. The regularly collected data through the monitoring activities would help with the decision-making process and provide the patient's EHR with regular updates. This technology can be integrated into the standard cancer care protocols supporting both hospital-based care and home-based recovery. This hybrid approach takes the benefits of both worlds, the current cancer care methodologies, and takes into advantage the benefits of what these technologies can provide [28].

3.2 Role of Teleconsultation in Cancer Care

Teleconsultation constitutes a more direct way to establish remote communication between the patient and the expert physician, allowing the conduction of remote consultation sessions that can be established on top of the in-person visits. This method can reduce the commute costs for the patient needing to go to the hospital and enable patients to connect with their healthcare providers from the comfort of their homes. Cancer patients often undergo long, complex treatments that require frequent follow-up hospital visits, which can be burdensome and harmful especially for those with limited mobility or weakened immune systems due to treatment. Cancer care often requires the input of a multidisciplinary team of specialists including oncologists, radiologists, pathologists, and surgeons [29]. Teleconsultation significantly can improve access to specialist care, where doctors with different specialists can jointly connect to teleconsultation sessions for a specific patient to provide expert knowledge. These multidisciplinary sessions could be beneficial for all parties, allowing doctors to make faster and more informed decisions, that also need less time than frequent hospital visits. This can give the opportunity to the doctors to see more patients within a specific timeframe.

3.3 Merging Telemonitoring and Teleconsultation in Cancer Care

Telemonitoring and teleconsultation and two different technologies that are complementary in nature and both fall into the broader category of Telemedicine. Telemonitoring provides continuous, real-time data, whereas teleconsultation provides flexibility and accessibility. Merging the two, one can have a complete healthcare model that can drastically enhance patient care. This merge can enhance decision-making and drive data-driven decision-making for the expert clinicians, and the data production of the two can be embedded into advanced machine learning model for predictive analytics, or forecast, that can possibly track, predict, and prevent the evolution of cancer. Advanced models, along with expert knowledge of doctors, allows for a more proactive and personalized treatment that ultimately improves patient outcomes.

4 Existing Work and Case Studies

This area of cancer management has seen significant progress and development particularly concerning the use of telemonitoring and teleconsultation. Some eHealth, mHealth, IoT, and platform-based solutions have been designed and deployed around the world for enhancing patient's experiences, efficiency, and the effectiveness of care delivery processes and minimizing the pressure on the healthcare systems. This section presents brief information about the most significant case studies and solutions, emphasizing the outlook in oncological practice.

4.1 eHealth Solutions

eHealth involves the use of information and communication technologies (ICTs) within healthcare especially in the area of sharing of health information and in the delivery of healthcare information [30]. In cancer care eHealth solutions have played a significant role through the management of patient monitoring, communication and decision-making. A promising solution was developed through eCAN Joint Action (JA) EU-funded project [31] that allows for constant monitoring of the condition of cancer patients and making interventions based on collected data. The eCAN project provides a new model toward cancer treatment that stands as a comprehensive eHealth solution specifically designed for the continuous monitoring and support of cancer patients. This platform comprises telemonitoring, and teleconsultation services enabled by wearable, mobile and web-based technologies. The goal of eCAN is to enhance efficiency in data acquisition and reporting that will enable patients and health care practitioners to receive essential information regarding the need to intervene or alter treatment plans as and when required. eCAN is designed in a way that it can monitor the patients' vital signs, symptoms, treatment side effects in an ongoing and timely manner, which makes it applicable for use in cancer care settings. The eCAN platform monitors the physical status of patients with wearable devices to monitor their heart rates, sleep, and movement. Information from these wearables is synced to the eCAN server daily, ensuring that the health care professionals are constantly updated on the health status of their patients. Owing to the constant stream of information, health care professionals can easily notice signs of exacerbation or side effects of therapy, thereby providing more effective treatment. eCAN utilizes two categories which are broken down into: patient-reported outcome measures (PROMs) and patient-reported experience measures (PREMs). These measures are served to the patients through a mobile application where patients are reporting their health-related quality of life (HRQoL), pain and distress levels, and overall experience with the telemonitoring services. More specifically for measuring HRQoL, EORTC QLQ-C30 [30] is employed, where for distress and pain levels visual analog scale (VAS) [32] is utilized. For the project's pilots, PROMs are collected bi-weekly, while PREMs are gathered at the conclusion of the study from each patient. In addition, eCAN provides teleconsultation services through a web-based platform called "EduMeet" [33]. This reduces the trips to the doctor, which is particularly useful for patients with mobility problems or based in remote areas. This ensures that, upon remotely connecting patients to oncologists in real time, they continuously get support throughout their treatment. Through the platform, health care professionals can effectively monitor the results of the patients' PROMs and identify any deterioration in the patients. Pilot studies have demonstrated the platform's effectiveness and that patients have a great interest in the eCAN tools for teleconsultation and telemonitoring. It also encourages patients to stay engaged in their own care by giving them tools to track their health status, giving them the option of involvement and responsibility in managing their treatment. The data management in eCAN follows the highest standards of privacy and security from GDPR recommendations [16, 23] about data protection in the European Union. Data originating from wearables and PROMs are securely transmitted and stored on a cloud platform and are pseudonymized to maintain the confidentiality of the patient. In all, the eCAN platform represents an integrated state-of-the-art solution for remote care in cancer. This integrates continuous telemonitoring with patient centric tools and secure teleconsultation services, putting forth a comprehensive approach to cancer treatment management with patient-centricity and data-driven insights. This leads not only to quality care but also reduces the burden on healthcare systems by avoiding unnecessary hospital visits, hence increasing efficiency in cancer care delivery.

Besides eCAN, other eHealth initiatives in cancer care that have been developed over the years, besides increasing this potential, provide evidence of improved patient outcomes, especially for the underserved. Another solution is the

ONCOAssist [34] eHealth application built exclusively for the oncology profes-sional. In this app, the user has accessed the cancer treatment guidelines, calcula-tors, and drug dosing recommendations. It helps the oncologists to take quick and evidence-based decisions. The essential resources are combined into one easy-to-use app. The ONCOAssist is widely utilized in clinical settings to ensure the prac-tice of cancer treatment based on the latest research evidence and clinical guidelines for improved patient care.

4.2   mHealth Solutions

mHealth solutions have made cancer care portable, user-friendly, and essential tools in symptoms and health metric monitoring. The first example is MyCancerJourney [35], which is an advanced mobile phone application that empowers those with cancer to monitor their symptoms, medication adherence, and treatment side effects. This app records daily the pain level, fatigue, and other measurable symptoms of patients that are directly shared with healthcare professionals through secure mes-saging. These data enable specialist oncologists to identify trends and adjust treat-ment plans accordingly. There are studies that indicate that such an increase in involvement translates to a higher compliance with treatment programs and reduced health complications among the patients [36]. Noona [37] is a different mHealth platform that enables live interactions between patients and their care teams. Through the tracking of PROs, it detects early signals of complications and facili-tates timely interventions of healthcare providers. This implementation of a proac-tive symptom management approach guarantees the monitoring of patients over time, hence preventing the possibility of health complication associated with the treatments of cancers.

4.3   IoT Solutions

The role of the Internet of Things has become very important in cancer care; the concept of patient monitoring is no longer confined to a single physical location but is remotely accessible. Wearable sensors are part of IoT-enabled devices that can monitor data continuously and, in turn, feed the oncologist to help in the treatment of patients who are not physically present. Apple Watch, Fitbit, and fitness trackers from Garmin have become an indispensable part of daily life for many users who use them for monitoring constant heart rate, physical activity, and sleeping behavior. In the treatment of cancer, these wearables can prove to be more and more helpful in monitoring the recovery of a patient from an ongoing treatment process by detect-ing early signs of complications with ease. For example, wearable ECG monitors have often been used in the cardiac monitoring of cancer patients with underlying cardiovascular risks. More sophisticated IoT solutions include smart sensors that constantly track vital signs, such as oxygen saturation and blood pressure.

This technology can be easily embedded into telemonitoring platforms that will enable oncologists to evaluate the condition of a patient from a distance and take immediate action if required [38, 39].

4.4   Platforms

Remote patient monitoring (RPM) Platforms are the cornerstone of telemonitoring and teleconsultation in cancer care and integrate information coming from wearable devices, mobile apps, and clinical records into one platform available in real time to healthcare professionals. Examples include Vivify Health [40], is an RPM platform used within oncology care is Vivify Health. The platform allows health providers to remotely monitor patients with integrated data from several wearable devices and biosensors. Vivify also supports secure teleconsultations, allowing patients and oncologists to communicate through video conferencing and messaging. Further developing RPM, Medopad solution adds to its telemonitoring and teleconsultation capabilities an artificial intelligence backbone. The AI algorithms in Medopad analyze longitudinal patient data for predictive analytics on the outcomes of treatments and identify high-risk patients with need for extra interventions. It thus has become a strong partner for oncology with personalized and data-driven decision-making [41].

4.5   AI Tools in Cancer Care

Artificial intelligence (AI) tools are foreseen to usher in a new paradigm in cancer care through personalized care and intensive monitoring of changing treatments. AI can provide data-driven insights and decision support based on volume acquired directly from patient-health data that also enable predictions and improve the overall efficiency of patient care, tailored to the needs of each patient [42].

Sophisticated AI models can be developed with a vast majority of data from different sources and types, such as: medical imaging, teleconsultation notes, wearable data, patient-reported data, etc. AI can be utilized for predictions, recognizing patterns that no human could, based on volumes of data. In addition, it can assist the doctors with the design of treatment plans, and/or continuous monitoring while alerting patients and doctors of alarming situations before they happen. Some examples include the application of AI in medical practice at IBM Watson for Oncology; this AI analyzes structured and unstructured medical data from a vast array of sources, including clinical trials, medical literature, and patient records. This system allows an oncologist to identify the best treatment options very rapidly on the grounds of the medical profile of the patient. These AI algorithms from Watson have tended to increase accuracies of treatment plans and decrease manual data analysis time [43].

AI is revolutionizing medical practice, enhancing expert doctor's ability during diagnosis and treatment phases. This reduces the manual required analysis time, and at the same time enhances accuracy in finding tumors and abnormalities with predictions [44]. Some examples of applications include Google DeepMind and Zebra Medical Vision, that are pioneering AI in healthcare. DeepMind conducts research in breakthrough ML and AI models, focusing on creating algorithms that mimic the learning process of human brain. Some applications of their AI models include the diagnostic phases of diseases, such as eye diseases or Cancer. It is worth noting that according to Nature.com, this model was trained to analyze X-ray images of a large number of woman in the USA, achieving a reduction of 5.7% in false positives, where mammogram is diagnosed as abnormal, and also a reduction of 9.4% in false negatives, where cancer was missed. It is also worth mentioning that this model outperformed six radiologists in cancer detection [45]. Zebra Medical Vision, utilizing artificial intelligence and deep learning, has developed an imaging analytics platform. This platform allows healthcare institutions to identify patients at risk of disease and offer preventative treatment pathways to improve patient care [46]. These are just a few of the paradigms that exist, and just a glance at what is coming in the upcoming years in the research community. AI has set the cornerstone for excelling in bioinformatics, ultimately assisting doctors to provide better services for their patients.

5   Concluding Remarks and Future Research

The integration of telemonitoring and teleconsultation in cancer care has the potential to greatly enhance the way in which cancer patients are monitored and treated in the course of their medical treatment. The technologies outlined above are capable of establishing a data-driven cancer care model that meets the personalized needs of each patient. This enhances the quality of the attention given, enabling the monitoring of continuous parameters that are subject to early interventions, at the same time allowing easy access for patients to healthcare professionals and specialists, especially in cases where access is limited by geographical issues. The integration of real-time data collection through telemonitoring, and remote consultations through telemedicine, aim to accomplish what was lacking in conventional cancer treatment, hence offering a more personalized and effective management approach. While the obvious advantages, applications, and ongoing studies are present, several aspects do require further scrutiny if the effectiveness of telemonitoring and teleconsultation in oncology care is to be achieved. The foregoing domains include, but are not limited to, the following: Data privacy and security; as telemonitoring and teleconsultation both generate and collect large amounts of sensitive patient data, ensuring privacy and security of the developed platforms remain top priority. Moreover, the integration of Artificial Intelligence and predictive analytics into the telemonitoring systems brings tremendous opportunities for the possible delivery of real-time decision support or facilitating the prediction of treatment outcomes based on a patient's medical history. Development of artificial intelligence models requires large, real-world datasets obtained with the help of telemonitoring and teleconsultation programs. While AI holds immense promise, significant challenges remain regarding the complete integration of these tools into daily cancer management. Probably the greatest challenge that faces the application of AI in routine clinical care is ensuring the transparency and interpretability of the AI models, whereby health professionals understand why an AI approach makes a particular suggestion.

References

1. Lorenzini E, Boell JEW, Oelke ND, Rodrigues CD, Trindade LF, Winter VDB, Malkiewiez MM, Flores GC, Pluta P, Kolankiewicz ACB. Care transition from hospital to home: cancer patients' perspective. J Pain Symptom Manag. 2020; https://pmc.ncbi.nlm.nih.gov/articles/PMC7268360/. Accessed 21 Oct 2024.
2. Khan SA, Kukafka R, Bigger JT, Johnson SB. Re-engineering opportunities in clinical research using workflow analysis in community practice settings. J Am Med Inform Assoc. 2008; https://pubmed.ncbi.nlm.nih.gov/18999299/. Accessed 21 Oct 2024.
3. Paré G, Jaana M, Sicotte C. Systematic review of home telemonitoring for chronic diseases: the evidence base. J Am Med Inform Assoc. 2007;14(3):269–77. https://doi.org/10.1197/jamia.M2270. Accessed 21 Oct 2024.
4. Deldar K, Bahaadinbeigy K, Tara SM. Teleconsultation and clinical decision making: a systematic review. Acta Inform Med. 2016;24(4):286–92. https://doi.org/10.5455/aim.2016.24.286-292. Accessed 21 Oct 2024.
5. Martin S, Fritsch A, Jouannaud C, Sonntag C, Morel A, Barthelemy P, et al. Real-life clinical and organizational evaluation of telemonitoring and assisted telemonitoring in more than 1500 cancer patients. Ann Oncol. 2023; https://www.annalsofoncology.org/article/S0923-7534(23)02447-X/fulltext. Accessed 21 Oct 2024.
6. Shaffer KM, Turner KL, Siwik C, Gonzalez BD, Upasani R, Glazer JV, Ferguson RJ, Joshua C, Low CA. Digital health and telehealth in cancer care: a scoping review of reviews. Lancet Digit Health. 2023; https://pmc.ncbi.nlm.nih.gov/articles/PMC10124999/. Accessed 21 Oct 2024.
7. Kombathula SH, Pareek P, Srinivasan S, Harika KD, Solanki A, Vyas RK, Kamal M, Vishnoi JR, Bhardwaj P, Misra S. 1454P a prospective trial evaluating the impact of tele-palliative care in cancer patients: exploring opportunities in adversities. Ann Oncol. 2021;32(suppl_5):S1080. https://doi.org/10.1016/j.annonc.2021.08.219.
8. Velikova G, Awad N, Coles-Gale R, Wright EP, Brown JM, Selby PJ. The clinical value of quality of life assessment in oncology practice: a qualitative study of patient and physician views. Psycho-Oncology. 2008;17(7):690–8. https://doi.org/10.1002/pon.1295. https://pubmed.ncbi.nlm.nih.gov/18033733/.
9. Fitzsimmons D, Johnson CD, George S, Payne S, Andrén Sandberg A, Bassi C, Beger HG, Birk D, Büchler MW, Dervenis C, Fernandez Cruz L, Friess H, Grahm AL, Jeekel J, Laugier R, Meyer D, Singer MW, Tihanyi T, EORTC Study Group on Quality of Life. Development of a disease-specific quality of life (QoL) questionnaire module to supplement the EORTC core cancer QoL questionnaire, the QLQ-C30, in patients with pancreatic cancer. Eur J Cancer. 1999;35(7):939–41. https://www.ejcancer.com/article/S0959-8049(99)00047-7/abstract.
10. Lazzari C, Ceresoli GL, Bearz A, Ferreri AJ, Mandalá M, Cordio S, Aprile G, Ghio D, Ferrari Da Passano C, Gregorc V. PSC2.07 telemedicine: a new era for the treatment of patients with cancer. J Thorac Oncol. 2017;12(11):S2178. https://doi.org/10.1016/j.jtho.2017.09.406. https://www.jto.org/article/S1556-0864(17)30779-7/fulltext. Accessed 21 Oct 2024.
11. Mehta V. Artificial intelligence in medicine: revolutionizing healthcare for improved patient outcomes. J Med Res Innov. 2023;7(2):e000292. https://doi.org/10.32892/jmri.292. https://jmrionline.com/jmri/article/view/292. Accessed 21 Oct 2024.

12. Verma K, Preity P, Ranjan R. An insight into wearable devices for smart healthcare technologies. IEEE; 2023. https://doi.org/10.1109/JMRI.10048809. https://ieeexplore.ieee.org/document/10048809. Accessed 21 Oct 2024.
13. He T, Ogunti R, Puppala M, Chen S, Yu X, Mancuso JJ, Wong STC. A smartphone app framework for segmented cancer care coordination. IEEE; 2023. https://ieeexplore.ieee.org/document/10048809. Accessed 21 Oct 2024.
14. Pires ETC, Cheng C, Silva SLFC, Gois SR, Sabbadini FS, Gonçalves AA. The implementation of a mobile app for cancer care management at the Brazilian National Cancer Institute. Stud Health Technol Inform. 2021;289:353–6. https://doi.org/10.3233/SHTI210932. https://ebooks.iospress.nl/doi/10.3233/SHTI210932. Accessed 21 Oct 2024.
15. Haoues M, Mokni R, Sellami A. Machine learning for mHealth apps quality evaluation. Softw Qual J. 2023;31:1179–209. https://doi.org/10.1007/s11219-023-09630-8. Accessed 21 Oct 2024.
16. Ilioudis C, Pangalos G, Zafiropoulos E. Data protection aspects of telemedicine in Europe: the role of the GDPR. J Data Protect Priv. 2020;3(1):53–67.
17. Siddiqui J, Herchline T, Kahlon S, Moyer KJ, Scott JD, Wood BR, Young J. Infectious diseases Society of America position statement on telehealth and telemedicine as applied to the practice of infectious diseases. Clin Infect Dis. 2017;64(3):237–42. https://doi.org/10.1093/cid/ciw773.
18. Pramuka M, van Roosmalen L. Telerehabilitation technologies: accessibility and usability. Int J Telerehab. 2009;1(1) https://doi.org/10.5195/ijt.2009.6016. https://telerehab.pitt.edu/ojs/Telerehab/article/view/6016. Accessed 21 Oct 2024.
19. Barro SG, Kambire JG, Kantagba YMK, Karambiri D, Ouattara TA, Ougda CN, Staccini P. Setting up a video transmission tool for teleconsultation and tele-expertise in an African context: case of Burkina Faso. Stud Health Technol Inform. 2023;309:194–8. https://doi.org/10.3233/SHTI230777. https://ebooks.iospress.nl/doi/10.3233/SHTI230777. Accessed 21 Oct 2024.
20. Lee HK, Malkin T, Nahum E. Cryptographic strength of SSL/TLS servers: current and recent practices. IMC'07: Proceedings of the 7th ACM SIGCOMM conference on Internet measurement; 2007. p. 83–92. doi:https://doi.org/10.1145/1298306.1298318. Accessed 21 Oct 2024.
21. Maxhelaku S, Kika A. Improving interoperability in healthcare using HL7 FHIR. 47th international academic conference, Prague; 2019. https://www.researchgate.net/publication/335362287_IMPROVING_INTEROPERABILITY_IN_HEALTHCARE_USING_HL7_FHIR. Accessed 21 Oct 2024.
22. Rinehart-Thompson LA. Redefining the health information management privacy and security role. Perspect Health Inf Manag. 2009;6(Summer):1d.
23. Bakare SS, Adeniyi AO, Akpuokwe CU, Eneh NE. Data privacy laws and compliance: a comparative review of the EU GDPR and USA regulations. Comput Sci Inform Technol Res J. 2023;5(3) https://doi.org/10.51594/csitrj.v5i3.859. https://www.fepbl.com/index.php/csitrj/article/view/859. Accessed 21 Oct 2024.
24. Gijsbers H, Feenstra TM, Eminovic N, van Dam D, Nurmohamed SA, van de Belt T, Schijven MP. Enablers and barriers in upscaling telemonitoring across geographic boundaries: a scoping review. BMJ Open. 2022;12(4):e057494. https://doi.org/10.1136/bmjopen-2021-057494. https://bmjopen.bmj.com/content/12/4/e057494. Accessed 21 Oct 2024.
25. Shah SM, Khan RA. Secondary use of electronic health record: opportunities and challenges. IEEE; 2020. https://doi.org/10.1109/ACCESS.2020.9146114.
26. Marelli L, Stevens M, Sharon T, Van Hoyweghen I, Boeckhout M, Colussi I, Degelsegger-Márquez A, El-Sayed S, Hoeyer K, van Kessel R, Krekora Zając D, Matei M, Roda S, Prainsack B, Schlünder I, Shabani M, Southerington T. The European health data space: too big to succeed? Health Policy. 2023; https://www.sciencedirect.com/science/article/pii/S016885102300146X. Accessed 21 Oct 2024.
27. Majeed A, Lakhani M, Ashraf A, Grewal US, Thirunagari P, Wahab A, Hassan H, Faisal MS, Raziq FI, Anwer F. Teleoncology: prospects and challenges for cost-effective cancer care. J Clin Oncol. 2019;37(15_suppl):e23182. https://doi.org/10.1200/JCO.2019.37.15_suppl.e23182. Accessed 21 Oct 2024.

28. Fennell ML, Prabhu Das I, Clauser S, Petrelli N, Salner A. The organization of multidisciplinary care teams: modeling internal and external influences on cancer care quality. JNCI Monographs. 2010;2010(40):72–80. https://doi.org/10.1093/jncimonographs/lgq010. https://academic.oup.com/_ncimono/article/2010/40/72/894376. Accessed 21 Oct 2024.

29. Marchibroda JM. eHealth initiative: improving health care through information technology. J Oncol Pract. 2007;3(3):160–4. https://doi.org/10.1200/JOP.0738001. https://ascopubs.org/doi/10.1200/JOP.0738001. Accessed 21 Oct 2024.

30. EORTC Quality of Life Group EORTC QLQ-C30 English specimen; 2018. https://www.eortc.org/app/uploads/sites/2/2018/08/Specimen-QLQ-C30-English.pdf. Accessed 21 Oct 2024.

31. Pace A, Castaldo V, Paggi M, Kyriacou E, Plomariti C, Rosinska M, Schmitt T, Leclercq V. eCAN project: the EU joint action on strengthening eHealth including telemedicine and telemonitoring for cancer prevention and care. Cancer Res. 2024;84(7_Suppl):CT293. https://doi.org/10.1158/1538-7445.AM2024-CT293.

32. McMurray JJV, Cella DF, Kvien TK, Walsh PC. visual analog scale. Int J Surg Case Rep. 2021; https://www.sciencedirect.com/topics/medicine-and-dentistry/visual-analog-scale. Accessed 21 Oct 2024.

33. Heitmann N, Siewert H, Moog S, Somorovsky J. Security analysis of BigBlueButton and eduMEET. Applied Cryptography and Network Security (ACNS 2024). Lecture notes in computer science, vol. 14585; 2024. p. 190–216. https://doi.org/10.1007/978-3-031-54776-8_8. Accessed 21 Oct 2024.

34. Impact of digital tools in oncology: a global analysis of the adoption of ONCOassist and NCCN chemotherapy order templates (NCCN templates) in collaboration with OncoAlert. J Clin Oncol. 42(15_suppl):e13662. https://doi.org/10.1200/JCO.2024.42.16_suppl.e13662. Accessed 21 Oct 2024.

35. Piccirillo JF, Kallogjeri D, Kukuljan S, Palmer R. The development of MyCancerJourney and the incorporation of predictive analytics to improve cancer patient care. https://openurl.ebsco.com/EPDB%3Agcc%3A7%3A7352039/detailv2?sid=ebsco%3Aplink%3Ascholar&id=ebsco%3Agcd%3A110C87141&cr=c. Accessed 21 Oct 2024.

36. Prince V, Bellile EL, Sun Y, Wolf GT, Hoban CW, Shuman AG, Taylor JMG. Individualized risk prediction of outcomes for oral cavity cancer patients. Oral Oncol. 2016;61:85–93. https://doi.org/10.1016/j.oraloncology.2016.08.015. https://www.sciencedirect.com/science/article/pii/S1368837516302135. Accessed 21 Oct 2024.

37. Peltola MK, Poikonen-Saksela P, Mattson J, Parkkari T. A novel digital patient-reported outcome platform (Noona) for clinical use in patients with cancer: pilot study assessing suitability. JMIR Format Res. 2021;5(5):e16156. https://doi.org/10.2196/16156. https://formative.jmir.org/2021/5/e16156. Accessed 21 Oct 2024.

38. Sivaraman H. IoT-enabled healthcare monitoring: a systematic review of wearable devices. IT Industry. 2021;7(3) https://doi.org/10.17762/itii.v7i3.815. http://it-in-industry.org/index.php/itii/article/view/815. Accessed 21 Oct 2024.

39. Beg S, Handa M, Shukla R, Rahman M, Almalki WH, Afzal O, Altamimi ASA. Wearable smart devices in cancer diagnosis and remote clinical trial monitoring: transforming the healthcare applications. Drug Discov Today. 2022; https://doi.org/10.1016/j.drudis.2022.06.014. Accessed 21 Oct 2024.

40. Offodile AC 2nd, DiBrito SR, Finder JP, Shete S, Jain S, Delgado DA, Miller CJ, Davidson E, Overman MJ, Peterson SK. Active surveillance of chemotherapy-related symptom burden in ambulatory cancer patients via the implementation of electronic patient-reported outcomes and sensor-enabled vital signs capture: protocol for a decentralised feasibility pilot study. BMJ Open. 2022;12(4):e057693. https://doi.org/10.1136/bmjopen-2021-057693. https://bmjopen.bmj.com/content/12/4/e057693.abstract. Accessed 21 Oct 2024.

41. Xanthos D. Medopad. Lancet Oncol. 2015;16(8) https://doi.org/10.1016/S1470-2045(15)00150-3. https://www.thelancet.com/journals/lanonc/article/PIIS1470-2045(15)00150-3/abstract. Accessed 21 Oct 2024.

42. Tekkeşin Aİ. Artificial intelligence in healthcare: past, present and future. Anatol J Cardiol. 2019; https://doi.org/10.14744/anatoljcardiol.2019.28661.

43. Ferrucci D, et al. Building Watson: an overview of the DeepQA project. AI Mag. 2010;31(3):59–79. https://doi.org/10.1609/aimag.v31i3.2303.
44. Topol EJ. High-performance medicine: the convergence of human and artificial intelligence. Nat Med. 2019;25(1):44–56. https://doi.org/10.1038/s41591-018-0300-7.
45. Mahase E. AI system outperforms radiologists in first reading of breast cancer screening, study claims. BMJ. 2020a:m16. https://doi.org/10.1136/bmj.m16.
46. Kolanu N, Silverstone EJ, Ho BH, Pham H, Hansen A, Pauley E, Quirk AR, Sweeney SC, Center JR, Pocock NA. Clinical utility of computer-aided diagnosis of vertebral fractures from computed tomography images. J Bone Miner Res. 2020;35(12):2307–12.

Technological Innovations to Tackle Health Inequalities in Cancer Care

Grigorios Kotronoulas, Rebecca Marshall-Mckenna, Tongyao Wang, and Constantina Papadopoulou

1   Current State of Health Inequalities in Cancer Care

Approximately 53.5 million patients live with cancer across the world [1], with likely triple or quadruple numbers of people within the patient's support network also being affected. This translates into an additional 150–200 million individuals indirectly affected by the disease. Up to 10% of cancers are also hereditary [2], putting millions more at increased risk due to genetic factors such as BRCA mutations that significantly increase the risk for familial breast or ovarian cancer [3]. Lifestyle, environmental and work-related risk factors, including smoking, poor diet, physical inactivity, and exposure to carcinogens further contribute to approximately 50% of the global cancer burden [4].

Advancements in cancer prevention, such as vaccines for human papillomavirus (HPV) and hepatitis B, have shown significant efficacy in reducing cancer incidence [5]. Screening programmes, including mammography, colonoscopy, and low-dose computing tomography scans for lung cancer in some countries, have been critical in early detection, improving survival rates [6]. Modern treatments, such as targeted therapies and immunotherapies, have revolutionised cancer care by offering more personalised and effective treatment options [7]. Coordinated follow-up care,

G. Kotronoulas (✉) · R. Marshall-Mckenna
School of Medicine, Dentistry and Nursing, University of Glasgow, Glasgow, UK
e-mail: grigorios.kotronoulas@glasgow.ac.uk; Rebecca.Marshall@glasgow.ac.uk

T. Wang
School of Nursing, The University of Hong Kong, Pokfulam, Hong Kong
e-mail: tongyao1@hku.hk

C. Papadopoulou
School of Health and Life Sciences, University of the West of Scotland, Glasgow, UK
e-mail: Constantina.Papadopoulou@uws.ac.uk

including personalised survivorship and rehabilitation programmes, plays a vital role in improving the quality of life for cancer survivors and their support network [8–11]. These advancements have collectively contributed to a marked decrease in cancer morbidity and mortality globally [1].

To benefit from such advancements, people at risk of cancer or affected by cancer must be able to access health information and/or healthcare services in an equitable manner so that a timely response if brought about. Equitable access is critical to ensure that all individuals, irrespective of socioeconomic status, geography, or ethnicity, can benefit from the latest in cancer care and prevention. Unfortunately, such access is not equal across all communities, thus creating cancer health disparities that affect millions of people [12]. Cancer health disparities are evident in many forms, including limited access to quality healthcare, education, and socioeconomic opportunities [13–15]. Frequently inequitable access to healthcare is linked to greater disproportionate difficulties in obtaining support and worse health outcomes for a wide array of people including those of older age, from racial and ethnic minority groups, people in sexual orientation communities, from socioeconomically deprived areas, those facing financial distress, and those living in geographically marginalised areas [16]. For instance, African American patients have the shortest survival and highest mortality rates for most leading cancer types compared to any other racial or ethnic group [17].

Education, socioeconomic status, income, insurance, health literacy, and gender are important person-level factors and social determinants that have been linked to inequities in cancer prevention, screening, treatment, and follow-up care [18]. For example, people with higher education levels are more likely to participate in regular cancer screening [19], while those with lower socioeconomic status often face barriers to accessing healthcare services even in high-income countries [20]. At the provider level, unconscious bias and stereotyping exhibited by health professionals towards age, race, and type of cancer have been linked to inequalities in medical advice, case management, or clinical recommendations [21–23]. Evidence shows that Black women are less likely to receive prompt follow-up after an abnormal mammogram compared to White women [17]. At the health service level, the lack of specialist services within geographically remote and rural areas often translates into disproportionate access to cancer screening, testing, follow-up care, and adverse health outcomes [24]. For instance, rural patients diagnosed with cancer are less likely to receive the recommended standard of care and more likely to experience delays in diagnosis and treatment. Where considerable staff shortages are observed, the likelihood of exacerbating cancer-related health inequities for at-risk population groups' increases [25, 26].

At the country level, inequities exist in Europe in relation to spending on cancer care, prevention, and screening, with significant variations between countries [27]. Northern and Western European countries tend to have higher spending and better cancer outcomes compared to Eastern and Southern European countries. In low- and middle-income countries, lack of access to diagnosis and treatment is common [15] as well as access to trained staff [26], which collectively result in many patients presenting with late-stage disease. For example, in sub-Saharan Africa, access to radiotherapy, a critical component of cancer treatment and palliation, is hindered for many people due to barriers in funding, available technology and staff, and community populations [28]. Furthermore, socioeconomic disparities within countries exacerbate these issues, with poorer individuals less likely to receive timely and effective cancer care. The economic burden of cancer is also significant, with high out-of-pocket costs leading to financial hardship for many patients and their families [29, 30]. Addressing these disparities requires a multifaceted approach, including policy changes, increased funding, and targeted planning to improve health literacy and access to care for disadvantaged groups. One approach to address cancer health disparities is to leverage the power of technology to identify and implement innovative solutions and processes that can be customised to the needs and resources of people, providers, systems and countries.

2 Technological Innovation in Cancer

The Internet's reach and advances in data processing power have allowed for widespread growth opportunities in healthcare technology development and implementation [31]. Digital health technologies include computing platforms, software, digital infrastructure, Internet-connected devices and sensors as well as the processes involved to implement and interconnect them to support cancer prevention, screening, diagnosis, digital pathology, and monitoring, access to services, precision medicine, and survivorship care. Types of digital health technologies include smartphone applications, medical devices, network-connected wearable devices, web-based communication platforms, videoconferencing, artificial intelligence (AI) technology, and virtual reality technology [32]. Technological innovation in cancer refers to new or improved digital health technologies or processes that are implemented for health-related purposes, whose technological characteristics are significantly different from before, or their use is applied in novel ways to better support people at risk of or affected by cancer and cancer services [33–35].

Digital health technologies are developed to perform relatively simple or more complex tasks, and the level of technological innovation achieved signifies how efficiently these simple or complex tasks are delivered to effectively support their intended purpose. For instance, web-based tele-dermatology can enable faster screening for skin cancer [36], while web-based programmes can help increase knowledge about prostate cancer, thus helping men make decisions to take part in prostate cancer screening [37] An AI-powered chatbot was also developed to communicate with people during routine colonoscopy to determine whether screening heritable cancer syndrome is necessary [38].

Digital infrastructure systems are employed for telemedicine to enable remote delivery of medical treatment via videoconferencing and use of the electronic health record (EHR) [39]. EHR systems have evolved to sufficiently integrate more complex clinical decision support algorithms that aim to reduce medication errors and assist in the optimisation of therapy [40]. Moreover, deep learning-based technologies for speech recognition [41] can free healthcare providers from the need to manually enter patient information. The use of large datasets containing clinical, genetic, imaging, and molecular biomarkers has enabled the training of machine learning and deep learning models to achieve more precise and automated predictions in cancer risk assessment, digital pathology, prognosis determination, therapy selection, and drug discovery [42]. A promising application of generative AI, such as generative pre-trained transformers (GPTs), is in the advancement of adaptive cancer therapy [43], whereby medication doses are tailored for individual patients to prevent drug resistance.

Digital health technologies directed towards patients, such as smartphone health applications, enable access to remote symptom monitoring, patient-clinician communication, and self-management [44–47]. Patient-facing technologies, such as digital therapeutics, video gaming, telephone-based care, and web-based platforms, have been used as complementary therapies to promote health outcomes such as physical activity, access to psychological support, health management education, and survivorship care [48–53]. Conversational AI agents powered by large language models have demonstrated feasibility in the context of cancer patient education, providing tailored information and support to patients and caregivers [54–56].

Medical devices (e.g., smart weight scales) and non-medical devices (e.g., activity trackers, smartwatches) can allow for telemonitoring by gathering rich information from dispersed devices to provide a more comprehensive picture of a patient's health status, activity and functional status, and promote positive health behaviours [57]. Non-medical devices can track a range of health metrics, including physical activity, heart rate, sleep patterns, and even detect irregular heart rhythm. They can empower individuals to take a proactive role in managing their health and can be particularly useful in monitoring patients who have completed cancer treatment and are in the survivorship phase [58–61].

3 Thinking Outside the Box: Tackling Cancer Inequalities with Technological Innovation

Much progress has been made in identifying patient-, provider-, and health service-level interventions to reduce cancer health disparities. The challenge of implementation and dissemination remains for most of these interventions. Innovative technology can help tackle some of these barriers to provide scalable solutions that can benefit people, providers, systems and countries. However, increased adoption of technological innovation without consideration for historically underserved populations may exacerbate existing disparities [32]. Where cancer health disparities are most pronounced, technological innovation must be strategically developed and implemented to target the inequities themselves or their precipitating or perpetuating causes. We provide below exemplar technological innovations that specifically target cancer health disparities and disadvantaged populations at risk of cancer or affected by cancer.

3.1   Patient-Level Examples

Within primary care, several digital health strategies have been developed and tested to improve women's knowledge, awareness, and access to early screening for cervical cancer in low- and middle-income countries [62]. In Iran, Khademolhosseini et al. tested an educational intervention on the Pap smear test delivered via the instant messaging platform Telegram [63]. The researchers used a diverse range of content including text messages, posters, infographics, podcasts, and video tutorials. Three months after the training, 48% of participants in the intervention group had taken the Pap smear test compared to only 6% in the control group [63]. In Tanzania, cervical cancer represents 25% of all cancers and rates of cervical cancer screening are as low as 10% due to lack of awareness, affordability concerns and travel cost [64]. Erwin et al. ran a randomised controlled trial that tested the effectiveness of consecutive behaviour-change mobile text messages over a period of 21 days and either provided with or without transportation eVouchers delivered via text message, which covered return transportation to the nearest screening clinic [65]. Significantly more women attended screening in the behaviour-change text message plus eVoucher group (18%), followed by 13% in the behaviour-change text message only group, and 4.3% in the control group (three simple text messages). Intervention effects were more pronounced in the rural areas of Tanzania [65].

Technological innovation should be tailored to the cultural context and address the social determinants of health of the patient population just as they are tailored to cancer. The chatbot iDecide promotes informed prostate cancer screening decisions among racial minorities [66]. iDecide is a computer-based conversational agent designed to educate patients about prostate cancer screening and promote informed decision-making. It was shown to enhance African Americans' intentions to engage in shared decision-making, but there was no subsequent evidence that it increased their likelihood of actually discussing prostate cancer treatment with a provider or participating in shared decision-making [66].

Refugee populations are known to experience poorer health outcomes compared to non-refugee populations, which is often linked to language and financial barriers, biographical disruption, and lack of knowledge around primary and secondary care offered in the host country [67, 68]. Kizilkaya et al. identified fewer resources being available for refugee-focused public health initiatives related to cancer, and as such, developed a simple telephone-based, 1-hour education intervention for breast cancer awareness and screening uptake specifically targeting Afghan refugees in Türkiye [69]. Six months after the intervention, 99% of participants were able to correctly identify common signs, symptoms, and risk factors for breast cancer. Six months after the intervention, all participants had accepted an invitation to a screening mammogram [69].

Patients who are older, those of a lower socioeconomic status, and those from ethnic or racial minority groups are likely to face greater barriers to technology use [70, 71]. Barriers related to digital literacy can have a direct impact on actual use of any technological innovation and widen health disparities in vulnerable cancer population groups. In the USA, the Patient Empowerment Network the digital sherpa®

programme was launched to help people affected by cancer (mainly 65 and older) learn to use technology [72]. The programme runs workshops, whereby patients and their support network are paired with university students ('sherpas') who provide training in basic Internet and social media skills, and work as a team to learn new skills and access available resources in a supportive environment. The philosophy of the programme lies in bringing younger and older generations together to create a long-lasting supportive relationship and strengthen local communities [72]. The digital sherpas® programme is complemented by Digitally Empowered®, a 10-module online course, available in English and Spanish (particularly for Hispanic minority groups), that offers free access to training material on Internet and tele-health use to people affected by cancer [73].

In the field of cancer survivorship, SmartSurvivor is a mobile health app that enables remote, personalised care coordination for breast cancer survivors in rural areas in the USA [74]. The prototype app was developed with direct involvement of rural breast cancer survivors, primary care providers, and an oncologist. The intention was to directly address unique challenges that rural cancer survivors' face, including access to treatment, health information, psychosocial and mental health services, cancer support groups, and support with positive health behaviours. Portability, accessibility, and having one place for all contact were highly valued in a preliminary evaluation [74]. Important key features were identified for future development, including enabling linkages with the EHR and patient tracking tools such as Fitbit to provide clinicians with more comprehensive data for remote patient monitoring. Although evidence of effectiveness is yet to be published, SmartSurvivor is an example approach of patient-based use of smartphone apps to help close the urban–rural gap in survivorship care planning [74].

3.2   Provider-Level Examples

Smartphone-based, automated image classification methods that can run with high accuracy despite limited computation power and Internet access have been developed to enable point-of-care screening for oral cancer in resource-limited settings. Song et al. describe the development of a system for use in resource-constrained areas in India [75], where oral cancer is the second most prevalent type of cancer [1], thus making early screening and detection paramount. The researchers based their system on the use of convolutional neural networks (CNNs), i.e., a type of 'deep learning' artificial technology that can be trained to detect and classify patterns in images with high accuracy. The trained CNN platform was embedded in a simple Android smartphone application, which enabled local clinicians to perform real-time classification of images of clinically suspicious oral lesions, and obtain initial indication of malignancy or not, irrespective of Internet connection. The finalised system was only ~16.3 MB in size and processed one image pair in only ~300 ms, using an average performance Android smartphone, thus making it ideal for use in settings where trained specialists, health facilities, and Internet access are limited [75]. In addition to promising evidence on diagnostic accuracy (81%), real-world implementation of this innovative technology must be confirmed to show how it can address disparities in cancer screening for oral cancer. Similar applications of CNN have been used in the field of tele-cytology to improve early detection of oral cancer where resources are limited. A platform was developed and tested in India that enabled automated analysis of tele-cytology images of oral lesions via use of machine learning, specialised web-based servers, and iPad tablet computers to provide reliable, remote connectivity to frontline, non-specialist health workers in resource-challenged settings and countries, where trained specialists are not available [76].

Tele-mammography for breast cancer screening has been used in several high-income and low- and middle-income countries to overcome barriers to accessibility and lack of trained health providers in rural or resource-limited areas. Pascha et al. explore the cost-utility of tele-mammography for at-risk women over 40 years old in the highly fragmented healthcare system of Argentina [77]. Tele-mammography networks usually operate via clinician collaboration between a core centre and strategically located digital mammography facilities in remote or in-need areas. Mammography images are sent to the core centre for interpretation and sent back to the remote facility in less than 24 hours. It was estimated that 39% of new cases of breast cancer would be detected by tele-mammography compared to 31% by mammography. There was a 59% chance for tele-mammography to be more cost-effective compared to mammography [77], thus enabling early diagnosis and subsequent reduction of cancer morbidity and mortality among women in a country with high cancer health disparities.

To reduce racial screening disparities related to colorectal cancer, Cooks et al. conducted a pilot study of Meet ALEX (Agent Leveraging Empathy for eXams), whereby ALEX, a web-based interactive virtual clinician powered by interactive 3D technology with human voices and gestures engages in patient-clinician conversation in a digital exam room. In the study, the virtual clinician's race was matched to the patient's race, with a particular focus on increasing screening uptake among African American at-risk people [78]. Matching races was linked to a favourable but statistically non-significant influence on screening intention for Black participants, but not for White participants. In addition, Black participants who were matched to a Black virtual clinician perceived the technology more credible, attractive and relevant compared to White participants, and these parameters were strong mediators of screening intention [78]. This study shows how technological innovations can be easily adjusted (race-matching) to condone to heuristic cues (such as race) that may be linked to some people perceiving prevention messaging components as more personally relevant, and as such more convincing to undertake colorectal cancer screening.

HuroneAI (https://hurone.ai/) is an organisation that develops innovative digital tools to specifically reduce disparities in cancer care in low-income settings in sub-Saharan Africa (specifically in Nigeria, Kenya, and Rwanda) via an approach to the development and application of AI technology that takes into account the region's resources and cultural specificities [79]. Preliminary evidence showed that use of HuroneAI technology reduced off-duty oncology calls be almost 60% and saved

oncology teams time that would be traditionally required for specific care responsibilities, thus enabling more effective cancer treatment and follow-up to be provided
by healthcare teams in these low-resource countries.

Apart from the obvious reason of a lack of specialised workforce in remote and
low-resource regions, there is also limited access to health provider specialist education and training in cancer. A prime example of using technology to bring down
knowledge barriers in the community is the Extension for Community Healthcare
Outcomes (ECHO) tele-mentoring programme (https://projectecho.unm.edu/).
Project originally started in New Mexico, USA, and currently has 113 hubs across
25 countries (including low- and middle-income countries) to educate primary care
providers in specialised fields, including cancer (https://iecho.org/echo-initiatives/
cancer). Project ECHO uses video conferencing to connect specialist teams with
primary care providers in remote areas, enabling knowledge sharing and improving
care delivery for patients in underserved regions [80]. Project ECHO is different
from telemedicine, where the specialist assumes the care of the patient. Instead,
with tele-mentoring, the community clinician retains responsibility for managing all
patient cases, operating with increasing independence [81]. Project evaluations
reveal widespread participation, improved learning, and changes in health providers' practices in relation to cancer care [82].

3.3   Health Service-Level Examples

At the health service level, leveraging digital innovative tools allows healthcare
providers to optimise patient outcomes, streamline care processes, and facilitate
more personalised treatment plans to tackle inequalities in accessing cancer care
services. Heifetz et al. established a telehealth oncology programme in rural and
mountain communities of California, USA, whereby underserved communities
without oncology services were partnered with a major urban cancer centre [83]. A
synaptic knowledge network was put in place via daily participation of rural clinicians in virtual tumour boards (videoconferencing) and remote telemedicine clinics
for the four most prevalent cancers, i.e., lung, colorectal, breast, and prostate. The
programme was evaluated between 2006 and 2018 to show expansion: new medical
staff were accrued in the rural communities, patient visits, and referrals of patients
from outside the main catchment area increased, and the number of eligible rural
patients who enrolled to clinical trials also increased [83]. The authors considered
synaptic knowledge networks a vital strategy to tackle rural–urban disparities in
cancer care.

In Queensland, Australia, the Townsville Cancer Centre has employed videoconferencing technology since 2007 to oversee the management of medical oncology
patients from rural and remote towns in this vast geographical area of
1200×1200 km². Medical oncologists consult with patients who may be supported
during the videoconference by local health care professionals, depending on the
complexity of the case [84]. Consultations may involve review of new cases, follow-
up of existing cases or urgent review for acutely ill patients. The telemedicine model

was adopted for its potential to minimise the need for distant travel for the patient, which can lead to reduction in burden and costs, and increased patient satisfaction. Indeed, evaluation of this model showed that high satisfaction among both patients and health workers, due to effective communication between patients and specialists, reduced travel time and money expenditure, and superior specialist support for the rural health providers [84]. Adoption of the model resulted in a net saving of AUS\$320,118, which could be redirected to enhance rural resources and service capabilities [85]. Subsequent investigation concluded with no concerns over safety to administer chemotherapy to rural patients under remote supervision by medical oncologists from the urban cancer centre, and no evidence of compromise in dose intensity and therapeutic benefit, thus pointing to clinical comparability between tele-oncology and standard practice [86].

Inequalities in the treatment of breast and lung cancer have been consistently documented for Black patients, leading to suboptimal care and mortality [87]. In response, five health organisations in the USA joined a consortium that developed a multifaceted, systems-based intervention to enhance racial equity in the completion of cancer treatment. The ACCURE intervention uses real-time data from electronic health records to monitor and address treatment delays [88]. At the same time, it disseminates race- and ethnic-specific feedback to clinical teams in relation to treatment completion rates, while a nurse navigator trained in antiracism principles monitors the real-time warning system and informs the wider team of treatment delays and identifies barriers to patient care. ACCURE was associated with overall improvements in care quality and reductions in racial and ethnic inequities treatment completion for early-stage breast and lung cancer [88].

The COVID-19 pandemic helped progress the acceptance and use of digital health technology by patients as cancer consultations moved from face-to-face to remote appointments, which has progressed into mixed models of consultations in hospitals today. This has addressed some of the health inequalities associated with financial toxicity and time costs as well as the additional impact on ability to work, loss of income, family commitments and childcare costs. Miziara et al. tested integration and feasibility of tele-oncology orientation embedded within a government health system in Brazil for low-income patients with breast cancer during the pandemic [89]. Telephone consultations were conducted via an application that allowed free-of-charge conversation and involved real-time interaction between the patient and the surgeon. Target patients lacked basic access to technology, had low levels of education, and poor financial resources. Despite these challenges, a relatively satisfactory 71% of patients managed to successfully engage with this low-resource tele-oncology orientation model. The researchers reported slightly negative impressions among the involved breast surgeons who were not experienced in virtual care [89].

Another example of technological innovation embedded within a national health system comes from the United Kingdom. The Dorset Integrated Care System Cancer Programme, Wessex Cancer Alliance, NHS Innovation support organisation Wessex Academic Health Science Network, and NHS England Innovation for Healthcare Inequalities Programme have partnered with 'C the Signs' to improve cancer survival and tackle inequalities in Dorset, England, particularly in relation to colorectal cancer and Faecal Immunochemical Test (FIT) kit completion [90]. C the Signs is an early cancer detection system that employs an AI-powered clinical decision support tool for cancer screening, referral, and monitoring (https://www.cthesigns.com/). C the Signs is used across GP practices in Dorset (including more and less deprived areas) to help identify patients at risk of cancer, and help patients access more specialist cancer services through their GPs and enable communities to receive equal access to timely healthcare and anticancer treatment [90]. While feedback from GP practices was overall positive, preliminary analyses based on limited data suggested no significant observable impact of C the Signs on FIT kit completion rates when compared with GP practices without C the Signs deployment [91]. Longer term evaluation is under way.

4   The Dark Side of the Moon? Tackling Inequalities Caused or Exacerbated by Technology

Even for technologies designed for underserved populations, developers and researchers must be critical of their efficacy and fitness to purpose [32]. Inequalities caused or exacerbated by digital health technologies stem from several factors. Country-wide implementation challenges in resource-limited settings can also be unique with higher training requirement, greater challenges in the procurement and roll-out of technology, insufficient network coverage, and unintended inequitable access to technology [62]. Limited network infrastructure and device availability contribute to digital exclusion, while disparities in access lead to varied health outcomes, including differences in disease incidence and mortality rates [92]. Technical challenges, such as continuous software development and maintenance (fixing software bugs and login problems), further hinder adoption. Concerns about cybersecurity and legal issues also present significant barriers that require planning and vigilance. Organisational barriers include difficulties in the smooth integration of these platforms into existing systems as well as the allocation of time and resources [93]. Key influencing factors also include age, race, socioeconomic status, health conditions, health literacy, and digital literacy [94]. Patients' potential struggles to understand medical information can lead to increased anxiety. Where population health literacy and educational attainment are low, mistrust in technology may be highly prevalent, which can lead to rejection or low uptake even where technological innovations have been carefully developed for the underserved target population. This makes the wider buy-in process particularly important. Health providers may even report worsened communication with automatic electronic report releases, thus discouraging the use of online health resources due to misinformation [95, 96]. It is not surprising that some health providers may advise against online health resources because of increased doubts, confusion, and emotional distress [97].

The digital divide, i.e., the 'inequitable distribution of digital technologies' [98] can further exacerbate health disparities by unevenly distributing digital health technologies, particularly affecting traditionally disadvantaged groups, or putting additional population groups in a disadvantaged position. Imbalances between offer, demand, and ability to absorb may occur where no strategic development of new technology products is noted. Intention to use health technology is a key starting point for many and may influence subsequent outcomes of actual use and successful use. Significant existing social disparities in smartphone usage, Internet access, and broadband subscriptions mean that digital health technologies do not automatically democratise information for everyone [99]. It is often the middle-upper classes that have unrestricted access to extensive health information through various tools and methods. Additionally, telecommunication providers tend to increase privileges for high-volume users while reducing those of low-volume users, who are often low-income individuals. This information gap can exacerbate disparities in access to health information, affecting people's ability to self-manage their health and ultimately resulting in varying health outcomes. There has been work in the USA to tackle the major barrier of inadequate broadband infrastructure in the provision of telehealth services and remote learning in rural areas with the Affordable Connectivity Program (ACP) [100]. This programme provided eligible households with discounted broadband services and discounts towards the purchase of computing devices, including tablet computers. Drawing on the ACP, an innovative model was devised that aimed to reduce cancer care's digital divide by providing broadband-enabled tablets preloaded with education and support resources to people affected by cancer within partner sites of the nonprofit Cancer Support Community network, thus benefitting hundreds of individuals [101]. Having run for 3 years, the ACP was forced to an end in June 2024 due to lack of additional funding from Congress. A formal evaluation of the ACP would be crucial to provide hard evidence on the programme's impact on the 23 million supported households across the USA, evaluate its cost-utility, and devise sustainable plans to inform a potential second launch.

There is rising concern that innovations in technology may worsen existing inequalities in cancer care due to lack of proficiency in operating intricate digital gadgets, issues related to cost, inconsistent access among different regions, and biased AI and machine learning models [102]. AI and machine learning models rely heavily on extensive training datasets obtained from past medical information, and as such, they are limited by the quality of their training data. A comprehensive understanding of these limitations is important primarily among health providers, who should use caution when interpreting these models' outcomes and how they apply to certain population groups. Interacting with technology at a high frequency requires mental effort, including higher cognitive functions such as concentration, multitasking, and memory [103]. This information overload can lead to cognitive overload, with increased feelings of exhaustion and lack of engagement. Mental fatigue due to technology use demands can create disparities for certain population groups, including older patients, patients with chemotherapy-related cognitive impairment, those with mental health comorbidities, and those with intellectual disabilities. Accessibility is a key parameter, and patient-facing technological innovations should be made more inclusive, e.g., by offering multilingual, culturally appropriated content, particularly in countries whereby people from ethnic minority communities require support. Forty percent of cancer information available on social media and the Internet can be confusing, misleading, or not from reliable sources [104]. This may widen the gap for populations (older, younger, less educated), who may not have the knowledge or skills to cross-check reliability of published information about cancer [105].

5   Conclusions: The Way Forward

It is essential to remember that using technology should be an individual's choice, so efforts must be made to ensure that no one is left behind. To address the growing divide that digital technologies bring, efforts must be made to engage more with people who are known to be prone to cancer health disparities [106]. Public involvement and engagement is recognised for the many benefits it brings to the quality improvement in healthcare [107] and is critical for obtaining successful funding for developing digital health innovations. However, public involvement is sometimes suboptimal, and there are numerous barriers to its implementation in co-production in the cancer health disparities landscape, perhaps because of limited frequency, duration, and quality of input required in the developmental stages to make technological innovations meaningful for real-world use in cancer care [108]. Bold and strategic initiatives from government bodies and large telecommunications companies will be required to enable equitable, long-term technological solutions for population groups at risk of cancer health disparities. We have discussed several key initiatives in this chapter, including programmes that provide affordable Internet connection and digital equipment, programmes that offer free digital education and navigation, and programmes that enable remote supportive interconnectedness. Sustaining and expanding such initiatives will be key to make technological innovations for cancer accessible, appealing and implementable for all.

References

1. Ferlay J, Ervik M, Lam F, Laversanne M, Colombet M, Mery L, Piñeros M, Znaor A, Soerjomataram I, Bray F. Global cancer observatory: cancer today. Lyon: International Agency for Research on Cancer; 2024. GLOBOCAN 2020. https://gco.iarc.fr/en. Accessed 22 Jul 2024.
2. Cancer Research UK. Family history and inherited cancer genes. Cancer Research UK; 2021. https://www.cancerresearchuk.org/about-cancer/causes-of-cancer/inherited-cancer-genes-and-increased-cancer-risk/family-history-and-inherited-cancer-genes. Accessed 22 Jul 2024.
3. Cancer Research UK. Inherited genes and cancer types. Cancer Research UK; 2021. https://www.cancerresearchuk.org/about-cancer/causes-of-cancer/inherited-cancer-genes-and-increased-cancer-risk/inherited-genes-and-cancer-types. Accessed 22 Jul 2024.
4. International Agency for Research on Cancer (IARC). Environment and lifestyle epidemiology branch (ENV). World Health Organisation; 2024. https://www.iarc.who.int/branches-env/. Accessed 22 Jul 2024.
5. Valle I, Tramalloni D, Bragazzi NL. Cancer prevention: state of the art and future prospects. J Prev Med Hyg. 2015;56:E21–7.

6. Moleyar-Narayana P, Leslie S, Ranganathan S. Cancer Screening [Updated 2024 May 31]. In: StatPearls [Internet]. Treasure Island: StatPearls Publications; 2024. https://www.ncbi. nlm.nih.gov/books/NBK563138/. Accessed 22 Jul 2024.

7. Debela DT, Muzazu SG, Heraro KD, Ndalama MT, Mesele BW, Haile DC, Kitui SK, Manyazewal T. New approaches and procedures for cancer treatment: current perspectives. SAGE open Med. 2021;9:20503121211034370.

8. Halpern M, Mollica MA, Han PKJ, Tonorezos ES. Myths and presumptions about cancer survivorship. J Clin Oncol. 2023;42:134–9.

9. Vaz-Luis I, Masiero M, Cavaletti G, et al. ESMO expert consensus statements on cancer survivorship: promoting high-quality survivorship care and research in Europe. Ann Oncol. 2022;33:1119–33.

10. Kobayashi LC, Westrick AC, Doshi A, Ellis KR, Jones CR, LaPensee E, Mondul AM, Mullins MA, Wallner LP. New directions in cancer and aging: state of the science and recommendations to improve the quality of evidence on the intersection of aging with cancer control. Cancer. 2022;128:1730–7.

11. Hart NH, Nekhlyudov L, Smith TJ, et al. Survivorship care for people affected by advanced or metastatic cancer: MASCC-ASCO standards and practice recommendations. Support Care Cancer. 2024;32:313.

12. Marmot M. Social inequalities, global public health, and cancer. In: Vaccarella S, Lortet-Tieulent J, Saracci R, et al., editors. Reducing social inequalities in cancer: evidence and priorities for research. Lyon: International Agency for Research on Cancer; 2019.

13. So WKW, Chan RJ, Truant T, Trevatt P, Bialous SA, Barton-Burke M. Global perspectives on cancer health disparities: impact, utility, and implications for cancer nursing. Asia-Pacific J Oncol Nurs. 2015;3:316–23

14. Minas TZ, Kiely M, Ajao A, Ambs S. An overview of cancer health disparities: new approaches and insights and why they matter. Carcinogenesis. 2021;42:2–13.

15. Dos-Santos-Silva I, Gupta S, Orem J, Shulman LN. Global disparities in access to cancer care. Commun Med. 2022;2:31.

16. Green B, Davis J, Rivers D, Buchanan K, Rivers B. Cancer health disparities. In: Alberts D, Hess L, editors. Fundam. Cancer Prev. 4th ed. Cham: Springer; 2019. p. 199–246.

17. American Cancer Society. Cancer disparities in the black community. American Cancer Society; 2024. https://www.cancer.org/about-us/what-we-do/health-equity/cancer-disparities-in-the-black-community.html. Accessed 22 Jul 2024.

18. Green B, Davis J, Rivers D, Buchanan K, Rivers B. Cancer health disparities. In: Alberts D, Hess L, editors. Fundamentals of cancer prevention. 4th ed. Cham: Springer; 2019. p. 199–246.

19. Willems B, Bracke P. Participants, physicians or programmes: participants' educational level and initiative in cancer screening. Health Policy (New York). 2018;122:422–30.

20. Bourgeois A, Horrill T, Mollison A, Stringer E, Lambert LK, Stajduhar K. Barriers to cancer treatment for people experiencing socioeconomic disadvantage in high-income countries: a scoping review. BMC Health Serv Res. 2024;24:670.

21. Liang J, Wolsiefer K, Zestcott CA, Chase D, Stone J. Implicit bias toward cervical cancer: provider and training differences. Gynecol Oncol. 2019;153:80–6.

22. Neal D, Morgan JL, Kenny R, Ormerod T, Reed MWR. Is there evidence of age bias in breast cancer health care professionals' treatment of older patients? Eur J Surg Oncol. 2022;48:2401–7.

23. Penner LA, Dovidio JF, Gonzalez R, et al. The effects of oncologist implicit racial bias in racially discordant oncology interactions. J Clin Oncol. 2016;34:2874–80.

24. Bhatia S, Landier W, Paskett ED, Peters KB, Merrill JK, Phillips J, Osarogiagbon RU. Rural-urban disparities in cancer outcomes: opportunities for future research. J Natl Cancer Inst. 2022;114:940–52.

25. Griffin S. Cancer care: staff shortages are limiting progress in England, says expert panel. BMJ. 2022;376:o852.

26. Trapani D, Murthy SS, Boniol M, Booth C, Simensen VC, Kasumba MK, Giuliani R, Curigliano G, Ilbawi AM. Distribution of the workforce involved in cancer care: a systematic review of the literature. ESMO Open. 2021;6:100292.
27. Pousette A, Hofmarcher T. Tackling inequalities in cancer care in the European Union. IHE Lund, Sweden; 2024. https://efpia.eu/media/cnygfywo/tackling-inequalities-in-cancer-care-in-the-european-union.pdf. Accessed 21 Mar 2024.
28. Beltrán Ponce SE, Abunike SA, Bikomeye JC, et al. Access to radiation therapy and related clinical outcomes in patients with cervical and breast cancer across sub-Saharan Africa: a systematic review. JCO Glob Oncol. 2023;9:e2200218.
29. Pauge S, Surmann B, Mehlis K, Zueger A, Richter L, Menold N, Greiner W, Winkler EC. Patient-reported financial distress in cancer: a systematic review of risk factors in universal healthcare systems. Cancers (Basel). 2021;13(19):5015. https://doi.org/10.3390/cancers13195015.
30. Ngan TT, Tien TH, Donnelly M, O'Neill C. Financial toxicity among cancer patients, survivors and their families in the United Kingdom: a scoping review. J Public Health (Bangkok). 2023;45:e702–13.
31. Amjad A, Kordel P, Fernandes G. A review on innovation in healthcare sector (telehealth) through artificial intelligence. Sustainability. 2023;15(8):6655. https://doi.org/10.3390/su15086655.
32. Briggs LG, Labban M, Alkhatib K, Nguyen D-D, Cole AP, Trinh Q-D. Digital technologies in cancer care: a review from the clinician's perspective. J Comp Eff Res. 2022;11:533–44.
33. Honeyman M, Maguire D, Evans H, Davies A. Digital technology and health inequalities: a scoping review. Cardiff: Public Health Wales NHS Trust; 2020. https://phw.nhs.wales/publications/publications1/digital-technology-and-health-inequalities-a-scoping-review/. Accessed 22 Jul 2024.
34. Badr J, Motulsky A, Denis J-L. Digital health technologies and inequalities: a scoping review of potential impacts and policy recommendations. Health Policy (New York). 2024;146:105122.
35. Flessa S, Huebner C. Innovations in health care—a conceptual framework. Int J Environ Res Public Health. 2021;18(19):10026. https://doi.org/10.3390/ijerph181910026.
36. Finnane A, Dallest K, Janda M, Soyer HP. Teledermatology for the diagnosis and management of skin cancer: a systematic review. JAMA Dermatol. 2017;153:319–27.
37. Baptista S, Teles Sampaio E, Heleno B, Azevedo LF, Martins C. Web-based versus usual care and other formats of decision aids to support prostate cancer screening decisions: systematic review and meta-analysis. J Med Internet Res. 2018;20:e228.
38. Heald B, Keel E, Marquard J, Burke CA, Kalady MF, Church JM, Liska D, Mankaney G, Hurley K, Eng C. Using Chatbots to screen for heritable cancer syndromes in patients undergoing routine colonoscopy. J Med Genet. 2021;58:807–14.
39. Patel S, Goldsack JC, Cordovano G, et al. Advancing digital health innovation in oncology: priorities for high-value digital transformation in cancer care. J Med Internet Res. 2023;25:e43404.
40. Armando LG, Miglio G, de Cosmo P, Cena C. Clinical decision support systems to improve drug prescription and therapy optimisation in clinical practice: a scoping review. BMJ Health Care Inform. 2023;30(1):e100683. https://doi.org/10.1136/bmjhci-2022-100683.
41. Xia X, Ma Y, Luo Y, Lu J. An online intelligent electronic medical record system via speech recognition. Int J Distrib Sens Networks. 2022;18:15501329221134480.
42. Perez-Lopez R, Reis-Filho JS, Kather JN. A framework for artificial intelligence in cancer research and precision oncology. npj Precis Oncol. 2023;7:43.
43. Derbal Y. Adaptive cancer therapy in the age of generative artificial intelligence. Cancer Control. 2024;31:10732748241264704.
44. Charbonneau DH, Hightower S, Katz A, Zhang K, Abrams J, Senft N, Beebe-Dimmer JL, Heath E, Eaton T, Thompson HS. Smartphone apps for cancer: a content analysis of the digital health marketplace. Digit Health. 2020;6:2055207620905413.

45. Maguire R, McCann L, Kotronoulas G, et al. Real time remote symptom monitoring during chemotherapy for cancer: European multicentre randomised controlled trial (eSMART). BMJ. 2021;374:n1647. https://doi.org/10.1136/bmj.n1647.
46. Basch E, Deal AM, Dueck AC, Scher HI, Kris MG, Hudis C, Schrag D. Overall survival results of a trial assessing patient-reported outcomes for symptom monitoring during routine cancer treatment. JAMA. 2017;318:197–8.
47. Lim DSC, Kwok B, Williams P, Koczwara B. The impact of digital technology on self-management in cancer: systematic review. JMIR Cancer. 2023;9:e45145.
48. Iivanainen S, Ekstrom J, Virtanen H, Kataja VV, Koivunen JP. Electronic patient-reported outcomes and machine learning in predicting immune-related adverse events of immune checkpoint inhibitor therapies. BMC Med Inform Decis Mak 2021;21:205.
49. Acuna N, Vento I Alzate-Duque L, Valera P. Harnessing digital videos to promote cancer prevention and education: a systematic review of the literature from 2013–2018. J Cancer Educ Off J Am Assoc Cancer Educ. 2020;35:635–42.
50. Sabel M, Sjölund A, Broeren J, Arvidsson D, Saury J-M, Blomgren K, Lannering B, Emanuelson I. Active video gaming improves body coordination in survivors of childhood brain tumours. Disabil Rehabil. 2016;38:2073–84.
51. Marzorati C, Renzi C, Russell-Edu SW, Pravettoni G. Telemedicine use among caregivers of cancer patients: systematic review. J Med Internet Res. 2018;20:e223.
52. Kim AR, Park H-A. Web-based self-management support interventions for cancer survivors: a systematic review and meta-analyses. Stud Health Technol Inform. 2015;216:142–7.
53. Ream E, Hughes AE, Cox A, Skarparis K, Richardson A, Pedersen VH, Wiseman T, Forbes A, Bryant A. Telephone interventions for symptom management in adults with cancer. Cochrane Database Syst Rev. 2020;6:CD007568.
54. Chaix B, Bibault J-E, Pienkowski A, Delamon G, Guillemassé A, Nectoux P, Brouard B. When Chatbots meet patients: one-year prospective study of conversations between patients with breast cancer and a Chatbot. JMIR Cancer. 2019;5:e12856.
55. Görtz M, Baumgärtner K, Schmid T, Muschko M, Woessner P, Gerlach A, Byczkowski M, Sültmann H, Duensing S, Hohenfellner M. An artificial intelligence-based Chatbot for prostate cancer education: design and patient evaluation study. Digit Health. 2023;9:20552076231173304.
56. Bibault J-E, Chaix B, Guillemassé A, Cousin S, Escande A, Perrin M, Pienkowski A, Delamon G, Nectoux P, Brouard B. A Chatbot versus physicians to provide information for patients with breast cancer: blind, randomized controlled noninferiority trial. J Med Internet Res. 2019;21:e15787.
57. Valle CG, Deal AM, Tate DF. Preventing weight gain in African American breast cancer survivors using smart scales and activity trackers: a randomized controlled pilot study. J Cancer Surviv. 2017;11:133–48.
58. Hedrick TL, Hassinger TE, Myers E, Krebs ED, Chu D, Charles AN, Hoang SC, Friel CM, Thiele RH. Wearable technology in the perioperative period predicting risk of postoperative complications in patients undergoing elective colorectal surgery. Dis Colon Rectum. 2020;63:538–44.
59. Patel Y, Hylton D, Rok M, et al. MA16.05 wearable technology for preconditioning before thoracic surgery: a feasibility study. J Thorac Oncol. 2019;14:S314.
60. Ma X, Zhang J, Zhong W, Shu C, Wang F, Wen J, Zhou M, Sang Y, Jiang Y, Liu L. The diagnostic role of a short screening tool—the distress thermometer: a meta-analysis. Support Care Cancer. 2014;22:1741–55.
61. Hooke MC, Gilchrist L, Tanner L, Hart N, Withycombe JS. Use of a fitness tracker to promote physical activity in children with acute lymphoblastic leukemia. Pediatr Blood Cancer. 2016;63:684–9.
62. Rossman AH, Reid HW, Pieters MM, Mizelle C, von Isenburg M, Ramanujam N, Huchko MJ, Vasudevan L. Digital health strategies for cervical cancer control in low- and middle-income countries: systematic review of current implementations and gaps in research. J Med Internet Res. 2021;23:e23350.

63. Khademolhosseini F, Noroozi A, Tahmasebi R. The effect of health belief model-based education through telegram instant messaging services on pap smear performance. Asian Pac J Cancer Prev. 2017;18:2221–6.
64. Cunningham MS, Skrastins E, Fitzpatrick R, Jindal P, Oneko O, Yeates K, Booth CM, Carpenter J, Aronson KJ. Cervical cancer screening and HPV vaccine acceptability among rural and urban women in Kilimanjaro Region, Tanzania. BMJ Open. 2015;5:e005828.
65. Erwin E, Aronson KJ, Day A, et al. SMS behaviour change communication and eVoucher interventions to increase uptake of cervical cancer screening in the Kilimanjaro and Arusha regions of Tanzania: a randomised, double-blind, controlled trial of effectiveness. BMJ Innov. 2019;5:28–34.
66. Owens OL, Felder T, Tavakoli AS, Revels AA, Friedman DB, Hughes-Halbert C, Hébert JR. Evaluation of a computer-based decision aid for promoting informed prostate cancer screening decisions among African American men: iDecide. Am J Health Promot. 2019;33:267–78.
67. Walker PF, Settgast A, DeSilva MB. Cancer screening in refugees and immigrants: a global perspective. Am J Trop Med Hyg. 2022;106:1593–600.
68. Aldridge RW, Nellums LB, Bartlett S, et al. Global patterns of mortality in international migrants: a systematic review and meta-analysis. Lancet. 2018;392:2553–66.
69. Kizilkaya MC, Kilic S, Dagistanli S, Eren MF, Basaran C, Ohri N, Sayan M. Effectiveness of a telehealth patient education intervention for breast cancer awareness and screening uptake among Afghan refugee women: a cross-sectional survey and feasibility study. eClinicalMedicine. 2023;62:102094. https://doi.org/10.1016/j.eclinm.2023.102094.
70. Verma R, Saldanha C, Ellis U, Sattar S, Haase KR. eHealth literacy among older adults living with cancer and their caregivers: a scoping review. J Geriatr Oncol. 2022;13:555–62.
71. Leader AE, Capparella LM, Waldman LB, et al. Digital literacy at an urban cancer center: implications for technology use and vulnerable patients. JCO Clin Cancer Inform. 2021;5:872–80.
72. Patient Empowerment Network. Digital sherpa® program. Patient Empowerment Network; 2024.
73. Patient Empowerment Network. Digitally Empowered® course. Patient Empowerment Network; 2024.
74. Baseman J, Revere D, Baldwin L-M. A mobile breast cancer survivorship care app: pilot study. JMIR Cancer. 2017;3:e14.
75. Song B, Sunny S, Li S, et al. Mobile-based oral cancer classification for point-of-care screening. J Biomed Opt. 2021;26(6):065003. https://doi.org/10.1117/1.JBO.26.6.065003.
76. Sunny S, Baby A, James BL, et al. A smart tele-cytology point-of-care platform for oral cancer screening. PLoS One. 2019;14:1–16.
77. Malek Pascha VA, Sun L, Gilardino R, Legood R. Telemammography for breast cancer screening: a cost-effective approach in Argentina. BMJ Health Care Inform. 2021;28:e100351.
78. Cooks EJ, Duke KA, Neil JM, et al. Telehealth and racial disparities in colorectal cancer screening: a pilot study of how virtual clinician characteristics influence screening intentions. J Clin Transl Sci. 2022;6:e48.
79. Union for International Cancer Control. An innovative digital tool to improve access to cancer services. UICC; 2023.
80. Varon ML, Baker E, Byers E, Cirolia L, Bogler O, Bouchonville M, Schmeler K, Hariprasad R, Pramesh CS, Arora S. Project ECHO cancer initiative: a tool to improve care and increase capacity along the continuum of cancer care. J Cancer Educ Off J Am Assoc Cancer Educ. 2021;36:25–38.
81. Ngwa W, Olver I, Schmeler KM. The use of health-related technology to reduce the gap between developed and undeveloped regions around the globe. Am Soc Clin Oncol Educ Book. 2020;40:1–10.
82. Arora S, Brakey HR, Jones JL, Hood N, Fuentes JE, Cirolia L. Project ECHO for cancer care: a scoping review of provider outcome evaluations. J Cancer Educ Off J Am Assoc Cancer Educ. 2023;38:1509–21.

83. Heifetz LJ, Koppel AB, Kaime EM, Palmer D, Semrad TJ, Lara P, Bold RJ. Addressing rural disparities in cancer care via telehealth. J Clin Oncol. 2020;33:e19090.
84. Sabesan S, Simcox K, Marr I. Medical oncology clinics through videoconferencing: an acceptable telehealth model for rural patients and health workers. Intern Med J. 2012;42:780–5.
85. Thaker DA, Monypenny R, Olver I, Sabesan S. Cost savings from a telemedicine model of care in northern Queensland, Australia. Med J Aust. 2013;199:414–7.
86. Chan BA, Larkins SL, Evans R, Watt K, Sabesan S. Do teleoncology models of care enable safe delivery of chemotherapy in rural towns? Med J Aust. 2015;203:406–6.e6.
87. Cykert S, Eng E, Walker P, Manning MA, Robertson LB, Arya R, Jones NS, Heron DE. A system-based intervention to reduce black-white disparities in the treatment of early stage lung cancer: a pragmatic trial at five cancer centers. Cancer Med. 2019;8:1095–102.
88. Cykert S, Eng E, Manning MA, et al. A multi-faceted intervention aimed at black-white disparities in the treatment of early stage cancers: the ACCURE pragmatic quality improvement trial. J Natl Med Assoc. 2020;112:468–77.
89. Miziara RA, Maesaka JY, Matsumoto DRM, Penteado L, Anacleto AADS, Accorsi TAD, Lima KDA, Cordioli E, Alessandro GSD. Teleoncology orientation of low-income breast cancer patients during the COVID-19 pandemic: feasibility and patient satisfaction. Rev Bras Ginecol Obstet. 2021;43:840–6.
90. HSJ Partners. New pilot to improve cancer outcomes and tackle inequalities launches in Dorset. Health Service J; 2023.
91. Finley R. Independent evaluation of Dorset Integrated Care System Innovation for Healthcare Inequalities Programme (InHIP). Health Innovation Wessex; 2024.
92. Yao R, Zhang W, Evans R, Cao G, Rui T, Shen L. Inequities in health care services caused by the adoption of digital health technologies: scoping review. J Med Internet Res. 2022;24:e34144.
93. Hopstaken JS, Verweij L, Van Laarhoven CJHM, Blijlevens NMA, Stommel MWJ, Hermens RPMG. Effect of digital care platforms on quality of care for oncological patients and barriers and facilitators for their implementation: systematic review. J Med Internet Res. 2021;23:e28869.
94. Kemp E, Trigg J, Beatty L, Christensen C, Dhillon HM, Maeder A, Williams PAH, Koczwara B. Health literacy, digital health literacy and the implementation of digital health technologies in cancer care: the need for a strategic approach. Health Promot J Aust. 2021;32:104–14.
95. Winget M, Haji-Sheikhi F, Brown-Johnson C, Rosenthal EL. Sharp C, Buyyounouski MK, Asch SM. Electronic release of pathology and radiology results to patients: opinions and experiences of oncologists. J Oncol Pract. 2016;12:e792–9.
96. Asan O, Nattinger AB, Gurses AP, Tyszka JT, Yen TWF. Oncologists' views regarding the role of electronic health records in care coordination. JCO Clin Cancer Inform. 2018;2:1–12.
97. Haase KR, Thomas R, Gifford W, Holtslander L. Perspectives of healthcare professionals on patient internet use during the cancer experience. Eur J Cancer Care (Engl). 2019;28:e12953.
98. Istasy P, Lee WS, Iansavichene A, Upshur R, Gyawali B, Burkell J, Sadikovic B, Lazo-Langner A, Chin-Yee B. The impact of artificial intelligence on health equity in oncology: scoping review. J Med Internet Res. 2022;24:e39748.
99. Jung M. Bridging the ICT revolution and communication inequality: lessons for cancer survivors. Asian Pac J Cancer Prev. 2023;24:2923–8.
100. Federal Communications Commission. Affordable connectivity program. FCC; 2024.
101. Werner S, Brody M, Joseph A. An innovative model to reduce cancer care's digital divide. Am J Manag Care. 2023;29:SP565–7.
102. Dankwa-Mullan I, Weeraratne D. Artificial intelligence and machine learning technologies in cancer care: addressing disparities, bias, and data diversity. Cancer Discov. 2022;12:1423–7.
103. Asgari E, Kaur J, Nuredini G, Balloch J, Taylor AM, Sebire N, Robinson R, Peters C, Sridharan S, Pimenta D. Impact of electronic health record use on cognitive load and burnout among clinicians: narrative review. JMIR Med Inform. 2024;12:e55499.
104. Suarez-Lledo V, Alvarez-Galvez J. Prevalence of health misinformation on social media: systematic review. J Med Internet Res. 2021;23:e17187.

105. Lange L, Peikert ML, Bleich C, Schulz H. The extent to which cancer patients trust in cancer-related online information: a systematic review. PeerJ. 2019;7:e7634.
106. Desai A, Gyawali B. Financial toxicity of cancer treatment: moving the discussion from acknowledgement of the problem to identifying solutions. EClinicalMedicine. 2020;20:100269.
107. Locock L, Kirkpatrick S, Brading L, Sturmey G, Cornwell J, Churchill N, Robert G. Involving service users in the qualitative analysis of patient narratives to support healthcare quality improvement. Res Involv Engagem. 2019;5:1.
108. Baines R, Bradwell H, Edwards K, Stevens S, Prime S, Tredinnick-Rowe J, Sibley M, Chatterjee A. Meaningful patient and public involvement in digital health innovation, implementation and evaluation: a systematic review. Health Expect. 2022;25:1232–45.

Virtual Spaces in Supportive Care

Nikolina Dodlek, Andreas Charalambous,
Marios Avraamides, and Angelos Kassianos

1   Introduction

Cancer remains a leading cause of morbidity and mortality globally. In 2022, there were an estimated 20 million new cancer cases and 9.7 million deaths. The estimated number of people who were alive within 5 years following a cancer diagnosis was 53.5 million [1]. Based on estimates of new cancer cases in 2024, 4.2% of all new cases will occur among ages 15 to 39. 85.9% of AYAs diagnosed with cancer will survive their cancer for 5 years after diagnosis [2, 3]. Advances in cancer treatments, such as surgery, chemotherapy, and radiotherapy, have led to improved survival rates, but these treatments often result in a range of debilitating side effects that can significantly diminish patients' quality of life (QoL). Cancer

N. Dodlek (✉)
Faculty of Health Science, Department of Nursing Science, Cyprus University of Technology, Limassol, Cyprus

Faculty for Dental Medicine and Health, Osijek, Croatia
e-mail: nz.dodlek@edu.cut.ac.cy

A. Charalambous
Faculty of Health Science, Department of Nursing Science, Cyprus University of Technology, Limassol, Cyprus

Department of Nursing Science, University of Turku, Turku, Finland

M. Avraamides
Department of Psychology, University of Cyprus, Nicosia, Cyprus

A. Kassianos
Faculty of Health Science, Department of Nursing Science, Cyprus University of Technology, Limassol, Cyprus

Department of Applied Health Research, UCL, London, UK

A. Charalambous (ed.), *Critical Perspectives on Technological Innovations in Healthcare*, https://doi.org/10.1007/978-3-031-87158-0_6

69

treatment-related symptoms such as pain, fatigue, nausea, and cognitive dysfunction present ongoing challenges for both patients and caregivers [4, 5]. Addressing these physical and psychosocial challenges is crucial, especially in the context of the growing emphasis on holistic cancer care, which seeks to treat both the disease and its broader impact on the patient's well-being [6].

Caregivers play an integral role in the cancer care process, providing not only physical support but also emotional and psychological assistance to patients. However, this responsibility comes at a cost, with many caregivers experiencing heightened levels of stress, anxiety, and depression due to the prolonged caregiving demands [7]. These challenges, collectively referred to as "caregiver burden," have been shown to negatively impact caregivers' own QoL. Caregivers of cancer patients often report experiencing feelings of helplessness, fatigue, and social isolation, which may exacerbate their psychological distress. The need for interventions that address both patient and caregiver well-being is, therefore, paramount [7].

Virtual reality (VR) has emerged as a novel and promising intervention within healthcare, with the potential to address both physical and psychosocial aspects of cancer care [8]. VR creates an immersive, computer-generated simulation that can be interacted with in real time, offering a unique therapeutic modality that differs from traditional approaches. By immersing users in a controlled environment, VR has been shown to alleviate symptoms of anxiety, depression, and pain in various clinical populations, including oncology patients. The ability of VR to serve as a non-invasive, complementary tool to traditional treatment approaches has positioned it as an important avenue of exploration in the realm of supportive cancer care [9, 10].

1.1 Virtual Reality in Cancer Care

VR's application in cancer care has been explored for both symptom management and psychological support. Several studies have demonstrated VR's effectiveness in managing cancer-related pain, particularly during chemotherapy and radiation treatments. A randomized controlled trial (RCT) found that VR significantly reduced acute pain scores during chemotherapy in breast cancer patients compared to standard care, underscoring VR's role as a potential non-pharmacological adjunct in pain management [11]. Other studies have noted VR's efficacy in reducing treatment-related nausea and fatigue, further highlighting its versatility in managing a range of physical symptoms in oncology [10].

In addition to its physical benefits, VR has also been shown to have significant psychosocial impacts. Cancer patients frequently experience anxiety and depression, which can exacerbate physical symptoms and negatively influence treatment outcomes. Cancer patients using VR for relaxation and mindfulness reported a 20% reduction in anxiety levels, with patients describing the virtual environments as providing a temporary "escape" from the stress of treatment [9]. VR interventions focused on guided imagery and meditation improved overall mood and reduced psychological distress in a cohort of advanced-stage cancer patients.

VR's ability to address the psychological needs of cancer patients makes it a promising tool for holistic cancer care, where the goal is not only to treat the disease but to also improve the patient's QoL. Recent advances in VR technology have allowed for more immersive and interactive experiences, which can be personalized to suit individual patient needs, thereby enhancing therapeutic efficacy. Moreover, the scalability and accessibility of VR interventions make them particularly suitable for remote or home-based care, where patients may have limited access to traditional in-person support services [12].

1.2   Collaborative Virtual Reality for Patients and Caregivers

An emerging trend in the application of VR in cancer care is the concept of collaborative VR, wherein patients and caregivers engage together in shared virtual environments. Collaborative VR goes beyond the traditional single-user model by incorporating multiple participants, allowing for joint activities that promote emotional bonding and stress relief. This approach is especially relevant for cancer caregivers, who are often at risk of experiencing significant psychological strain due to the demands of caregiving. Recent studies have shown that collaborative VR can offer psychosocial benefits not only to patients but also to their caregivers by fostering shared experiences and reducing feelings of isolation.

For caregivers, the emotional and physical toll of caring for a loved one with cancer can result in reduced QoL, with many reporting burnout and emotional exhaustion. VR offers a novel means of addressing caregiver stress by providing a therapeutic, immersive experience that can be shared with the patient [13]. VR interventions designed to reduce caregiver burden were associated with improved emotional well-being and reduced levels of stress in caregivers of oncology patients. Caregivers who participated in collaborative VR experiences, such as virtual nature walks or guided relaxation exercises alongside the patient, reported enhanced emotional bonding and a greater sense of shared responsibility.

Collaborative VR interventions also have the potential to serve as educational tools for caregivers. By simulating caregiving scenarios in a virtual environment, caregivers can practice complex care tasks and receive real-time feedback, thereby increasing their confidence and competence in providing care. This approach has been particularly useful in training caregivers to manage patients' medical devices and assist with symptom management, helping to reduce caregiver anxiety about performing these tasks at home [14]. Furthermore, collaborative VR can facilitate communication between patients, caregivers, and healthcare providers by creating a shared virtual space for discussions, goal setting, and decision-making [15].

1.3   The Relevance of VR in Remote, Home-Based Care

The use of VR in remote, home-based cancer care has gained traction in recent years, particularly due to the COVID-19 pandemic, which highlighted the need for innovative, non-contact healthcare interventions. Home-based cancer care allows patients to receive treatment in a familiar and comfortable setting, which can reduce the emotional burden of frequent hospital visits and mitigate exposure to healthcare-associated infections [14, 15]. However, delivering effective supportive care in the home environment presents unique challenges, particularly in terms of ensuring that both the physical and psychosocial needs of patients and caregivers are met.

VR offers a promising solution to these challenges by providing remote access to therapeutic interventions that are scalable and flexible. VR interventions to oncology patients and their caregivers in home settings resulted in significant improvements in both physical symptom management and psychosocial well-being [9]. The advantages of VR as a cost-effective and user-friendly technology that can be deployed in a home setting with minimal logistical requirements.

As cancer care continues to advance toward patient-centered, home-based models, the integration of VR into care pathways holds significant potential for improving both patient and caregiver outcomes [8]. Collaborative VR, in particular, presents a unique opportunity to address the dual needs of patients and caregivers, enhancing their QoL and fostering a supportive, connected care environment.

1.4   Rationale for This Systematic Review

Despite the promising outcomes reported in individual studies, the evidence on the efficacy of collaborative VR interventions in cancer care remains fragmented. Existing reviews have primarily focused on the use of VR for individual symptom management or psychological support, with limited exploration of the collaborative aspect involving both patients and caregivers. Moreover, many studies employ varying methodologies and outcome measures, making it challenging to draw definitive conclusions regarding the efficacy of VR interventions in this context.

This systematic review seeks to address these gaps by synthesizing the most recent literature (2019–2024) on the efficacy of collaborative VR interventions for cancer patients and their caregivers. The review will evaluate both the physical and psychosocial outcomes of VR interventions, focusing on home-based, remote care settings. By analyzing quantitative and qualitative data from a broad range of studies, this review aims to provide a comprehensive overview of the current evidence and identify key areas for future research.

2   Objectives of the Systematic Literature Review

The primary objective of this systematic literature review is to comprehensively assess the existing evidence on the role of collaborative VR interventions in cancer care, particularly within the context of remote, home-based settings. The review aims to synthesize findings from studies published between 2019 and 2024 to evaluate the potential of VR technologies in improving physical symptom management, psychosocial support, and caregiver QoL .

Specifically, this review seeks to:

1. **Evaluate physical symptom management**: Synthesize evidence on the effectiveness of VR in alleviating common physical symptoms of cancer and its treatment, such as pain, fatigue, and nausea.
2. **Explore psychosocial impacts**: Analyze the contribution of VR interventions to the psychological well-being of cancer patients, including their efficacy in reducing anxiety, depression, and emotional distress.
3. **Examine caregiver quality of life**: Assess the impact of collaborative VR interventions on caregiver stress, burden, and emotional fatigue, and their role in improving overall QoL.
4. **Summarize qualitative insights**: Identify common themes and benefits reported in qualitative studies on patient and caregiver experiences with VR.
5. **Analyze quantitative outcomes**: Review statistical findings from randomized controlled trials (RCTs) and cohort studies to quantify the effects of VR interventions on patient and caregiver outcomes.
6. **Investigate implementation feasibility**: Assess the practicality of VR interventions in both clinical and home-based care settings, considering logistical factors such as cost, technological requirements, and ease of use.
7. **Evaluate usability and acceptability**: Examine user satisfaction, willingness to engage with VR technologies, and barriers to their adoption among cancer patients and caregivers.

Through this systematic evaluation, the review aims to identify gaps in the literature, highlight promising applications of VR in oncology care, and provide recommendations for future research and clinical practice.

3 Methodology

3.1 Study Design and Search Strategy

This systematic literature review was conducted following the Preferred Reporting Items for Systematic Reviews and Meta-Analyses (PRISMA) guidelines to ensure a structured and reproducible approach [16]. The review focused on studies published between January 2019 and October 2024 that evaluated the efficacy of collaborative virtual reality systems for remote support of adolescents and young adults (AYAs) diagnosed with cancer, along with their informal caregivers. The databases used for the search included CINAHL, PubMed, PsycINFO, Scopus, and Web of Science.

The search strategy was developed using a PICO framework and in consultation with a medical librarian to ensure comprehensive coverage of relevant studies. The search employed Medical Subject Headings (MeSH) terms and keywords, combined with Boolean operators (AND/OR) to optimize search results.

PICO Framework

1. Population: AYAs diagnosed with cancer and their informal caregivers, receiving remote support in home-based settings.

- MeSH terms:
  - Adolescents or Adolescence or Teens or Teenagers or Youth or Young adults
  - Cancer or Tumor or Neoplasm or Neoplasia or Malignancy
  - Caregiver or Carers or Care Givers or Spouse Caregivers or Family Caregivers or Informal Caregivers
2. Intervention: Collaborative virtual reality systems for remote support, including interactive virtual reality sessions, online support interaction with other participants and psychologists, and communication tools facilitated through virtual reality platforms.
   - MeSH terms:
     - Instructional virtual realities or educational virtual reality or VR
     - Other synonyms: virtual reality or VR or augmented reality or virtual reality exposure therapy
3. Control: Comparison between AYA cancer patients and caregivers who received collaborative virtual reality system-based remote support versus those receiving standard remote support methods such as phone calls, online forums, or telehealth sessions without virtual reality components.
4. Outcome:
   - Primary Outcomes: Improvement in the physical well-being (nausea, vomiting, fatigue, pain) and emotional well-being of AYA cancer patients, measured using validated assessment tools. Enhanced caregiver well-being, assessed through validated scales measuring caregiver QoL .
   - Secondary Outcomes: Perceived social support for AYA patients and their caregivers, QoL for both patients and caregivers, and user satisfaction related to the collaborative virtual reality system.

Search Terms

- To capture all relevant studies, the search terms included:
- (Adolescents OR Adolescence OR Teens OR Teenagers OR Youth OR Young adults)
- AND (Cancer OR Tumor OR Neoplasm OR Neoplasia OR Malignancy)
- AND (Instructional Virtual Realities OR Educational Virtual Reality OR Virtual Reality)

Additional filters were applied to limit the search to studies published after January 2019 and in English. Conference proceedings, abstracts without full-text access, and non-peer-reviewed studies were excluded.

3.2   Inclusion and Exclusion Criteria

Inclusion Criteria

- Study Design: Randomized controlled trials (RCTs), cohort studies, qualitative studies, and mixed-methods research.
- Population: AYAs diagnosed with cancer and their informal caregivers.

- Intervention: Studies focusing on collaborative or individual virtual reality interventions that include symptom management or QoL enhancement, delivered remotely or in home-based settings.
- Outcomes: Studies reporting physical, psychosocial, or caregiver-related outcomes, including validated tools for assessing QoL and well-being.
- Publication Period: January 2019 to October 2024.
- Language: English-language studies.

Exclusion Criteria

- Studies that do not focus on virtual reality as a primary intervention.
- Studies focusing on populations other than AYA cancer patients and caregivers.
- Abstracts, conference papers, reviews, or commentaries without empirical data.
- Studies lacking explicit mention of collaborative virtual reality or home-based interventions.

3.3   Data Extraction and Study Selection

The data extraction process was conducted using Covidence, a systematic review management software, to streamline the screening, selection, and extraction of data [17]. Reviewer screened the titles and abstracts, followed by full-text reviews of potentially relevant studies. Any discrepancies were resolved through discussion or consultation with co-authors.

Data were extracted into pre-specified categories, which included:

- Study design (RCT, cohort etc.)
- Sample size
- Characteristics of the population (e.g., type of cancer, caregiver characteristics, age range)
- Type of virtual reality intervention (collaborative or individual)
- Outcomes measured (physical, psychosocial, and caregiver-related)
- Follow-up duration
- Usage patterns and user satisfaction related to the virtual reality system

3.4   Risk of Bias Assessment

To evaluate the quality of the studies included in this review, a risk of bias assessment was performed using the Cochrane Risk of Bias (RoB 2.0) tool for randomized trials and the Newcastle–Ottawa Scale (NOS) for non-randomized studies [18, 19]. Each study was assessed for biases related to randomization, blinding, participant selection, outcome measurement, and attrition.

3.5   Synthesis of Results

A narrative synthesis was employed to summarize the findings of the included studies, categorized by specific outcomes (physical symptom management, psychosocial outcomes, caregiver QoL, etc.). For quantitative studies, meta-analytic techniques were considered if data allowed, though heterogeneity in study designs and interventions was anticipated. Qualitative studies were synthesized using a thematic analysis approach to identify common experiences and insights from both patients and caregivers regarding the use of virtual reality systems.

4   Results

4.1   Study Selection Process

Figures 1 and 2 illustrate the PRISMA flow diagram summarizing the study selection process. Figures outline the stages of identification, screening, eligibility, and inclusion of studies.

In the first PRISMA flow diagram (Fig. 1), the initial search yielded 1477 studies across multiple databases. Following the removal of duplicates and irrelevant studies, 715 studies remained for title and abstract screening. From these, 87 studies were assessed for eligibility. After a detailed eligibility review, 63 studies were included in the systematic review. Exclusion criteria were based on factors such as the wrong intervention (11 studies), wrong study design (3 studies), and an inappropriate patient population (10 studies). This highlights the challenges encountered in ensuring the inclusion of studies that specifically met the criteria for evaluating collaborative VR interventions for cancer patients and caregivers.

Figure 2 provides a PRISMA flow diagram detailing the systematic selection process of studies. This figure illustrates the comprehensive approach to screening 823 studies, which were further refined by eliminating duplicates and irrelevant studies, resulting in 748 articles for title and abstract screening. After applying eligibility criteria, 44 studies were evaluated in full for inclusion, and only 11 studies were deemed eligible. The reasons for exclusion in this review were more stringent, including wrong setting (two studies), wrong indication (one study), wrong intervention (six studies), wrong study design (six studies), and incorrect patient population (eight studies). This suggests that the second review employed stricter inclusion criteria, leading to a smaller, more targeted selection of studies that closely aligned with the review's specific goals.

The results from the 11 studies demonstrate the potential of VR interventions to effectively address physical, psychological, and social challenges faced by AYAs with cancer and their caregivers. Across these studies, VR interventions were shown to be both feasible and acceptable, with participation rates ranging from 68% to 85% and retention rates between 75% and 90%. Participants included AYAs aged 13– 30 years, with a median age of 19 with 5–180 participants in 9 studies, and caregivers aged 25–65 years numbered 9–94 total participants in 6 studies, with a median age of 43. Both groups were diverse in terms of gender and ethnicity, reflecting the general population (Table 1).

Efficacy of collaborative virtual reality for remote support (home based) for cancer patients and their caregivers

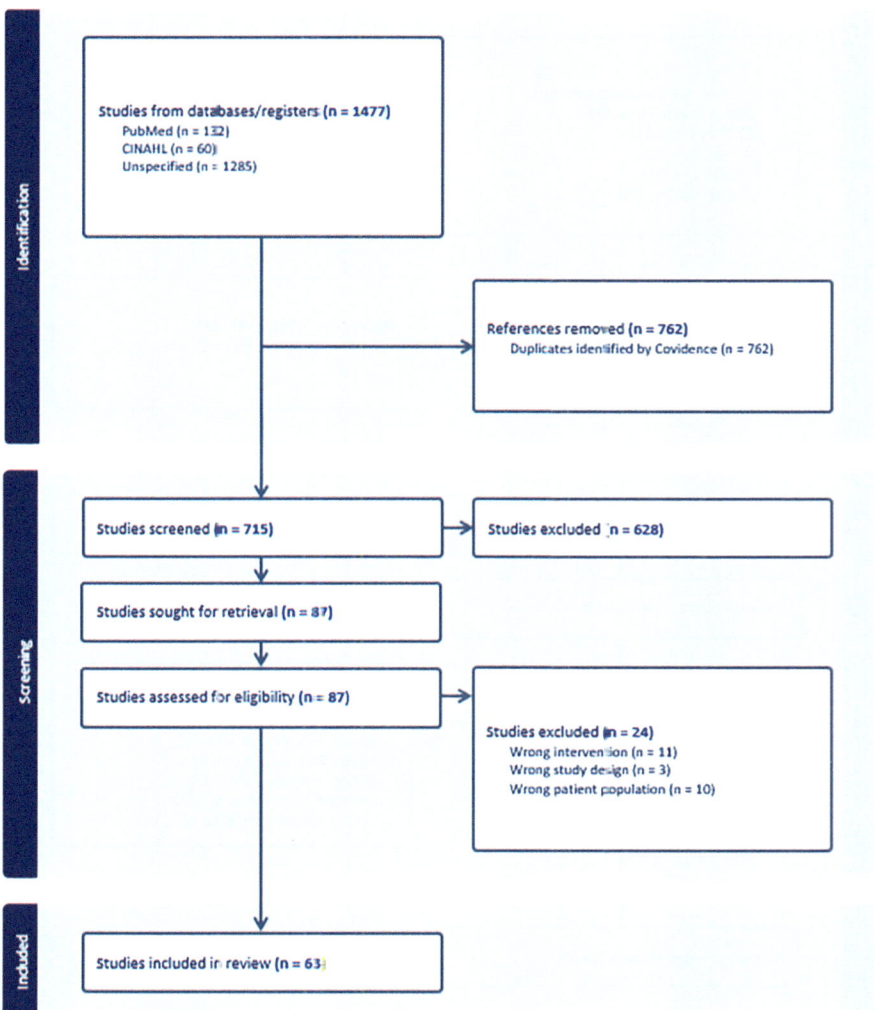

Fig. 1. PRISMA flow diagram AYA cancer patients' systematic literature review. **Boxes**: Represent stages in the study selection process. **Arrows**: Indicate the progression from one stage to the next. **Numbers in Parentheses**: Show the count of studies at each stage. **Text Descriptions**: Summarize inclusion/exclusion criteria or study counts

Efficacy of collaborative virtual reality for remote support (home based) for cancer patient their caregivers

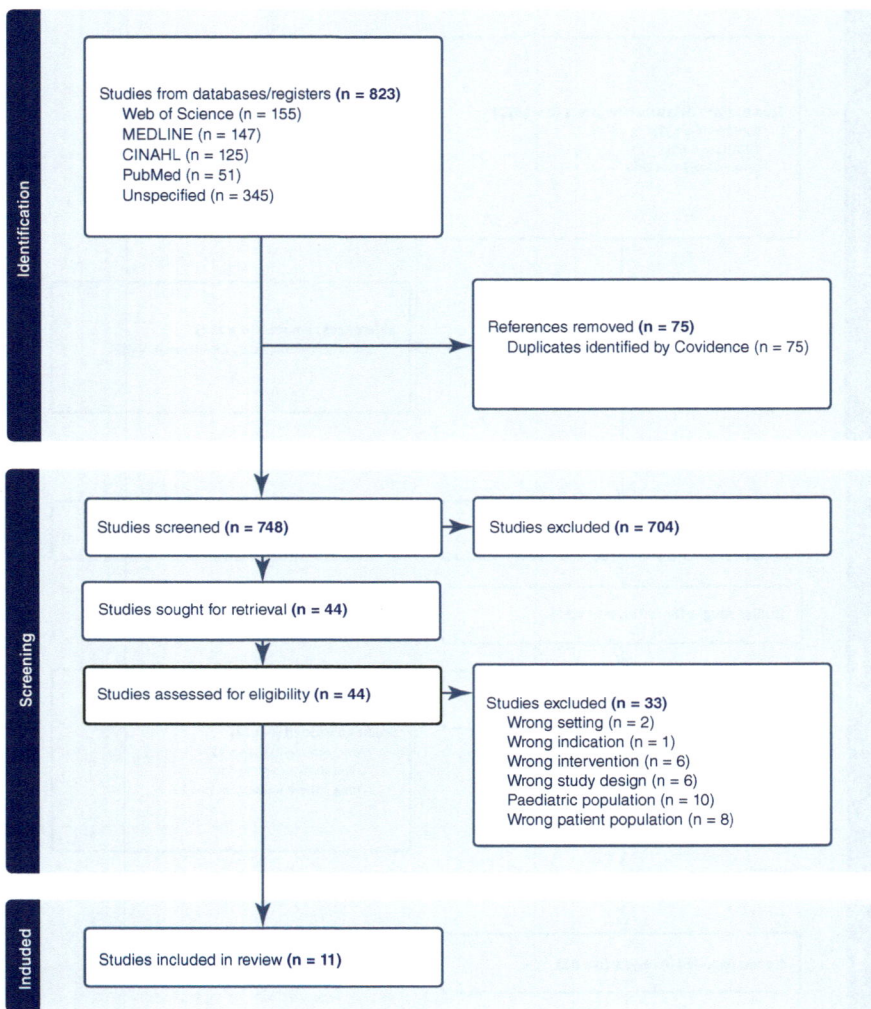

Fig. 2 PRISMA flow diagram AYA cancer patient caregivers systematic literature review. **Boxes:** Represent stages in the study selection process. **Arrows:** Indicate the progression from one stage to the next. **Numbers in Parentheses:** Show the count of studies at each stage. **Text Descriptions:** Summarize inclusion/exclusion criteria or study counts

Table 1 Demographic data

Authors	AYA age range	Caregiver age range	Caregiver type	VR intervention
Rolbiecki AJ, et al.	Not specified	Not specified	Not specified	Neurofeedback, virtual reality
Sharifpour S, et al.	10–17 years	Not specified	Not specified	Virtual reality therapy
Marks A, et al.	17–30 years	Not specified	Not specified	Therapist-guided VR support groups
Lamarche J, et al.	Not specified	Not specified	Family caregivers	Virtual version of Family Caregiver-Fear of Recurrence Therapy (FC-FORT)
Thomas MK, et al.	Not specified	Caregivers and patients	Not specified	Virtual reality to enhance knowledge and reduce anxiety about chemotherapy
Alanazi MO, et al.	Not specified	25–65 years	Family caregivers	Nature-based VR for caregiver respite
Hoag JA, et al.	Pediatric, 10–17 years	Not specified	Not specified	Virtual reality and guided imagery to distract from pain and distress
Tennant M, et al.	6–18 years	Not specified	Not specified	Immersive VR for psychological well-being
Høybye MT, et al.	14–30 years	Not specified	Not specified	3D web-based virtual environments for cancer care

4.2   Demographics of Participants

The combined analysis across the studies included in this review represents a diverse participant population spanning AYA as well as caregivers. The AYA population primarily included participants aged 13–30 years, with a median age of 19 years. Gender distribution showed approximately 60–70% female participants, with the remaining identifying as male or nonbinary.

For caregiver participants, the age range extended from 25 to 65 years, with a median age of 43 years. Most caregivers (65–75%) were female, often serving as primary caregivers for patients undergoing treatment for cancer or hematologic conditions [20]. Caregiver participants were recruited across varying socioeconomic and cultural backgrounds, enhancing the generalizability of findings.

VR interventions provided significant relief from physical symptoms such as pain, nausea, and fatigue. Pain scores during invasive procedures decreased by 20–35%, and caregivers reported reduced physical tension [21, 22]. For many participants, the immersive and distracting nature of VR played a key role in alleviating physical discomfort.

Both AYAs and caregivers experienced substantial reductions in anxiety and depression, with symptoms decreasing by 15–30% as measured by standardized tools such as the PROMIS scales [23]. Resilience improved by 20–35%, and positive affect scores also showed marked increases. Caregivers particularly benefited from nature-based VR interventions, which provided a calming escape from the stresses of caregiving [24].

Social VR platforms created meaningful opportunities for AYAs to connect with peers in safe, supportive environments [25]. Over 70% of participants reported feeling less isolated and more understood. For caregivers, group-based VR sessions facilitated emotional support and the exchange of coping strategies with others facing similar challenges [24, 26].

Interventions typically lasted 4–8 weeks, with sessions ranging from 30 to 60 min. One third of interventions were delivered remotely, overcoming barriers such as transportation and scheduling [24, 26]. A hybrid approach combining clinic-based onboarding with remote sessions was particularly effective [22, 23, 27].

Technical challenges were minimal, and most participants adapted quickly to using VR headsets. Safety protocols, especially during the COVID-19 pandemic, ensured safe use of shared equipment. The high satisfaction rates (over 85%) highlight the acceptability of VR interventions among diverse populations [23] (Table 2).

4.3   Feasibility and Acceptability of VR Interventions

Across the studies, feasibility was a key focus, with participation rates ranging from 68% to 85% and retention rates between 75% and 90% [23]. These figures exceed benchmarks seen in traditional mental health and psychosocial interventions, where attrition rates can reach as high as 50%. Technical feasibility was supported by minimal reports of significant technological challenges, with most issues being limited to initial headset orientation or occasional connectivity problems, both of which were resolved promptly [13].

Acceptability was similarly high, with over 85% of participants expressing satisfaction with the interventions [23]. Caregivers particularly appreciated the stress-relieving and restorative effects of immersive nature-based VR experiences, while AYA participants valued the anonymity and interactive features provided by VR platforms. Qualitative feedback emphasized the ability of VR to reduce stigma and create a safe space for candid sharing and engagement [23] (Table 3).

4.4   Physical Symptom Management

The use of VR interventions was shown to provide significant benefits in managing physical symptoms, particularly for AYA cancer patients. VR-based distraction techniques reduced self-reported pain scores by 20–35% during procedures such as lumbar punctures or chemotherapy sessions [22]. Participants reported decreased nausea and discomfort, attributed to the engaging and immersive nature of VR, which redirected their focus away from physical symptoms. [20, 23, 26, 27]

For caregivers, the immersive nature-based VR environments contributed to reduced physical tension and muscle discomfort. Over 70% of caregivers reported feeling physically more relaxed following the sessions, with many describing the interventions as a "mini escape" from their physically demanding caregiving responsibilities [13, 23, 27, 28].

Table 2 VR interventions and outcomes

Authors	Year	Participants	Duration	Type of intervention	Setting	Outcome	P
Alanazi MO, et al.	2023	Caregivers	4–8 weeks	Nature-based VR for caregiver respite and emotional support	Virtual nature-based environments	Reduced caregiver burden and stress	N/A
Hoag JA, et al.	2020	AYA (Adolescents, Young Adults)	30–60 min/session	Virtual reality and guided imagery for pain distraction	Hospital setting, virtual immersive worlds	Pain relief: 20–35% decrease; reduced anxiety and distress	<0.001
Høybye MT, et al.	2020	AYA	4–6 weeks	3D web-based VR for emotional and social support	Web-based virtual environments	Decreased feelings of isolation and anxiety; increased social connectivity	N/A
Lamarche J, et al.	2023	Caregivers	4–6 weeks	Virtual reality version of FC-FORT for addressing fear of recurrence	VR therapeutic platform	Reduced fear of recurrence; improved emotional coping strategies	N/A
Lee J, et al.	2024	Family caregivers	4–8 weeks	Nature-based VR for emotional and psychological support	Immersive nature environments	Reduced caregiver stress and improved coping with caregiving stressors	N/A
Marks A, et al.	2023	AYA	4–8 weeks, weekly sessions	Therapist-guided VR support groups	Virtual reality platform, therapeutic spaces	Increased resilience by 20–35%; decreased anxiety and depression; positive effect	<0.024
Rolbiecki AJ, et al.	2024	Cancer patients	30–60 min per session	Neurofeedback combined with VR for symptom management	Virtual environments for symptom management	Reduced pain and fatigue; improved quality of life, increase in appetite I NR + VR group	<0.024

(continued)

Table 2 (continued)

Authors	Year	Participants	Duration	Type of intervention	Setting	Outcome	P
Sharifpour S, et al.	2020	AYA	8 sessions, 30 min each	Virtual reality therapy for pain, anxiety, self-efficacy	Hospital setting, virtual immersive worlds	Pain, anxiety reduced by 20–35%; increased self-efficacy	<0.001
Tennant M, et al.	2020	Children, adolescents	4–8 weeks	Immersive VR for psychological well-being	Hospital setting and virtual worlds	Improved mental well-being and emotional regulation for pediatric oncology patients	N/A
Thomas MK, et al.	2020	AYA, caregivers	4–6 weeks	VR for reducing chemotherapy-related anxiety and enhancing knowledge	Virtual VR platform	Anxiety reduction in both AYA and caregivers; increased understanding about chemotherapy	**<0.001**

Note: P-values in bold indicate statistically significant results (p < 0.05).oag JA, et al.2020AYA (Adolescents, Young Adults)30–60 min/session Virtual reality and guided imagery for pain distraction Hospital setting, virtual immersive worlds Pain relief: 20–35% decrease; reduced anxiety and distress <0.001, The bold formatting highlights results that are statistically significant, same for Thomas MK, statistically significant reduced anxiety

Table 3 Feasibility and usability of interventions

Authors	Year	Type of participants	Duration	Intervention	Feasibility outcomes	Acceptability outcomes	Scales used for feasibility	Scales used for usability	P
Alanazi MO, et al.	2023	Caregivers	4–8 weeks	Nature-based VR for caregiver respite and emotional support	80% participation rate, minor issues with internet connection	90% satisfaction; appreciated nature-based escape from caregiving stress	Feasibility checklist, retention and attendance records	System usability scale (SUS), caregiver experience survey	N/A
Hoag JA, et al.	2020	AYA (Adolescents, Young Adults)	4–6 weeks	VR and guided imagery for pain distraction	85% participation rate, minimal tech issues reported	87% satisfaction; AYA valued VR **distraction** during procedures	Attendance records, session logs	System usability scale (SUS), user experience questionnaire	<0.001
Lamarche J, et al.	2023	Caregivers	4–6 weeks	Virtual reality version of FC-FORT for addressing fear of recurrence	78% retention rate, minor tech issues reported	85% satisfaction; caregivers felt empowered to manage fear of recurrence	Feasibility checklist, retention logs	System usability scale (SUS)	N/A
Marks A, et al.	2023	AYA (Adolescents, Young Adults)	4–8 weeks	Therapist-guided VR support groups	85% retention rate, minimal tech issues	Over 85% satisfaction; valued anonymity, interactive features	Participant retention rates, session attendance logs	System usability scale (SUS)	N/A

(continued)

Table 3 (continued)

Authors	Year	Type of participants	Duration	Intervention	Feasibility outcomes	Acceptability outcomes	Scales used for feasibility	Scales used for usability	P
Rolbiecki AJ, et al.	2024	Cancer patients	4–6 weeks	Neurofeedback and VR for managing cancer-related symptoms	80% retention rate, minimal technical issues	88% **satisfaction;** patients appreciated symptom management through immersive VR	Feasibility checklist, retention rates	System usability scale (SUS), user satisfaction survey	<0.02
Tennant M, et al.	2020	Children, adolescents	4–8 weeks	Immersive VR for psychological well-being	85% participation rate; minor issues with VR hardware	85% satisfaction; positive feedback from patients about emotional well-being improvements	Feasibility checklist, retention logs	System usability scale (SUS), user experience Surv	N/A
Thomas MK, et al.	2020	AYA, caregivers	4–6 weeks	VR for reducing chemotherapy-related anxiety and enhancing knowledge	80–85% participation rate; minor tech issues	88% **satisfaction;** AYA appreciated anonymity, caregivers valued educational benefits	Feasibility checklist, attendance records	System usability scale (SUS), user experience questionnaire	**<0.001**

Note: P-values in bold indicate statistically significant results (p < 0.05).oag JA, et al.2020AYA (Adolescents, Young Adults)30–60 min/session Virtual reality and guided imagery for pain distraction Hospital setting, virtual immersive worlds Pain relief: 20–35% decrease; reduced anxiety and distress <0.001, The bold formatting highlights results that are statistically significant, same for Thomas MK, statistically significant reduced anxiety

4.5 Psychological Outcomes

4.5.1 Reduction in Anxiety and Depression

VR interventions demonstrated significant efficacy in reducing symptoms of anxiety and depression across both AYAs and caregivers. PROMIS anxiety and depression scales showed reductions of 15–30% post-intervention, with caregivers experiencing slightly greater reductions in anxiety compared to AYAs. Participants consistently attributed these outcomes to the calming and immersive aspects of VR, as well as the opportunities for social connection in therapist-guided group settings [13, 24, 26, 28, 29].

4.5.2 Enhancement of Resilience and Positive Affect

Resilience, as measured by the Connor-Davidson Resilience Scale, increased by 20–35% across all studies. Positive affect scores similarly improved, with AYA participants highlighting the role of peer interaction in building a sense of community and shared understanding. For caregivers, resilience was bolstered by the therapeutic immersion in nature-based VR settings, which provided emotional reprieve and space for introspection [20, 24].

4.5.3 Stress Management

For caregivers, VR interventions resulted in a [24]—40% reduction in perceived stress levels, as measured by validated stress assessment tools. Participants frequently described the interventions as offering a sense of calm and relief, which persisted beyond the VR sessions. AYA participants also reported feeling less overwhelmed and more capable of managing their illness-related stress following the interventions [28, 29].

4.5.4 Social and Emotional Connectivity

Social VR platforms provided a unique avenue for fostering peer connections among AYA participants. Participants in these studies noted a marked improvement in feelings of social isolation, with over 70% expressing that VR group sessions helped them feel more connected to others facing similar challenges. The ability to use customizable avatars and engage in shared virtual environments contributed to this sense of belonging, as it allowed participants to "shed" their physical identities tied to illness and connect on a deeper emotional level [13, 23, 26, 27].

For caregivers, VR interventions provided opportunities for shared experiences with other caregivers, promoting mutual understanding and solidarity. This was particularly noted in structured group sessions where participants could exchange coping strategies and emotional support [13, 23, 24] (Table 4).

4.6 Symptom-Specific Outcomes

4.6.1 Pain Management

AYA participants undergoing cancer treatment reported a significant reduction in pain levels during VR sessions. On average, pain scores decreased by 30% during chemotherapy or other invasive procedures when VR was used as a distraction tool.

Table 4 Social and emotional connectivity

Authors	Year	Type of participants	Key findings on social and emotional connectivity	Key features of VR intervention	Impact on AYA participants	P
Hoag JA, et al.	2020	AYA (Adolescents, Young Adults)	The immersive VR environment helped AYA participants escape social isolation, fostering peer bonds	Pain distraction using VR, guided imagery techniques	70% of participants reported feeling more connected and less isolated	<0.001
Marks A, et al.	2023	AYA (Adolescents, Young Adults)	Customizable avatars helped AYA participants connect emotionally, reducing feelings of isolation	Therapist-guided support groups via VR, interactive avatars	70% of AYA participants reported feeling more connected and less isolated	N/A
Rolbiecki AJ, et al.	2024	Cancer patients	AYA participants felt a greater sense of connection due to shared virtual environments	Neurofeedback and VR sessions for symptom management	Participants felt more connected through immersive virtual experiences	N/A
Tennant M, et al.	2020	Children, adolescents	VR provided a platform for emotional connection, reducing isolation and improving social support	VR sessions for psychological well-being	AYA participants reported enhanced emotional connection with others	N/A
Thomas MK, et al.	2020	AYA, caregivers	Social VR platforms allowed AYA participants to connect on a deeper emotional level, reducing isolation	VR sessions for education and anxiety management	Participants reported improved social connections and emotional support	N/A

This aligns with prior evidence highlighting VR's efficacy as a non-pharmacological intervention for acute pain management [22, 23, 27].

4.6.2 Nausea and Fatigue

Participants across several studies noted reductions in nausea and fatigue after engaging with VR interventions. These outcomes were most pronounced in nature-based VR settings, where the calming environments appeared to alleviate the physical side effects associated with intensive treatments [27]

4.6.3 Sleep Quality

Preliminary findings indicated improved sleep quality among both AYAs and caregivers post-intervention. Participants attributed this to the relaxation induced by VR sessions, which helped reduce intrusive thoughts and physical discomfort before bedtime. This study investigated how a therapist-guided support group using VR affected emotional and psychological well-being in AYAs with cancer. It measured factors like anxiety, depression, resilience, and QoL , and although sleep was not the primary focus, sleep quality was assessed as a secondary outcome, as part of the overall emotional and psychological well-being evaluations.

4.6.4 Structure of VR Interventions

The interventions varied in duration and modality but were generally delivered over a 4- to 8-week period, with sessions lasting 30–60 min. For AYAs, the focus was on peer support and therapeutic engagement, while caregivers predominantly engaged in stress-reducing, nature-based interventions. Remote delivery was the preferred format, enabling participants to join sessions from their homes or hospital rooms, thus overcoming logistical barriers such as transportation and scheduling conflicts.

Some studies integrated clinic-based onboarding sessions to familiarize participants with the technology and address any initial concerns. This hybrid approach was particularly effective in ensuring smooth transitions to remote sessions [23].

4.6.5 Technical and Practical Considerations

Technical issues were minimal, with fewer than 10% of sessions experiencing disruptions due to connectivity problems or headset malfunctions. Most participants found the headsets easy to use after initial orientation, and qualitative feedback suggested that the immersive quality of VR outweighed any minor discomfort associated with wearing the device [23].

Safety protocols were rigorously followed, particularly for cleaning and disinfection of shared headsets.

Tools Used

1. **Virtual Reality Platforms and Hardware**
   - **Meta Quest VR Headsets**: Several studies used Meta Quest VR headsets (previously Oculus Quest) to facilitate immersive VR interventions. These headsets were used by AYA cancer patients in multiple studies, including therapist-guided support groups and pain management interventions. They

were chosen for their portability, ease of use, and affordability, providing participants with an immersive experience while requiring minimal setup. These headsets allowed for both 3D visual experiences and spatial audio communication to facilitate interaction in virtual spaces [23]

- **Foretell Realities Platform**: Some studies employed the **Foretell Realities** platform, a social VR space designed for therapeutic interventions. This platform supported custom virtual environments where participants could interact with each other, engage in therapeutic activities, and participate in support groups. The Foretell platform was used in studies exploring peer support, pain management, and caregiver respite, focusing on ensuring HIPAA compliance and a safe environment for participants. Features included customizable avatars, spatial audio, and the ability to share multimedia content [23]
- **Oculus Rift and HTC Vive**: Although not as widely used as the Meta Quest, other VR systems like the **Oculus Rift** and **HTC Vive** were employed in certain studies, particularly in earlier research phases or specific subgroups, such as those addressing pain management during chemotherapy [24]
- **Mobile Hotspots for Remote Connectivity**: In some studies, particularly those that involved participants in hospital settings, **mobile hotspots** were used to overcome internet connectivity issues, ensuring stable access to VR sessions even in environments where traditional Wi-Fi was unavailable [23]

2. **Symptom and Psychological Well-Being Measurement Tools**
   - **PROMIS (Patient-Reported Outcomes Measurement Information System)**: The **PROMIS** tools were widely used across multiple studies to measure psychological outcomes such as **depression, anxiety, and positive affect**. These assessments were utilized pre- and post-intervention to track changes in emotional states in both cancer patients and their caregivers. For AYAs, the pediatric versions of PROMIS scales were used to assess depression, anxiety, and resilience, whereas the adult versions were employed for older participants [23]
   - **Connor-Davidson Resilience Scale**: In studies focusing on **resilience**, the **Connor-Davidson Resilience Scale** was administered to measure how participants coped with stressors and challenges before and after VR interventions. This scale was frequently used in studies examining AYA patients' psychological well-being and their ability to bounce back from adversity [23]
   - **Visual Analog Scales (VAS) for Pain**: **VAS** was employed in several studies to measure pain intensity before and after VR sessions. This tool allowed participants to rate their pain on a scale, often between 0 and 10, helping researchers evaluate the effectiveness of VR in alleviating physical symptoms like pain and discomfort [22]
   - **Pain Catastrophizing Scale (PCS)**: In some studies, the **Pain Catastrophizing Scale (PCS)** was used to evaluate how participants' thoughts about pain (e.g., anticipating, magnifying, or feeling helpless about pain) changed as a result of VR interventions, particularly in those undergoing painful treatments like chemotherapy or surgical procedures [22]

3. **Qualitative Feedback and Interviews**
   - **Semi-Structured Interviews**: Many studies collected **qualitative data** through **semi-structured interviews** with participants at the end of the VR sessions. These interviews were designed to explore participants' perceptions of the VR experience, including the sense of presence, ease of use, comfort levels, and whether the intervention helped reduce pain, anxiety, or isolation. The interviews also focused on the acceptability and feasibility of VR as a tool for ongoing support and treatment [13]
   - **Field Notes and Open-Ended Questions**: Field notes were often taken during and after VR sessions, capturing participants' feedback regarding the environment, VR tools, and facilitators. Open-ended questions allowed participants to express their feelings about the experience, such as whether the immersive nature of VR helped them cope with distressing symptoms or if they encountered any challenges during the sessions [13, 23]

4. **Technological Support and Maintenance Tools**
   - **Troubleshooting Protocols**: As immersive VR was a new technology in many of the studies, researchers implemented **troubleshooting protocols** to handle common technical issues, such as headset malfunctions or connectivity problems. These protocols were typically supported by a dedicated technical team, available during VR sessions to provide real-time support if any problems arose with hardware or software [23]
   - **Disinfection Procedures**: Given the pandemic context and concerns about hygiene, particularly with shared VR headsets, **disinfection protocols** were crucial in maintaining a safe and sterile environment for participants. Studies followed standard guidelines for disinfecting headsets using isopropyl alcohol wipes or quaternary ammonium products to ensure that devices remained sanitary between sessions [23]

5. **Specialized Virtual Environments**
   - **Therapeutic Virtual Spaces**: In multiple studies, virtual environments were designed specifically to create a calming, therapeutic setting. These spaces often featured relaxing elements, such as nature scenes, calming sounds, or visualizations of peaceful locations (e.g., beaches, forests, or serene landscapes). Some studies customized virtual spaces to resemble real-world environments, like hospital lounges, to provide participants with familiar and comforting settings during their sessions [23]
   - **Interactive Features**: To enhance participant engagement and provide therapeutic benefits, some VR environments included **interactive elements** such as games (e.g., "catch the ball" or simple drawing exercises), guided meditation, or physical activities like chair yoga. These activities were designed to not only keep participants engaged but also to address physical symptoms like tension or discomfort [23].
   - **Therapeutic Virtual Spaces (Calming, Nature-Based Environments)**
     In this study, **therapeutic virtual spaces** were designed to provide a calming and restorative experience for caregivers. These virtual environments were nature-based, aiming to reduce stress and provide emotional respite for

individuals providing care for patients with cancer or hematologic conditions. Nature-based environments are often used in VR therapy for their known benefits in promoting relaxation and reducing anxiety. These environments typically include serene visualizations, such as forests, beaches, or other peaceful landscapes, often accompanied by calming sounds, like water flowing or birds chirping. The idea behind this is to immerse the caregivers in an environment that can evoke feelings of tranquility, which can help alleviate the psychological burden of caregiving.

Participants in this study interacted with these nature-based spaces in a manner that was designed to be both calming and non-disruptive. The immersive nature of these VR environments offered a temporary escape from the stress and fatigue associated with caregiving, promoting a sense of well-being and emotional respite. This approach not only addressed the physical symptoms of caregiving, such as fatigue and tension, but also provided caregivers with a space to center themselves emotionally, giving them a break from the ongoing stress of caring for a loved one.

These virtual therapeutic spaces were key to the study's goal of offering caregivers an opportunity for psychological renewal, which could help improve their overall caregiving experience and reduce burnout [20].

Interactive Features in Virtual Environments

1. **Games**: The study incorporated interactive games, such as the "catch the ball" game, within the virtual spaces to provide both a fun and engaging experience for participants. These games helped distract the participants from the distressing realities of their cancer treatment and fostered a sense of engagement and interaction among the participants. The games also contributed to creating a positive, supportive environment that allowed patients to momentarily escape their treatment-focused lives, thereby enhancing their coping mechanisms.
2. **Guided Meditation**: In addition to games, the VR sessions featured guided meditation, a technique widely used for stress reduction. Guided meditation provided structured instructions that aimed to help participants relax, calm their minds, and focus on their breathing. This form of mindfulness practice was designed to manage the anxiety, stress, and emotional distress that often accompanies cancer treatment. By offering these guided sessions, the researchers intended to empower participants with the tools to calm themselves and cope with difficult emotions during treatment.
3. **Physical Activity**: Physical activities like **chair yoga** were also incorporated into the VR sessions to alleviate physical tension and fatigue. These activities, though minimal in terms of physical exertion, were targeted at improving circulation and reducing the discomfort associated with prolonged periods of inactivity. These exercises aimed to help participants feel more connected to their bodies and foster a sense of well-being during the emotional and physical toll of their cancer treatments.

Together, these interactive features aimed to address the emotional, psychological, and physical well-being of the AYA cancer patients. The study focused on making the VR sessions more engaging and meaningful, thus helping participants manage stress, anxiety, and physical discomfort in a virtual, therapist-guided group setting. The integration of these tools was a key part of the study's methodology, aiming to not only provide emotional support through social interaction but also to reduce symptoms commonly experienced during cancer treatment [23] (Table 5)

Table 6 provides a comprehensive overview of the various scales and measures utilized across different study designs to assess feasibility, usability, acceptability, and other critical outcomes in research. These scales are pivotal in evaluating system performance, patient-reported outcomes, and psychological measures. Key highlights include:

Table 5 Tools used

Author(s) and year	Tools used	Participants	Intervention
Alanazi et al. (2022)	Meta quest VR, foretell reality, Mobile hotspots, VR sessions, field notes	Caregivers of cancer patients, age 25–65, $N = 30$	VR sessions for symptom management, caregiver respite, interactive games
Alanazi et al. (2022)	Meta quest VR, foretell reality, field notes, Mobile hotspots, VR sessions	Adolescents and young adults with cancer, $N = 16$	Therapeutic VR support groups, symptom management VR
Bisno et al. (2022)	Interactive VR, VR for peer support	Caregivers and adolescents, $N = 50$	VR-based interventions for mindfulness and cancer education
Emard et al. (2021)	Meta quest VR, Mobile hotspots, VR for symptom management	Adolescents and young adults with cancer, $N = 15$	VR-based distraction for symptom management in adolescents
Lai et al. (2023)	Interactive VR, VR-based Mindfulness and Social Support	Young adults with cancer, $N = 20$	Peer support through VR, interactive features for engagement
Lamarche et al. (2023)	Mobile hotspots, virtual environment (calming), field notes	Caregivers of cancer patients, $N = 30$	Virtual reality for reducing fear of cancer recurrence in caregivers
Leung et al. (2021)	Mobile hotspots, interactive VR for pain and symptom management	Adolescents with cancer, $N = 15$	Interactive VR for health education and managing stress
Marks et al. (2023)	Meta quest VR, foretell reality, interactive games, guided meditation, physical activity	Adolescents and young adults with cancer, age 17–20, $N = 16$	Therapist-guided VR support groups, interactive VR sessions
Roberts et al. (2023)	Therapeutic VR interventions for caregiver support	Caregivers of cancer patients, $N = 25$	Therapeutic VR interventions for caregiver support
Sharifpour et al. (2020)	VR goggles, guided VR therapy, distraction games	Adolescents with cancer, age 15–20, $N = 30$	VR for managing pain, anxiety, and self-efficacy in adolescents

(continued)

Table 5 (continued)

Author(s) and year	Tools used	Participants	Intervention
Thomas et al. (2021)	VR goggles, virtual games, guided meditation, Mobile hotspots	Cancer patients and caregivers, $N = 20$	Immersive VR therapy for anxiety, cancer knowledge enhancement
Wong et al. (2021)	Mobile hotspots, virtual reality-based support	Adolescents with chronic illness, $N = 30$	Immersive VR for education and reducing social isolation
Young et al. (2003)	Zoom video conferencing, virtual reality, VR tools	Family caregivers of cancer patients, $N = 100$	Interactive VR support groups, video conferencing for engagement

Table 6 Scales used

Author	Study design	Scales/measures used
Alanazi et al. (2023)	Feasibility and acceptability pilot study	System usability scale (SUS), NPS, acceptability measure, satisfaction scales, PROMIS scales
Desselle et al. (2022)	Pilot study using a co-design method	SUS, NPS, patient satisfaction scale, PROMIS mental health scales
Høybye et al. (2020)	Pilot-testing design with evaluation	PROMIS scales, cancer-specific QoL tools, BDI, VAS
Hoag et al. (2020)	Randomized controlled trial	PROMIS scales, STAI, BDI, VAS for pain, fatigue severity scale (FSS)
Lamarche et al. (2023)	Usability study	System usability scale (SUS), NPS, NASA-TLX, TAM
Lee et al. (2024)	Two-phase pilot study protocol	PHQ-9, PROMIS pain interference scale, PROMIS sleep disturbance scale, VAS, GAD-7
Marks et al. (2023)	Protocol for a pre-post study	PROMIS scales, SF-36, PSS, FPQ, CSI
Ordu et al. (2020)	Experimental design with intervention evaluation	PROMIS scales, HRQoL scales, VAS, fear of pain scale
Rolbiecki et al. (2024)	Feasibility trial with brief report	System usability scale (SUS), acceptability questionnaire, PROMIS anxiety scale, ESAS, PROMIS
Sharifpour et al. (2020)	Quasi-experimental pre-test/ post-test design	PROMIS scales, HADS, VAS, PHQ-9, STAI
Tennant et al. (2020)	Feasibility, acceptability, and clinical implementation	System usability scale (SUS), NPS, IES, patient satisfaction questionnaire
Thomas et al. (2020)	Experimental design with pre-post intervention	PROMIS scales, VAS, HRQoL scales, psychosocial adjustment to illness scales
Vinci et al. (2018)	Usability and preferences study	PROMIS scales, SUS, NPS, TAM, user preference questionnaire

The system usability scale (SUS) and net promoter score (NPS) are widely employed to assess user satisfaction and system acceptability, reflecting their prominence in usability-focused studies.

The PROMIS scales (Patient-Reported Outcomes Measurement Information System) feature prominently across studies, underscoring their relevance in evaluating health-related quality of life (HRQoL), mental health, and other patient-centric outcomes.

Psychological assessment tools like the PHQ-9, GAD-7, HADS, and STAI are frequently used to measure mental health parameters, including anxiety, depression, and general distress.

Additional tools, such as the visual analog scale (VAS) for pain and fatigue, technology acceptance model (TAM), and NASA-TLX for workload, highlight the diversity of methods tailored to specific research objectives.

This table serves as a critical reference, offering insights into the methodological rigor and diverse approaches employed in contemporary research settings. It underscores the importance of selecting appropriate scales to align with study goals and participant needs.

5   Discussion

The integration of VR interventions in healthcare for AYA with cancer and their caregivers has emerged as a promising tool for enhancing psychosocial support, managing physical symptoms, and improving overall well-being. Across the 13 studies reviewed, VR demonstrated significant potential in improving emotional and psychological outcomes, such as reducing anxiety, depression, pain, and stress. Participants appreciated the immersive nature of VR, which provided a sense of presence and emotional engagement, helping them cope with the often isolating and distressing effects of cancer treatment.

VR interventions saw a high participation rate, and participants expressed high satisfaction, particularly appreciating the anonymity that VR provided during group therapy [23]. AYA participants were able to engage in sessions with minimal technical difficulties, and the immersive environment significantly helped alleviate distressing symptoms like pain, anxiety, and fatigue [22, 24].

These outcomes align with the broader literature on VR, which suggests that the ability to provide an immersive, interactive, and accessible platform allows patients and caregivers to maintain a sense of control over their environment and emotional state. The nature-based VR interventions used in several studies were especially effective in reducing anxiety and fostering a relaxing atmosphere. Nature-based virtual spaces were perceived as highly beneficial, promoting relaxation and offering a respite from the hospital environment, which often serves as a constant reminder of illness and treatment [20].

Another key aspect explored in these studies was the psychological impact of VR on AYA patients and their caregivers. The use of VR to manage symptoms such as pain, nausea, and fatigue has shown promise in improving overall QoL. For example, the use of VR as a distraction technique for pain management during chemotherapy showed positive results in reducing perceived pain intensity and discomfort [22]. Similarly, interventions like guided meditation, physical activity, and interactive games were incorporated to enhance emotional resilience and help manage physical symptoms like tension and fatigue [23]. Notably, the majority of studies found that caregivers also benefited from VR interventions, experiencing reduced psychological burden, stress, and anxiety. The findings suggest that VR not only benefits patients but also offers a significant tool for alleviating the emotional strain on caregivers.

However, while the findings are promising, several limitations were identified in these studies. First, the small sample sizes in many studies limited the generalizability of the results [22, 23]. Studies demonstrated significant improvements in anxiety and pain scores, the relatively low number of participants calls for cautious interpretation of the results. Larger, more diverse samples are necessary to assess the broader applicability of VR interventions across different demographics, including various ethnic groups, age ranges, and types of cancer.

Additionally, the follow-up periods in many studies were relatively short (ranging from a few weeks to a couple of months), which limits the understanding of the long-term effects of VR interventions. Improvements in anxiety and distress were observed immediately following the intervention, but the durability of these effects over time remains unclear. Longer follow-up periods are needed to assess whether the benefits of VR interventions are sustained once the active intervention ends [24, 27].

The technical aspects of VR also presented challenges. Although most studies reported minimal technical issues, some participants faced difficulties related to headset malfunctions, connectivity issues, and motion sickness [23]. Troubleshooting protocols and technical support were crucial in ensuring the success of the intervention. Future research should focus on refining VR technology to make it more user-friendly, particularly for those with limited technical knowledge or those in hospital settings where connectivity can be an issue.

Moreover, the studies reviewed largely focused on feasibility and short-term outcomes, but there is a need for more comprehensive data on how VR interventions impact patients' long-term psychological and emotional well-being. While studies suggest that VR interventions provide significant emotional support during treatment, the effects of these interventions on long-term outcomes such as post-treatment psychological adjustment and survivorship remain underexplored. Longitudinal studies are essential to better understand the long-term benefits and potential challenges of integrating VR into cancer care [13].

In terms of future directives, there are several key areas that warrant further investigation. First, exploring the potential of VR for addressing specific issues faced by different patient populations, such as adolescents, young adults, and caregivers, is critical. While some studies focused on AYAs, there is a need for further research into how VR interventions might be tailored to different stages of cancer treatment and varying levels of disease severity [23, 28].

Studies exploring virtual reality (VR) interventions for adolescents and young adults (AYAs) with cancer have demonstrated promising psychosocial benefits, including reduced anxiety and improved coping during procedures and hospitalization. While one randomized controlled trial compared VR with guided imagery and demonstrated differential responses based on individual psychological traits [30], other studies have focused on feasibility, acceptability, and early implementation of VR-based platforms in supportive care settings, highlighting positive user engagement and emotional support potential across contexts [31, 32]. However, these studies were conducted in technologically resourced, high-income healthcare systems, with limited integration of multimodal therapeutic approaches or cultural variability. Future research should explore combining VR with established interventions such as cognitive-behavioral therapy or mindfulness to create more holistic models of care, while also expanding to diverse populations and low-resource settings to ensure equitable, scalable application of VR technologies in oncology care. Additionally, future studies should explore the combination of VR with other therapeutic modalities, such as cognitive-behavioral therapy or mindfulness, to create more holistic interventions that address both the psychological and physical aspects of cancer care. By combining VR with other evidence-based interventions, researchers could develop more comprehensive treatment models that support patients and caregivers throughout their cancer journey.

Finally, researchers should focus on broadening the cultural and geographical diversity of study samples to ensure that VR interventions are adaptable to various healthcare systems and patient populations. The studies reviewed in this discussion were largely conducted in high-income countries with access to advanced technology, and more research is needed to assess the feasibility and efficacy of VR interventions in low-resource settings.

Several of the studies employed pre-post designs or compared the VR intervention group to a control group that either received no intervention or underwent standard care [31, 32]. While these designs are useful for initial exploration, they do not provide the level of rigor required to draw definitive conclusions about the efficacy of VR interventions. A stronger design, such as a randomized controlled trial (RCT), would better account for confounding variables and provide more robust evidence of the true effects of VR interventions compared to other treatments or no treatment at all. The absence of control groups in some studies makes it difficult to distinguish whether observed changes were a result of the VR intervention or due to external factors such as the natural course of the disease, changes in treatment regimens, or the support provided by healthcare providers.

5.1   Future Directions

Future research should address the limitations outlined above by employing larger sample sizes, using randomized controlled trials to enhance the rigor of the findings, and exploring long-term follow-up data to assess the sustainability of VR interventions. Additionally, studies should expand to include more diverse populations and consider the development of tailored VR interventions for specific subgroups, including caregivers, older adults, and individuals with different types of cancer

Technological advancements should also be explored to minimize technical issues, improve the user experience, and ensure that VR interventions are accessible to participants in various settings, including at home and in healthcare facilities. Further investigation into the long-term efficacy, cost-effectiveness, and scalability of VR interventions will be essential for integrating this technology into routine clinical practice for cancer care.

5.2   Strengths and Limitations

5.2.1   Strengths

Innovative Intervention: The use of VR offers a novel, immersive, and interactive approach to addressing the physical, emotional, and psychosocial challenges faced by AYAs with cancer and their caregivers.

High Feasibility and Acceptability: Participation rates ranged from 68% to 85%, with over 85% of participants reporting high satisfaction. This suggests that VR interventions are practical and well-received across diverse populations.

Diverse Outcomes Addressed: The review highlighted VR's potential to alleviate pain, reduce anxiety and depression, improve resilience, and enhance social connectivity. Caregivers also experienced reduced stress and emotional fatigue.

Broad Range of Tools and Approaches: The studies included various therapeutic modalities within VR, such as guided meditation, interactive games, and nature-based environments, catering to diverse participant needs.

Remote Access Capability: VR's ability to be delivered remotely overcomes logistical barriers, such as transportation and scheduling, making it a flexible option for home-based care.

Comprehensive Methodology: The review followed PRISMA guidelines and included diverse study designs, providing a thorough synthesis of available evidence.

5.2.2   Limitations

Small Sample Sizes: Many studies included a limited number of participants, which restricts the generalizability of the findings.

Short Follow-Up Periods: Most studies only assessed outcomes immediately after the intervention or within a few weeks, leaving the long-term efficacy of VR interventions unclear.

Limited Diversity: The studies were predominantly conducted in high-income settings, with limited exploration of how VR might function in low-resource or culturally diverse environments.

Technical Challenges: While generally minimal, some participants reported issues such as motion sickness, headset malfunctions, and connectivity problems, which could affect the user experience.

Absence of Rigorous Study Designs: Some studies lacked control groups or used quasi-experimental designs, reducing the ability to establish causal relationships between VR interventions and observed outcomes.

Underexplored Subgroups: While the review focused on AYAs and caregivers, it did not delve deeply into tailored interventions for specific demographic or clinical subgroups.

Cost and Scalability: Although feasibility was high, the review did not address the cost-effectiveness or scalability of implementing VR interventions in routine cancer care.

6 Conclusion

VR interventions show significant promise in addressing the physical, psychological, and emotional needs of AYAs with cancer and their caregivers. The studies reviewed demonstrate that VR can effectively reduce pain, anxiety, depression, and social isolation, while also enhancing resilience and social connectivity. Caregivers benefit from reduced stress and emotional fatigue, highlighting the dual impact of these interventions.

Despite these promising findings, limitations such as small sample sizes, short follow-up durations, and technical challenges underscore the need for further research. Future studies should prioritize larger, more diverse populations, employ rigorous randomized controlled designs, and explore the long-term effects and cost-effectiveness of VR interventions.

By addressing these gaps, VR has the potential to become a transformative tool in cancer care, offering accessible, engaging, and effective support for patients and caregivers alike.

References

1. World Health Organization. Global cancer burden growing amidst mounting need for services [Internet]. Geneva: WHO; 2024. [cited 2024 Dec 7]. https://www.who.int/news/item/01-02-2024-global-cancer-burden-growing%2D%2Damidst-mounting-need-for-services.
2. Zhou Y, et al. Global burden of adolescent and young adult cancer in 2022: incidence, mortality, and disparities [Internet]. J Hematol Oncol. 2024; [cited 2024 Dec 7]. https://jhoonline.biomedcentral.com/articles/10.1186/s13045-024-01623-9.
3. Surveillance, Epidemiology, and End Results (SEER) Program. Adolescent and young adult cancer statistics [Internet]. National Cancer Institute; 2024. [cited 2024 Dec 7]. https://seer.cancer.gov/statfacts/html/aya.html.
4. National Cancer Institute. Fatigue (PDQ®)–Health Professional Version [Internet]. Bethesda, MD: NCI; 2024. [cited 2024 Dec 7]. https://www.cancer.gov/about-cancer/treatment/side-effects/fatigue/fatigue-hp-pdq.
5. National Cancer Institute. Cognitive Impairment (PDQ®)–Patient Version [Internet]. Bethesda, MD: NCI; 2024. [cited 2024 Dec 7]. https://www.cancer.gov/about-cancer/treatment/side-effects/memory/cognitive-impairment-pdq.
6. Coyne E, Dieperink KB, Voltelen B, da Silva BM, Garcia-Vivar C. Posttreatment health interventions for adult cancer survivors and their families: an integrated review. Support Care Cancer. 2024;32:712.

7. Cui P, Yang M, Hu H, Cheng C, Chen X, Shi J, et al. The impact of caregiver burden on quality of life in family caregivers of patients with advanced cancer: a moderated mediation analysis of the role of psychological distress and family resilience. BMC Public Health. 2024;24(1):817.

8. Hao J, He Z, Li Y, Huang B, Remis A, Yao Z, et al. Virtual reality-based supportive care interventions for patients with cancer: an umbrella review of systematic reviews and meta-analyses. Support Care Cancer. 2024;32:603.

9. Reynolds LM, Cavadino A, Chin S, Little Z, Akroyd A, Tennant G, et al. The benefits and acceptability of virtual reality interventions for women with metastatic breast cancer in their homes: a pilot randomized trial. BMC Cancer. 2022;22(1):360.

10. Burrai F, Sguanci M, Petrucci G, De Marinis MG, Piredda M. Effectiveness of immersive virtual reality on anxiety, fatigue, and pain in patients with cancer undergoing chemotherapy: a systematic review and meta-analysis. Eur J Oncol Nurs. 2023;64:102340.

11. Bani Mohammad E, Ahmad M. Virtual reality as a distraction technique for pain and anxiety among patients with breast cancer: a randomized control trial. Palliat Support Care. 2019;17(1):29–34.

12. Shi C, Dumville J, Rubinstein F, Norman G, Ullah A, Bashir S, et al. Inpatient-level care at home delivered by virtual wards and hospital at home: a systematic review and meta-analysis of complex interventions and their components. BMC Med. 2024;22(1):145.

13. Patano A, Alanazi M, Lehto R, Goldstein D, Wyatt G. A nature-immersive virtual reality intervention to support hospice family caregivers: qualitative findings from a pilot study. Asia Pac J Oncol Nurs [Internet]. 2024;11:100616. https://linkinghub.elsevier.com/retrieve/pii/S2347562524002385.

14. Gautama MSN, Haryani H, Huang TW, Chen JH, Chuang YH. Effectiveness of smartphone-based virtual reality relaxation (SVR) for enhancing comfort in cancer patients undergoing chemotherapy: a randomized controlled trial. Support Care Cancer [Internet]. 2024;32(12):824. http://www.ncbi.nlm.nih.gov/pubmed/39589559.

15. Chiu M, Burhan AM. Virtual reality to provide caregiver skill development and problem solving. Int Psychogeriatr. 2023;35(S1):42–3.

16. Moher D, Liberati A, Tetzlaff J, Altman DG, PRISMA Group. Preferred reporting items for systematic reviews and meta-analyses: the PRISMA statement. PLoS Med. 2009;6(7):e1000097.

17. Covidence systematic review software, Veritas Health Innovation, Melbourne, Australia. www.covidence.org.

18. Higgins JPT, Savović J, Page MJ, Elbers RG, Sterne JAC. Assessing risk of bias in a randomized trial. In: Higgins JPT, Thomas J, Chandler J, Cumpston M, Li T, Page MJ, Welch VA, editors. Cochrane handbook for systematic reviews of interventions version 6.1 (updated September 2020). Cochrane; 2020.

19. Wells G, Shea B, O'Connell D, Peterson J, Welch V, Losos M, et al. The Newcastle-Ottawa scale (NOS) for assessing the quality of nonrandomized studies in meta-analyses. Ottawa: Ottawa Hospital Research Institute; 2000.

20. Alanazi MO, Patano A, Bente G, Mason A, Goldstein D, Parsnejad S, et al. Nature-based virtual reality feasibility and acceptability pilot for caregiver respite. Curr Oncol [Internet]. 2023;30(7):5995–6005. https://www.scopus.com/inward/record.uri?eid=2-s2.0-851658998 69&doi=10.3390%2fcurroncol30070448&partnerID=40&md5=6b18afa79b4bdb54c990488 7a29ce0b6.

21. Rolbiecki AJ, Froeliger B, Smith J, et al. Virtual reality and neurofeedback as a supportive approach to managing cancer symptoms for patients receiving treatment: a brief report of a feasibility trial. Palliat Support Care. 2024;22(4):811–7. https://doi.org/10.1017/S1478951524000385.

22. Sharifpour S, Manshaee GR, Sajjadian I. Effects of virtual reality therapy on perceived pain intensity, anxiety, catastrophising, and self-efficacy among adolescents with cancer. Couns Psychother Res. 2021;21(2):448–58. https://doi.org/10.1002/capr.12345.

23. Marks A, Garbatini A, Hieftje K, Puthenpura V, Weser V, Fernandes CSF. Use of immersive virtual reality spaces to engage adolescent and young adult patients with cancer in therapist-guided support groups: protocol for a pre-post study. JMIR Res Protoc. 2023;12:e48761. https://doi.org/10.2196/48761.

24. Lee LJ, Son EH, Farmer N, Gerrard C, Tuason RT, Yang L, et al. Nature-based virtual reality intervention to manage stress in family caregivers of allogeneic hematopoietic stem cell transplant recipients: a two-phase pilot study protocol. Front Psychiatry. 2024;15:1295097. https://www.scopus.com/inward/record.uri?eid=2-s2.0-85188174342&doi=10.3389%2ffpsyt.2024.1295097&partnerID=40&md5=fc1de6612b92c3f2a1dc2a614e28b795.

25. Desselle MR. "A Wanderer's Tale": the development of a virtual reality application for pain and quality of life in Australian burns and oncology patients. Cambridge University Press; 2022. https://doi.org/10.1017/S1478951522000201.

26. Lamarche J, Cussor A, Nissim R, Avery J, Wong J, Maheu C, Lambert SD, Laizner AM, Jones J, Esplen MJ, Lebel S. It's time to address fear of cancer recurrence in family caregivers: usability study of an virtual version of the Family Caregiver-Fear of Recurrence Therapy (FC-FORT). Front Digit Health. 2023;5:1129536. https://doi.org/10.3389/fdgth.2023.1129536.

27. Thomas MK, Jarrahi AA, Demmie L, Scott S, Lau T, Johnson A. Virtual reality in cancer care: enhancing knowledge and reducing anxiety about chemotherapy among patients and caregivers. Int J Environ Res Public Health. 2024;21(9):1163. https://doi.org/10.3390/ijerph21091163.

28. Ordu Y, Yilmaz S. The effect of using virtual reality goggles on psychological well-being and care burden of informal caregivers of patients hospitalized in a palliative care clinic. Eur J Oncol Nurs. 2024;73:102711. https://doi.org/10.1016/j.ejon.2024.102711.

29. Vinci C, Reblin M, Jim H, Pidala J, Bulls H, Cutolo E. Understanding preferences for a mindfulness-based stress management program among caregivers of hematopoietic cell transplant patients. Complement Ther Clin Pract. 2018;33:164–9. https://doi.org/10.1016/j.ctcp.2018.10.007.

30. Hoag JA, Karst J, Bingen K, Palou-Torres A, Yan K. Distracting through procedural pain and distress using virtual reality and guided imagery in pediatric, adolescent, and young adult patients: randomized controlled trial. J Pediatr Oncol Nurs. 2020;37(5):337–47. https://doi.org/10.1177/1043454220940531.

31. Tennant M, McGillivray J, Youssef GJ, McCarthy MC, Clark TJ. Feasibility, acceptability, and clinical implementation of an immersive virtual reality intervention to address psychological well-being in children and adolescents with cancer. J Pediatr Oncol Nurs. 2020;37(4):265–77. https://doi.org/10.1177/1043454220917859.

32. Høybye MT. Virtual environments in cancer care: pilot-testing a three-dimensional web-based platform as a tool for support in young cancer patients. Psychooncology. 2020;29(6):1076–84. https://doi.org/10.1002/pon.5292.

Virtual Reality in Stroke Rehabilitation and Treatment: Focusing on the Patient's Experience and Needs

Christos Hadjipanayi ⓘ, Domna Banakou ⓘ, and Despina Michael-Grigoriou ⓘ

1 Introduction

Stroke is one of the leading causes of death worldwide and its frequency among adults, especially those under 55 years of age, is projected to rise in the coming years [1]. Although not always fatal, stroke survivors often suffer from severe impairments due to neuronal damage, affecting both motoric and cognitive functions. These impairments can lead to emotional turmoil, further diminishing quality of life and overall well-being [2, 3]. Nevertheless, early exposure to rehabilitative interventions significantly enhances recovery prospects. This is because brain plasticity—the ability of the injured brain to generate new neuronal pathways in an attempt to compensate for the damaged ones—is heightened during the early post-stroke period [4]. Rehabilitation interventions, incorporating various therapeutic techniques, are critical for modulating plasticity [5]. When correctly applied, rehabilitation interventions enable the brain to generate neuronal pathways that assist in partially recovering lost motor and cognitive abilities [5, 6].

Brain plasticity, a complex phenomenon still under research [7, 8], activates within 48 h of brain injury and the reinforcement of synaptic connections between the new neuronal pathways can last from weeks to months. This process is likely influenced by various factors such as genetics, age, and activity, with activity being

C. Hadjipanayi · D. Michael-Grigoriou (✉)
GET Lab, Department of Multimedia and Graphic Arts, Cyprus University of Technology, Limassol, Cyprus
e-mail: despina.grigoriou@cut.ac.cy

D. Banakou
GET Lab, Department of Multimedia and Graphic Arts, Cyprus University of Technology, Limassol, Cyprus

Interactive Media, Arts and Humanities Division, New York University Abu Dhabi, Abu Dhabi, United Arab Emirates

© The Author(s), under exclusive license to Springer Nature Switzerland AG 2025
A. Charalambous (ed.), *Critical Perspectives on Technological Innovations in Healthcare*, https://doi.org/10.1007/978-3-031-87158-0_7

the most susceptible to environmental influence. Therapeutic approaches for rehabilitation mainly focus on the activity factor, emphasizing persistent and purpose-
driven physical training of varying difficulty. Key practices for enhancing
neuroplasticity and motor performance [9, 10] include but are not limited to occu-
pational therapy, mirror therapy, and constraint induced movement therapy. They
are often coupled with technological enhancements, such as robotic exoskeletons
and virtual reality (VR) applications as a means to increase therapeutic efficacy [4].
The reviews by Anwer et al. [5] and Deutsch and Westcott McCoy [8] provide
further insights into these therapeutic approaches and their application in
neurorehabilitation.

This chapter adopts an approach that, unlike the aforementioned reviews, is more
centered around the patients' experience with VR technology and less concerned
with its technical aspects. Even though these approaches are crucial for improving
current practices in the field, we argue that focusing on the patients' rehabilitation
experience in VR is less widespread in current literature, as it is codependent on and
often overshadowed by technical aspects. Thoroughly considering the patients'
experience within virtual environments merits more attention for facilitating patient
perseverance in rehabilitation. The content of this chapter can be particularly informative for product designers, healthcare practitioners, or other stakeholders who are
new to the field of physical rehabilitation.

This chapter is a brief overview of stroke rehabilitation VR interventions that
seek to facilitate the upper-limb rehabilitation process. There are various forms of
VR interventions in rehabilitation, both gamified and no-rule-based, which we discuss in this chapter. In this first section, we explain why VR technology, with
emphasis on immersive VR, can be a suitable rehabilitation tool. We explain this by
highlighting some of the psychological affordances of immersive VR which are
most likely to play a role in the induction of neuroplasticity. In the next section, we
introduce VR exergames and explain the distinction between different categories of
VR exergames in rehabilitation. This introduction lays the foundation for discussing
some critical perspectives on VR exergames in rehabilitation, namely, perspectives
pertaining to the role of VR exergames as a more entertaining alternative to traditional rehabilitation. This discussion leads to the importance of sustained player
engagement in VR rehabilitation and proposed techniques for prolonging patient
adherence and compliance in rehabilitation. We also address the fact VR exergames
can be incompatible with certain patient characteristics, in which case switching
over to no-rule-based VR interventions is advised. We dedicate a third chapter to
this topic, in which we focus on therapeutic artmaking, as a ludic activity that can
potentially integrate in immersive VR while configured for assisting rehabilitation
patients. We conclude this chapter with a summary of the current gaps in literature
and considerable challenges that seem to hinder the application of immersive VR in
stroke rehabilitation.

1.1 Suitability of VR Technology for Rehabilitation

Regarding technological enhancements for upper-limb stroke rehabilitation, VR technology stands out as particularly promising. Evidence shows that integrating digital exergame interventions (i.e., rule-based challenges in VR) into physical training practices can be an effective rehabilitation strategy [11]. This effectiveness stems from the ability of VR technology to provide patients with stimulating, interactive, and ecologically valid virtual environments, which can promote neuroplasticity [12]. Furthermore, VR enables the systematic collection of detailed data on motricity and performance, offering valuable feedback for both healthcare professionals and patients, as well as enhancing current diagnostic tools and treatment approaches [13, 14].

A further advantage of VR technology is its capacity for telerehabilitation, as affordable VR systems can be installed in patients' homes for personal use, allowing those with mobility impairments to continue their rehabilitation without needing to commute to rehabilitation centers on a regular basis [15]. In VR, users are immersed in virtual environments through computer-controlled display systems, allowing interaction with these environments [16]. Immersion, a key technical feature of VR systems, includes capabilities relevant to the system such as wide field-of-view displays and head tracking [17]. The degree of immersion experienced by users is determined by how accurately the VR system simulates the physical world in terms of sensorimotor contingencies [18]. For instance, head mount displays (HMDs) can fully envelop the user within virtual environments, creating a realistic experience perceived through the sensorimotor system, thus providing full immersion.

In fully immersive VR systems, when sensory input from the real world is successfully substituted by the virtual environment, the brain perceives virtual reality as genuine reality, despite users knowing it is only a simulation [17]. This leads to place illusion (PI), where users feel as though they are actually present in the virtual environment [19], and plausibility illusion (Psi), when users endorse the belief that events in the virtual environment are genuinely taking place, despite knowing that these events are computer-generated [20]. The combination of PI and Psi, referred to as presence [19, 21], is believed to be one of the factors that make VR technology particularly suitable for rehabilitation, as it engages cognitive resources crucial for motor control [22].

Beyond Pi and Psi, there is another illusion arising in VR which is one of the most highly regarded in rehabilitation—a body ownership illusion (BOI). VR offers the capability of substituting a user's real body with a life-sized, spatially coincident, and motorically synchronized virtual one, (also known as an avatar) that allows the user to view the virtual environment and their virtual body from a first-person perspective [23]. This process is referred to as VR embodiment [24]. Following successful multisensory integration [25–30], VR embodiment results in a BOI, where the user assumes ownership of the avatar's body (or body part), despite knowing it is a virtual construct [27, 31–35].

A BOI is crucial for rehabilitation as sensorimotor feedback from a body perceived to be owned by the patient has been shown to positively impact stroke recovery [36] (Fig. 1). For optimal rehabilitation outcomes, the patient's body awareness should be facilitated through visual input provided by embodied avatars [37]. These VR avatars primarily provide sensorimotor feedback, but their rehabilitative effectiveness becomes most pronounced when coupled with technologies such as brain-computer interface (BCI) and functional electrical stimulation (FES). In severe cases of paresis, a paretic limb might show no muscle contraction even if synaptic signals are attempting to activate the limb. In such cases, discerning whether the paretic limb is in a state of exercise or relaxation can be most effectively achieved through BCI. Subsequently, synaptic signaling data can be transmitted to the VR system, where the avatar visually represents the intended motor activation, projecting this representation as sensorimotor feedback [38].

This overt sensorimotor feedback derived from synaptic signaling data and VR technology, although not entirely accurate to real life, can enhance the rehabilitation process beyond merely interpreting the patient's intent. In other words, a virtual kinematic limb representation harmonized to the position and oftentimes covert movement of the paretic limb can facilitate neural modulation and aid in strengthening limb control [39, 40]. Neurons that specialize in mimicking observed actions, also known as the mirror neurons of the mirror neuron system (MNS), leverage this feedback to promote psychomotor learning, thus allowing neural modulation and fostering neuroplasticity [6]. Measurable changes in structural brain plasticity before and after VR interventions can be confirmed through MRI [41].

It is noteworthy that knowledge regarding the impact of the MNS on neuroplasticity precedes the advent of VR technology. For example, mirror therapy, a viable rehabilitation approach based on MNS activation, involves placing a mirror between the patient's limbs to cover the paretic limb. The sensorimotor feedback from the reflected movement of the contralateral limb creates the illusion of regained functionality in the paretic limb, similar to the effect achieved with VR through a virtual body and synaptic signaling data. This approach is applicable even for stroke patients with acute paresis [42]. However, the VR embodiment approach is deemed a more favorable alternative to traditional mirror therapy because looking through a tilted mirror for extended periods is uncomfortable for the patient's posture [40]. Additionally, VR technology can enhance mirror therapy by incorporating gamification techniques, making exercises more engaging and less monotonous [43].

1.2   VR Exergames in Rehabilitation

Serious games are a distinct category of games designed to facilitate behaviors beyond mere gameplay. Like entertainment games, serious games are available on various devices, including smartphones, smartwatches, gaming consoles, and desktop computers. Exergames, specifically, a sub-category of serious games, are designed to covertly make players enjoy physical exercise by integrating physical activity into their gameplay mechanics [11].

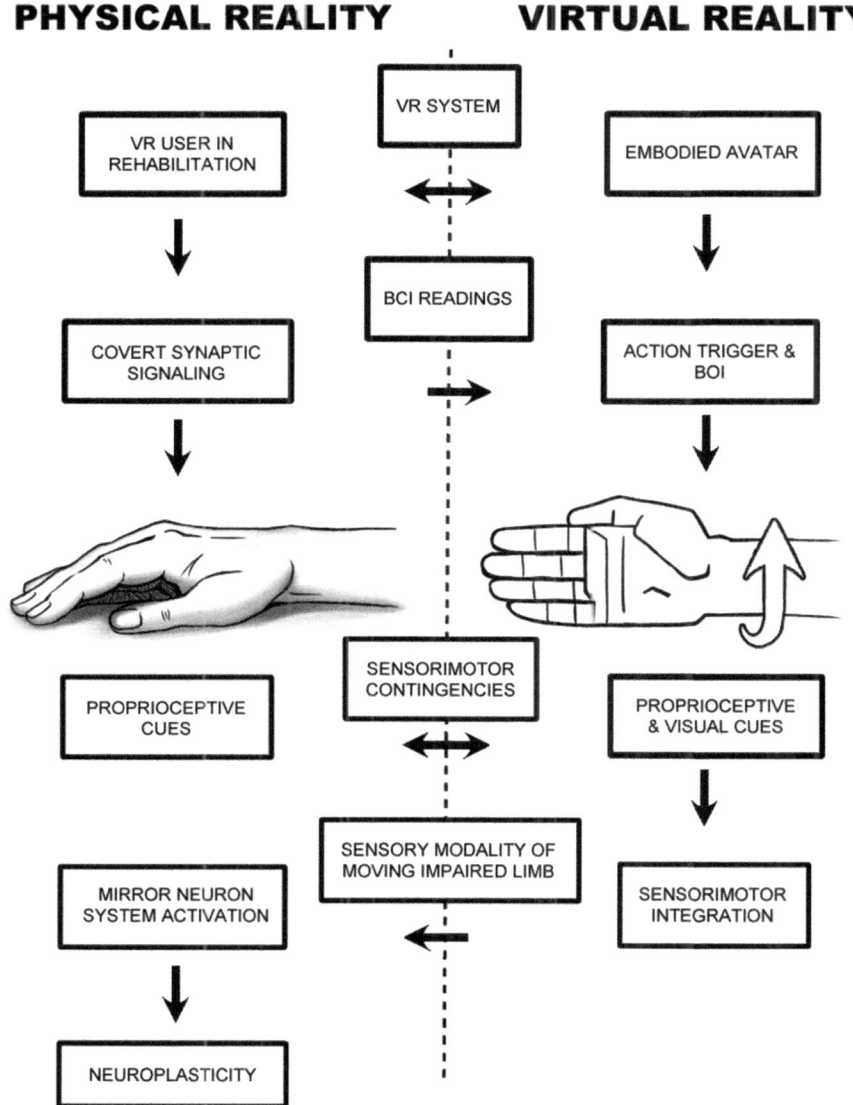

Fig. 1 Illustration of neurological mechanisms that interact with an input device (e.g., BCI in the case of severe paresis) and a fully immersive VR system to promote neuroplasticity in upper-limb stroke rehabilitation. The VR user presumes ownership of the embodied avatar (BOI) by familiarizing themself with a motorically coincident anthropomorphic avatar. Subsequently, attempts to change the position of the impaired upper limb can be visually adjusted through the visual output device. When proprioceptive and visual cues are repeatedly reinforced by the VR user's expectations and returned as sensorimotor feedback, the brain can use this feedback to relearn the repeated actions and reorganize neuronal pathways accordingly

Commercial exergames, such as *Beat Saber*[1] and *Ring Fit Adventure,*[2] emphasize entertainment and are typically marketed toward able-bodied individuals who enjoy physically active gaming, without being strictly limited to this group. In contrast, purpose-designed exergames focus on improving the physiological, motor, and sometimes cognitive condition of paraplegic patients during rehabilitation [44]. They are often less focused on enjoyment and entertainment associated with gaming, prioritizing clinical outcomes, rendering them more akin to therapeutic interventions than recreational activities.

Purpose-designed rehabilitation exergames are commonly characterized by constant performance feedback and body positioning information, aiming to enhance visuomotor coordination, spatial reasoning, and offer high customizability in order to accommodate the diverse requirements of patients [45–48]. Moreover, purpose-designed exergames are designed with consideration for the cognitive load capacity of brain-injured patients, integrating uncomplicated gameplay mechanics, minimalist graphics, and a simplified user interface [43].

Exergames of various designs are often used in healthcare for patient rehabilitation, provided that the individual's motor and cognitive functionality allow for their use. As postulated by Rizzo and Kim [49], the clinical value of these games lies in their immersive and interactive nature, which has the potential to transform repetitive exercise into enjoyable activities. However, a longstanding debate persists regarding the effectiveness of purpose-designed exergames compared to mainstream commercial exergames for rehabilitation. Some researchers argue that off-the-shelf entertainment exergames may prove too challenging for rehabilitation patients, as they may not cater to the specific needs of individuals with impairments. Patients testing these games can easily recognize that they are designed for an able-bodied demographic and do not consider their own challenges [50]. In contrast, purpose-designed exergames are tailored to accommodate the constraints imposed by neurocognitive disabilities [51, 52].

Mura et al. [53] conducted a meta-analysis of 13 studies comparing the rehabilitation efficacy of commercial entertainment exergames (primarily titles of the Nintendo Wii platform), to conventional rehabilitation. They concluded that entertainment exergames were effective in improving executive functions in patients with neurocognitive disorders. On the other hand, Doumas et al. [51] conducted a meta-analysis of 42 clinical trials comparing purpose-designed exergames to conventional therapy, concluding that purpose-designed exergames yielded superior results in terms of motor functionality for stroke patients. Another meta-analysis by Lohse et al. [54] compared the rehabilitation efficacy of commercial entertainment exergames and purpose-designed (custom) ones across 26 relevant studies. No significant differences were found between the two types regarding motor improvement in populations with neurocognitive disorders. However, it is acknowledged that a larger sample of studies is needed to draw more accurate conclusions.

---

[1] https://beatsaber.com/

[2] https://ringfitadventure.nintendo.com/

2   Critical Perspectives on VR Exergames for Rehabilitation

The gamification of rehabilitation exercises emerged primarily due to patients' aversion toward the monotonous nature of traditional rehabilitation practices [55, 56]. Although purpose-designed exergames can be more patient-friendly, they often lack the playfulness and appeal of entertainment exergames, which are designed to make players feel excited about playing. In other words, purpose-designed exergames are highly effective for rehabilitation, whereas entertainment exergames excel in maintaining patient adherence. Adherence, the quality of staying motivated and committed, is critical for rehabilitation success [57]. A rehabilitation exergame may be deemed ineffective if it consistently fails to improve rehabilitation outcomes over time. However, it would certainly be ineffective if it failed to motivate patients to adhere to rehabilitation training in the first place. Consequently, designing a serious game that considers the intrinsic motivation of stroke patients beyond their willingness to improve their quality of life can be far more complex than creating an entertainment game. This complexity arises mainly because the concept of gaming as a fun activity is rarely associated with undergoing therapy for brain injury treatment.

In the context of games, "fun" emerges from striving toward mastery of an in-game task, purely for the satisfaction this activity brings [58]. However, in purpose-designed exergames, patients engage while fully aware that this is an intervention administered by a healthcare professional to address a debilitating, non-fictional problem. Patients who can cognitively engage in rehabilitation exergames are also aware of the therapeutic context, which can diminish the fun factor and replace it with a determination to improve motor functions. While this determination can sustain adherence [10], it does not address the issue of boredom and monotony during exercise, potentially undermining one of the main goals of the purpose-designed exergaming intervention.

Efforts to employ more effective techniques of immersing patients in purpose-designed exergames, aiming to prolong player engagement, appear to be promising. Increased task engagement over a period of 3–4 weeks in VR rehabilitation exergames has been shown to support both motor (body function) and cognitive (participation) improvements in children with hemiplegia, as evidenced by four case studies [59]. However, maintaining sustained player engagement poses several challenges. Exergames are intended to be enjoyable, thanks to their gamification component, but researchers suggest that enjoyment is highly subjective and varies among patients [13]. Indeed, even when exergames adhere to established principles, their success in providing an engaging experience lies in the configuration of its comprising elements [60] as well as individual player characteristics. As Novak et al. [61] highlight, a patient's engagement with an exergame is influenced by their personality as well as occasional preferences. Customization of both the utility and esthetics of the experience can be crucial for overcoming this challenge. Even so, there are current technological limitations to the quality of personalization in rehabilitation exergames, and there are instances when rehabilitation patients are simply not in the mood to play, despite customization efforts. Depressive symptoms, which are common among rehabilitation patients, can lead to resistance against exergame interventions [62, 63].

2.1 Sustaining Player Engagement

Designing exercise regimens that not only consider individual traits and disabilities but also strike a balance between repetitive movements and sustained long-term motivation, while accounting for patients' individual traits and disabilities, is a significant challenge. Individual disabilities encompass varying degrees of both motor and cognitive deficiencies. Cognitive deficiencies, in particular, introduce specific design limitations that mainly pertain to audiovisual cues and game mechanics. For neurocognitively compromised patients, low-poly, simplistic 3D graphics, and straightforward game mechanics are highly recommended to prevent cognitive overload and adverse emotional effects [64]. Moreover, the design of highly engaging, purpose-designed exergames is complicated by the focus of scientific literature on the heuristic value of applications. While robust functionality and user comfort are undoubtedly significant reinforcers of the long-term use of VR applications, researchers often neglect secondary yet important aspects that further contribute to ensuring sustained use over time [65]. Therefore, our understanding on sustained player engagement in purpose-designed exergames remains limited.

Notwithstanding, our knowledge on sustained player engagement and long-term motivation in rehabilitation exergames is derived from disciplines that are only indirectly related to rehabilitation. Positive psychology and ludology introduce the theory of flow, which posits that a state of deep concentration, known as "the flow zone," allows an individual to effortlessly engage in an activity for extended periods when the challenge level aligns with their skill level. Entering this state alters perception in the sense that some difficult tasks which would otherwise be perceived as onerous, frustrating, and time-consuming can appear intriguing, pleasant, and fleeting [66, 67]. While being in the flow zone is not equivalent to having fun, the two experiences can often coincide [58]. The association between rehabilitation exercise regimens and the transformations of difficult tasks into pleasant experiences through the flow state is evident. Acknowledging this association is crucial, as aiming to enter the flow zone through rehabilitation exergames can be a worthwhile strategy for reducing adverse emotions (e.g., monotony), prolonging motivation, and increasing therapeutic outcomes [64].

3   Sustained User Engagement in VR Rehabilitation Beyond Exergames

The critical factor in triggering a flow state in rehabilitation training is how well the challenge level of an exergame matches the player's skill level. However, exergaming represents only a small fraction of activities where the flow state can occur in the context of VR rehabilitation. The nature of a meaningful challenge and a person's skillset can vary significantly among individuals. Jung et al. [64] explored the diverse reactions patients demonstrate after being introduced to rehabilitation exergames, categorizing them into four groups based on their attitudes toward exergames in their therapy. These include patients who respond positively to the administered exergame, those who prefer (and insist on) playing other games than the exergame relevant to their therapy, those who favor traditional rehabilitation methods, and those who reject exergames due to personal reasons. It is evident that there are rehabilitation patients who are not suited for rehabilitation exergames as a therapeutic practice, regardless of the exergame's design and quality. This seems to be especially true for the third and fourth categories, but less clear for the second category of patients, whose aversion toward the administered exergame might stem from a mismatch between preferred playstyle and gameplay (though other factors such as graphics could also influence this).

A common issue in gamification is that game designers predominantly focus on the achiever playstyle, which emphasizes earning points and medals, and aligns with the challenge and skill dynamic of those who enjoy such achievements. However, achievers may lose interest and underperform once achievements become routine, or their symbolic value becomes demystified, which becomes more likely with every new achievement unlocked [68]. This achiever-centric playstyle is also observed in rehabilitation exergames, aligning with the outcome-driven structure of rehabilitation programs [66]. Yet, this game design approach can be limiting for the player's sense of autonomy, as the rules that heavily favor the achiever playstyle tend to be quite rigid regarding the correctness of player actions. Other playstyles (e.g., socializer, explorer, and so on) exist and can be integrated into an exergame to benefit rehabilitation patients who are less focused on game mastery through achievement. Additionally, Pyae et al. [69] identified motivational factors for playing exergames, emphasizing social interaction, the therapeutic relationship between therapist and patient, the rehabilitative environment, and efficient human-computer interaction [70] as interconnected parts of gameplay design. Each of these factors poses various challenges for patients (e.g., learning game controls, receiving positive feedback from the therapist, and so on), which can also contribute to triggering the flow state despite them being peripheral to the main game.

3.1   Therapeutic Artmaking in VR Rehabilitation

Therapeutic artmaking is an example of a ludic activity distinct from rule-based activities like exergaming, but which aligns with the achiever playstyle and can serve a similar purpose of introducing pleasant challenges to rehabilitation exercises. Unlike more structured activities like exergames, therapeutic artmaking involves recreational experimentation with art materials, as described by Angheluta and Lee [71]. It encompasses multiple cognitive processes such as problem-solving, decision making, and differentiation [72]. Additionally, it offers valuable opportunities for self-expression, particularly for rehabilitation patients with speech impairments [73, 74]. The psychomotor and affective aspects of artmaking, including the exploration of painting tools and empathy elicited by interpreting the posture of painted figures, can positively impact rehabilitation [75, 76]. These benefits are further enhanced by VR technology. For instance, exaggerating the movement range of a virtual avatar's arm allows patients with limited arm mobility to effortlessly perform expansive brush strokes in the virtual environment using simple gestures [77].

Furthermore, artmaking in the form of drawing can be categorized into two types: creative self-expression (free drawing) and visual (rote) tracing. Creative self-expression can be used for recreational purposes but also as a form of neurocognitive test. Therapists use free drawing tasks that involve real-life objects to gather neurocognitive data on visuospatial reasoning and hand-eye coordination [78]. Current VR technology, with painting applications designed for creative self-expression such as *Tilt Brush*,[3] can be adapted to meet the needs of mildly to moderately impaired rehabilitation patients. However, significant modifications are required to make these applications more accessible for people with disabilities. Alex et al. [73] demonstrated this by exposing stroke patients to a 3D environment of a VR painting application and recorded their activity. The proposed improvements pertain to factors such as the complexity of controls and the ease of perspective-taking for reflecting on the artwork, among others.

Data collection for rehabilitation through artmaking can also be enhanced with VR technology, thanks to its high precision in tracking movements and translating them into the three-dimensional (3D) or two-dimensional (2D) space. This capability makes it possible to incorporate rote tracing tasks—where the hand must follow the exact trajectory of a guideline—into VR settings, as a combination of therapeutic artmaking and exergaming. An example is the *Painting Discovery* serious game, designed to track hand movements and measure hand jerks in rehabilitation patients through a painting simulation task [79]. In this game, patients are required to draw over a guideline on a desk pad with their impaired arm. Besides data collection, visual tracing tasks in virtual environments, like the VR game *Trajectory Trace* [80], can be administered as exercises to improve upper limb stability and control. While visual tracing exergames focus more on motor rehabilitation, creative self-expression artmaking emphasizes the enjoyment of the therapeutic process without undermining physical or cognitive healing [81]. These differences between creative self-expression and visual rote tracing in VR have also been observed through fNIRS prefrontal cortex activations in healthy adults [82].

4   Discussion and Conclusion

Although we previously mentioned some caveats of VR exergames, a more extensive critique of VR technology in rehabilitation interventions is warranted. The scoping review by Hadjipanayi et al. [83] examined the disadvantages of

---

[3] https://www.tiltbrush.com/

no-rule-based (i.e., art-based) VR interventions in therapeutic practices, including rehabilitation. In this context, significant limitations include the social isolation of patients in virtual environments and the fact that VR technology primarily favors tech-savvy patients with mild neurological conditions. Alex et al. [73] suggest that sensory alienation caused by the lack of physical substance in digital brush strokes and the unfamiliarity of navigating virtual environments can be mitigated by patients' exposure to VR technology through time. However, the sensory barrier separating patients from their social environment during VR interventions requires the attention of therapy practitioners. This issue is critical because, as mentioned earlier, social interaction can be a key motivating factor for rehabilitation perseverance. One of the most crucial aspects of social interaction during rehabilitation is the interpersonal bond between the patient and the therapist, a fundamental component of the therapeutic alliance in ample forms of therapy [84, 85]. Currently, designers of VR rehabilitation interventions are working toward promoting the virtual representation of therapists and eliminating the communication barriers between patients and therapists in VR. Nevertheless, the impact of the virtual therapist on motor rehabilitation requires further research [86].

In conclusion, this chapter introduces VR stroke rehabilitation and treatment from a patient-centric perspective. As the use of both immersive and non-immersive VR in stroke rehabilitation gains increasing validation, this chapter outlines VR illusions most compatible with stroke rehabilitation, namely place illusion, plausibility, and body ownership. Body ownership, in particular, can be quite impactful for stroke rehabilitation patients, whose physical body is neurologically deficient. Using VR technology to experience using a neurologically efficient and motorically coincident body can aid in rehabilitation, despite the lack of physicality of the virtual body. This is mainly due to the skill transference that can occur from VR-based rehabilitation training to real-life scenarios. VR training can take various forms, with exergames being among the most popular.

Exergames combine gamification techniques and rehabilitation practices, making them particularly effective for enhancing patient adherence and compliance with their rehabilitation regimen thanks to their motivating and entertaining nature. However, designing exergames presents challenges pertaining to the patients' sense of autonomy, sustained engagement, and long-term motivation. These challenges can be addressed by focusing on (a) placing patients in the flow zone, (b) considering individual patient characteristics, including both pathologies and personal preferences, (c) considering the rehabilitation setting with respect to its technical and social components, and (d) configuring these exergame elements accordingly. Similar design principles can also be applied to no-rule-based VR interventions, such as VR therapeutic artmaking. The chapter concludes by critiquing current VR technology in rehabilitation for being inapplicable to some patients due to a technological divide, sensory alienation, and communication barriers that must be addressed moving forward.

References

1. Feigin VL, Owolabi MO, Feigin VL, Abd-Allah F, Akinyemi RO, Bhattacharjee NV, et al. Pragmatic solutions to reduce the global burden of stroke: a World Stroke Organization–Lancet Neurology Commission. Lancet Neurol. 2023;22(12):1160–206.
2. Shahmoradi L, Almasi S, Ahmadi H, Bashiri A, Azadi T, Mirbagherie A, et al. Virtual reality games for rehabilitation of upper extremities in stroke patients. J Bodyw Mov Ther [Internet]. 2021;26:113–22.
3. Stone KD, Chris Dijkerman H, Bekrater-Bodmann R, Keizer A. Mental rotation of feet in individuals with body integrity identity disorder, lower-limb amputees, and normally-limbed controls. PLoS One. 2019;14(8):1–21.
4. Ferreira B, Menezes P. Gamifying motor rehabilitation therapies: challenges and opportunities of immersive technologies. Information. 2020;11(2):88.
5. Anwer S, Waris A, Gilani SO, Iqbal J, Shaikh N, Pujari AN, et al. Rehabilitation of upper limb motor impairment in stroke: a narrative review on the prevalence, risk factors, and economic statistics of stroke and state of the art therapies. Healthcare. 2022;10(2):1–20.
6. Demarin V, Morović S, Béné R. Demarin. Period Biol. 2014;116(2):209–11.
7. Puderbaugh M, Emmady PD. Neuroplasticity [Internet]. In: StatPearls [Internet]. Treasure Island (FL): StatPearls Publishing; 2023.
8. Deutsch JE, Westcott McCoy S. Virtual reality and serious games in neurorehabilitation of children and adults: prevention, plasticity, and participation. Pediatr Phys Ther. 2017;29:S23–36.
9. Bressi F, Santacaterina F, Cricenti L, Campagnola B, Nasto F, Assenza C, et al. Robotic-assisted hand therapy with Gloreha Sinfonia for the improvement of hand function after pediatric stroke: a case report. Appl Sci. 2022;12(9):4206.
10. Standen PJ, Threapleton K, Connell L, Richardson A, Brown DJ, Battersby S, et al. Innovative technologies special series. Phys Ther. 2015;95(3):406–14.
11. Ning H, Wang Z, Li R, Zhang Y, Mao L. A review on serious games for exercise rehabilitation. J Latex Class Files. 2022;14(8):1–14.
12. Cheung KL, Tunik E, Adamovich SV, Boyd LA. Neuroplasticity and virtual reality. In: Weiss P, Keshner E, Levin M, editors. Virtual reality for physical and motor rehabilitation virtual reality technologies for health and clinical applications. Springer; 2014. p. 5–24.
13. Maier M, Ballester BR, Verschure PFMJ. Principles of neurorehabilitation after stroke based on motor learning and brain plasticity mechanisms. Front Syst Neurosci. 2019;13(December):1–18.
14. Maier M, Rubio Ballester B, Duff A, Duarte Oller E, Verschure PFMJ. Effect of specific over nonspecific VR-based rehabilitation on poststroke motor recovery: a systematic meta-analysis. Neurorehabil Neural Repair. 2019;33(2):112–29.
15. Laver KE, Adey-Wakeling Z, Crotty M, Lannin NA, George S, Sherrington C. Telerehabilitation services for stroke. Cochrane Database Syst Rev. 2020;1(1):CD010255.
16. Sanchez-Vives MV, Slater M. From presence to consciousness through virtual reality. Nat Rev Neurosci [Internet]. 2005;6(4):332–9.
17. Slater M, Sanchez-Vives M. Enhancing our lives with immersive virtual reality. Front Robot AI [Internet]. 2016;3(December):74.
18. O'Regan K, Noe A. What it is like to see: a sensorimotor theory of perceptual experience. Synthese. 2001;129:79–103.
19. Slater M. Place illusion and plausibility can lead to realistic behaviour in immersive virtual environments. Philos Trans R Soc Lond B Biol Sci [Internet]. 2009;364(1535):3549–57.
20. Slater M, Banakou D, Beacco A, Gallego J, Macia-Varela F, Oliva R. A separate reality: an update on place illusion and plausibility in virtual reality. Front Virtual Real. 2022;3(June):1–16.
21. Riva G, Mantovani F, Capideville CS, Preziosa A, Morganti F, Villani D, et al. Affective interactions using virtual reality: the link between presence and emotions. Cyberpsychology Behav. 2007;10(1):45–56.

22. Slobounov SM, Ray W, Johnson B, Slobounov E, Newell KM. Modulation of cortical activity in 2D versus 3D virtual reality environments: an EEG study. Int J Psychophysiol [Internet]. 2015;95(3):254–60.

23. Petkova VI, Ehrsson HH. If I were you: perceptual illusion of body swapping. PLoS One. 2008;3(12):e3832.

24. Kilteni K, Groten R, Slater M. The sense of embodiment in virtual reality. Presence 2012;21(4):373–87.

25. Petkova VI, Khoshnevis M, Ehrsson HH. The perspective matters! Multisensory integration in ego-centric reference frames determines full-body ownership. Front Psychol [Internet] 2011;2(March):35.

26. Slater M, Perez-Marcos D, Ehrsson HH, Sanchez-Vives MV. Inducing illusory ownership of a virtual body. Front Neurosci [Internet]. 2009;3(2):214–20.

27. Slater M, Perez-Marcos D, Ehrsson HH, Sanchez-Vives MV. Towards a digital body: the virtual arm illusion. Front Hum Neurosci. 2008;2(August):6.

28. Maselli A, Slater M. The building blocks of the full body ownership illusion. Front Hum Neurosci [Internet]. 2013;7(March):83.

29. Slater M, Spanlang B, Corominas D. Simulating virtual environments within virtual environments as the basis for a psychophysics of presence. ACM Trans Graph [Internet]. 2010;29(4):1.

30. Perez-Marcos D, Sanchez-Vives MV, Slater M. Is my hand connected to my body? The impact of body continuity and arm alignment on the virtual hand illusion. Cogn Neurodyn. 2012;6(4):295–305.

31. Slater M, Spanlang B, Sanchez-Vives MV, Blanke O. First person experience of body transfer in virtual reality. PLoS One. 2010;5(5):e10564. https://doi.org/10.1371/journal.pone.0010564.

32. Christofi M, Michael-Grigoriou D, Kyrlitsias C. A virtual reality simulation of drug users' everyday life: the effect of supported sensorimotor contingencies on empathy. Front Psychol. 2020;11(June):1–12.

33. Christou C, Michael D. Aliens versus humans: do avatars make a difference in how we play the game? 2014 6th Int Conf Games Virtual Worlds Serious Appl VS-GAMES 2014. 2014;1–7.

34. Banakou D, Groten R, Slater M. Illusory ownership of a virtual child body causes overestimation of object sizes and implicit attitude changes. Proc Natl Acad Sci U S A. 2013;110(31):12846–51.

35. Banakou D, Beacco A, Neyret S, Blasco-Oliver M, Seinfeld S, Slater M. Virtual body ownership and its consequences for implicit racial bias are dependent on social context. R Soc Open Sci. 2020;7(12):201848.

36. Warland A, Paraskevopoulos I, Tsekleves E, Ryan J, Nowicky A, Griscti J, et al. The feasibility, acceptability and preliminary efficacy of a low-cost, virtual-reality based, upper-limb stroke rehabilitation device: a mixed methods study. Disabil Rehabil [Internet]. 2019;41(18):2119–34.

37. Benrachou DE, Masmoudi M, Djekoune O, Zenati N, Ousmer M. Avatar-facilitated therapy and virtual reality: next-generation of functional rehabilitation methods. CCSSP 2020—1st Int Conf Commun Control Syst Signal Process. 2020;298–304.

38. Cho W, Heilinger A, Xu R, Zehetner M, Schobesberger S, Murovec N, et al. Hemiparetic stroke rehabilitation using avatar and electrical stimulation based on non-invasive brain computer interface. Int J Phys Med Rehabil. 2017;05(04) https://doi.org/10.4172/2329-9096.1000411.

39. Rong J, Ding L, Xiong L, Zhang W, Wang W, Deng M, et al. Mirror visual feedback prior to robot-assisted training facilitates rehabilitation after stroke: a randomized controlled study. Front Neurol. 2021;12(July):1–10.

40. Choi HS, Shin WS, Bang DH. Mirror therapy using gesture recognition for upper limb function, neck discomfort, and quality of life after chronic stroke: a single-blind randomized controlled trial. Med Sci Monit. 2019;25:3271–8.

41. Keller J, Štětkářová I, MacRi V, Kühn S, Pětioký J, Gualeni S, et al. Virtual reality-based treatment for regaining upper extremity function induces cortex grey matter changes in persons with acquired brain injury. J Neuroeng Rehabil. 2020;17(1):1–11.

42. Gandhi DBC, Sterba A, Khatter H, Pandian JD. Mirror therapy in stroke rehabilitation: current perspectives. Ther Clin Risk Manag. 2020;16:75–85.

43. Lew KL, Sim KS, Tan SC, Abas FS. Virtual reality post stroke upper limb assessment using unreal engine 4. Eng Lett. 2021;29(4):1511–23.
44. Aminov A, Rogers JM, Middleton S, Caeyenberghs K, Wilson PH. What do randomized controlled trials say about virtual rehabilitation in stroke? A systematic literature review and meta-analysis of upper-limb and cognitive outcomes. J Neuroeng Rehabil. 2018;15(1):1–24.
45. Standen PJ, Threapleton K, Richardson A, Connell L, Brown DJ, Battersby S, et al. A low cost virtual reality system for home based rehabilitation of the arm following stroke: a randomised controlled feasibility trial. Clin Rehabil. 2017;31(3):340–50.
46. Christou CG, Michael-Grigoriou D, Sokratous D. Virtual buzzwire: assessment of a prototype VR game for stroke rehabilitation. 25th IEEE conf virtual real 3D user interfaces, VR 2018—Proc. 2018;2(Median 34):531–2.
47. Almousa M, Al-Khalifa HS, Alsobayel H. Requirements elicitation and prototyping of a fully immersive virtual reality gaming system for upper limb stroke rehabilitation in Saudi Arabia. Mob Inf Syst. 2017;2017:507940.
48. Choi YH, Paik NJ. Mobile game-based virtual reality program for upper extremity stroke rehabilitation. J Vis Exp. 2018;2018(133):1–8.
49. Rizzo A, Kim GJ. A SWOT analysis of the field of virtual reality rehabilitation and therapy. Presence Teleoperators Virtual Environ. 2005;14(2):119–46.
50. Sevcenko K, Lindgren I. The effects of virtual reality training in stroke and Parkinson's disease rehabilitation: a systematic review and a perspective on usability. Eur Rev Aging Phys Act. 2022;19(1):1–16.
51. Doumas I, Everard G, Dehem S, Lejeune T. Serious games for upper limb rehabilitation after stroke: a meta-analysis. J Neuroeng Rehabil. 2021;18(1):1–16.
52. Holmes DE, Charles DK, Morrow PJ, McClean S, McDonough SM. Using fitt's law to model arm motion tracked in 3D by a leap motion controller for virtual reality upper arm stroke rehabilitation. Proc—IEEE Symp Comput Med Syst. 2016;2016(4):335–6.
53. Mura G, Carta MG, Sancassiani F, Machado S, Prosperini L. Active exergames to improve cognitive functioning in neurological disabilities: a systematic review and meta-analysis. Eur J Phys Rehabil Med. 2018;54(3):450–62.
54. Lohse KR, Hilderman CGE, Cheung KL, Tatla S, Van Der Loos HFM. Virtual reality therapy for adults post-stroke: a systematic review and meta-analysis exploring virtual environments and commercial games in therapy. PLoS One. 2014;9(3):e93318.
55. Pinto JF, Carvalho HR, Chambel GRR, Ramiro J, Gonçalves A. Adaptive gameplay and difficulty adjustment in a gamified upper-limb rehabilitation. In: 2018 IEEE 6th international conference on serious games and applications for health (SeGAH). IEEE; 2018. p. 1–8.
56. Najm A, Michael-Grigoriou D, Kyrlitsias C, Christofi M , Hadjipanayi C, Sokratous D. A virtual reality adaptive exergame for the enhancement of physical rehabilitation using social facilitation. ICAT-EGVE (Posters and Demos); 2020. p. 1–2.
57. Seo NJ, Arun Kumar J, Hur P, Crocher V, Motawar B, Lakshminarayanan K. Usability evaluation of low-cost virtual reality hand and arm rehabilitation games. J Rehabil Res Dev. 2016;53(3):321–34.
58. Koster R. A theory of fun for game design. Scottsdale, AZ: Paraglyph Press; 2005. p. 244.
59. Green D, Wilson PH. Use of virtual reality in rehabilitation of movement in children with hemiplegia—a multiple case study evaluation. Disabil Rehabil. 2012;34(7):593–604.
60. Mitgutsch K, Alvarado N. Purposeful by design? A serious game design assessment framework. Found Digit Games 2012, FDG 2012—Conf Progr; 2012. p. 121–128.
61. Novak D, Nagle A, Keller U, Riener R. Increasing motivation in robot-aided arm rehabilitation with competitive and cooperative gameplay. J Neuroeng Rehabil. 2014;11(1):1–15.
62. Burdea G, Kim N, Polistico K, Kadaru A, Grampurohit N, Hundal J, et al. Robotic table and serious games for integrative rehabilitation in the early poststroke phase: two case reports. JMIR Rehabil Assist Technol. 2022;9(2):e26990.

63. House G, Burdea G, Polistico K, Grampurohit N, Roll D, Damiani F, et al. A rehabilitation first—tournament between teams of nursing home residents with chronic stroke. Games Health J. 2016;5(1):75–83.

64. Jung HT, Park T, Mahyar N, Park S, Ryu T, Kim Y, et al. Rehabilitation games in real-world clinical settings: practices, challenges, and opportunities. ACM Trans Comput Interact. 2020;27(6):1–43.

65. Kniestedt I, Lefter I, Lukosch S, Brazier FM. Re-framing engagement for applied games: a conceptual framework. Entertain Comput [Internet]. 2022;October 2020(41):100475.

66. Charles D, Holmes D, Charles T. Rehabilitation. In: Rea PM, editor. Biomedical visualisation advances in experimental medicine and biology; 2020.

67. Csikszentmihalyi M. The collected works of Mihaly Csikszentmihalyi. 1st ed. Dordrecht: Springer; 2014. p. 600.

68. Groening C, Binnewies C. "Achievement unlocked!"—the impact of digital achievements as a gamification element on motivation and performance. Comput Human Behav. 2019;97:151–66.

69. Pyae A, Luimula M, Smed J. Rehabilitative games for stroke patients. EAI Endorsed Trans Game-Based Learn. 2015;1(4):e2.

70. Michael-Grigoriou D, Yiannakou P, Christofi M. Intuitive interaction for exploring human anatomy in a VR setup. Proc 2017 23rd Int Conf Virtual Syst Multimedia, VSMM 2017. 2018 January. p. 1–4.

71. Angheluta A, Lee BK. Art therapy for chornic pain: applications and future directions. Can J Couns Psychother [Internet]. 2011;45(2):112–31.

72. Rosal ML. Cognitive-behavioral art therapy from behaviorism to the third wave. 1st ed. New York: Routledge; 2018. p. 252.

73. Alex M, Wünsche BC, Lottridge D. Virtual reality art-making for stroke rehabilitation: field study and technology probe. Int J Hum Comput Stud. 2021;145:102481.

74. Zhang Y, Wang H, Shi BE. Gaze-controlled robot-assisted painting in virtual reality for upper-limb rehabilitation. Proc Annu Int Conf IEEE Eng Med Biol Soc EMBS. 2021:4513–7.

75. Haeyen S, Jans N, Glas M, Kolijn J. VR health experience: a virtual space for arts and psycho-motor therapy. Front Psychol. 2021;12(September):1–13.

76. Iosa M, Aydin M, Candelise C, Coda N, Morone G, Antonucci G, et al. The Michelangelo effect: art improves the performance in a virtual reality task developed for upper limb neurore-habilitation. Front Psychol. 2021;11(January):1–8.

77. Baron L, Wang Q, Segear S, Cohn BA, Kim K, Barmaki R. Enjoyable physical therapy experi-ence with interactive drawing games in immersive virtual reality. Proc–SUI 2021 ACM Spat User Interact 2021; 2021.

78. Jin R, Pilozzi A, Huang X. Current cognition tests, potential virtual reality applications, and serious games in cognitive assessment and non-pharmacological therapy for neurocognitive disorders. J Clin Med. 2020;9(10):1–19.

79. Viglialoro RM, Condino S, Turini G, Mamone V, Carbone M, Ferrari V, et al. Interactive seri-ous game for shoulder rehabilitation based on real-time hand tracking. Technol Heal Care. 2020;28(4):403–14.

80. Triandafilou KM, Tsoupikova D, Barry AJ, Thielbar KN, Stoykov N, Kamper DG. Development of a 3D, networked multi-user virtual reality environment for home therapy after stroke. J Neuroeng Rehabil. 2018;15(1):1–13.

81. Kaimal G, Carroll-Haskins K, Berberian M, Dougherty A, Carlton N, Ramakrishnan A. Virtual reality in art therapy: a pilot qualitative study of the novel medium and implications for prac-tice. Art Ther [Internet]. 2020;37(1):16–24.

82. Kaimal G, Carroll-Haskins K, Topoglu Y, Ramakrishnan A, Arslanbek A, Ayaz H. Exploratory fNIRS assessment of differences in activation in virtual reality visual self-expression including with a fragrance stimulus. Art Ther [Internet]. 2022;39(3):128–37.

83. Hadjipanayi C, Banakou D, Michael-Grigoriou D. Art as therapy in virtual reality: a scoping review. Front Virtual Real. 2023;4(February):1–16.

84. Bordin ES. The generalizability of the psychoanalytic concept of the working alliance. Psychother Theory, Res Pract. 1979;16(3):252–60.
85. Klonoff PS, Lamb DG, Henderson SW. Outcomes from milieu-based neurorehabilitation at up to 11 years post-discharge. Brain Inj. 2001;15(5):413–28.
86. Crowe SE, Yousefi M, Shahri B, Piumsomboon T, Hoermann S. Interactions with virtual therapists during motor rehabilitation in immersive virtual environments: a systematic review. Front Virtual Real. 2024;5(February):1284696.

The Use of Artificial Intelligence (AI) in Screening: The INCISIVE Project

Lithin Zacharias , Shereen Nabhani-Gebara ,
Ioanna Chouvarda , and Tatjana Loncar-Turukalo

1 Introduction

Cancer remains a major societal, public health, and economic problem in the twenty-first century [1]. The International Agency for Research on Cancer (IARC) reported that there were close to 20 million new cases of cancer in the year 2022 alongside 9.7 million deaths from cancer [2]. It was estimated that in a lifetime, one in five men or women develop cancer and one in nine men and one in 12 women die from it [2]. The most frequently diagnosed cancer in 2022 was lung, responsible for almost 2.5 million new cases, or one in eight cancers worldwide (12.4% of all cancers globally), followed by breast cancer in females (11.6%), colorectum (9.6%), prostate (7.3%), and stomach (4.9%) [2]. It is strikingly noted that 70% of cancer deaths occur in low- and middle-income countries often due to late diagnosis [3]. The demographics-based predictions indicate that the number of new cases of cancer will reach 35 million by 2050 [2].

A study conducted to understand the cancer care pathways across seven countries in Europe [4] revealed that, except the UK, none of the studied countries had established an organized national screening programme for cancer, despite strong evidence supporting the effectiveness of screening [5–7]. The study has also highlighted the inconsistent rollout of cancer screening programmes impacted the fair distribution of healthcare services and outcomes [4]. This indicates poor investment [4] in screening programmes.

L. Zacharias · S. Nabhani-Gebara (✉)
Kingston University London, London, UK
e-mail: S.Nabhani@kingston.ac.uk

I. Chouvarda
School of Medicine, Aristotle University of Thessaloniki, Thessaloniki, Greece

T. Loncar-Turukalo
University of Novi Sad, Novi Sad, Serbia

It is to be noted with utmost importance that cancer screening plays a vital role in early detection and improving survival rates [5, 8]. The body of research indicates that if the cancer disease is detected, diagnosed, and treated at an early stage, the survival of nearly all types of cancers can increase significantly [9–11]. This also helps in preventing lethality and progression of cancer development [9]. Existing studies confirm the relevance of early detection in varied stages [10] highlighting that people diagnosed with early (stage 1 or 2) cancers have a better 1-year survival than those diagnosed with late (stage 4) cancer. However, the bleak reality is the fact that 50% of cancers are diagnosed at an advanced stage [9]. This cancer burden can be reduced through early detection of cancer and appropriate treatment and care of patients [3]. Nevertheless, there are numerous challenges to making early detection a reality such as bottlenecks in the pathway due to the absence/low number of specialized healthcare professionals and limited equipment. The use of technology to support the early diagnosis of cancer has been proposed as an enabler [9].

To promote patient care, improve patient outcomes, and enhance workflow efficiencies the use of technologies in health care is indispensable [12, 13]. This also includes the use of automation, artificial intelligence (AI), and machine learning (ML) [12, 13]. The application of AI [12, 14–16] in cancer care has been profoundly impacting many cancer lives. However, the need for innovations and the development of early cancer detection approaches has been highlighted [9] as a priority. To address this issue, an integrated, interdisciplinary collaboration [9] was employed to bring possible solutions to early cancer detection with the help of an INCISIVE AI toolbox to deliver transformative progress in cancer care.

2   INCISIVE

INCISIVE is a European Union (EU) Horizon 2020-funded project that brings together 26 partners from across nine European countries [17–21]. One of the aims is to develop and validate an AI toolbox for the use of existing cancer imaging methods [17, 21]. INCISIVE employs data from the most common types of cancers: breast, prostate, lung, and colorectal cancer [17–21].

3   Role of AI in Screening

3.1   Definition

Artificial intelligence (AI) is a broad concept, concerned with generating machines that exhibit intelligence equivalent to humans, in the sense that they have the capacity to perform tasks that typically require human intelligence, such as planning, inference and reasoning, problem-solving, learning and adapting, or being creative.

Typically, there is a distinction between general and narrow AI [22]. General AI refers to machines that can think, understand, learn, respond, solve any problem in any situation, and even have a level of autonomy, e.g. robotic applications. Certain industry-driven general AI applications have found their way to a wide spectrum of uses and have greatly contributed to the public interest in AI.

Narrow AI corresponds to more focused applications that aim to solve specific problems and perform specific tasks. Machine learning, a subset of the overall AI field deals exactly with using data and algorithms, to solve specific problems by gradually gaining experience from data. Following a data-driven approach, these systems, often developed in the healthcare domain, start with an adequate amount of data, which are presented as inputs to machine learning algorithms, to allow them to get gradually trained on these data and capture from them the relevant information to generate a useful output on a well-defined problem, e.g., the diagnostic classification of a patient.

So, general AI encompasses the idea of a machine that can mimic human intelligence, while ML aims for a machine that accurately identifies patterns and provides accurate results in a specific problem. Deep learning (DL), a subcategory of ML, advances the work of ML, in the way that the large neural networks employed learn complex patterns and make predictions, with less or no human input to highlight the important features in data [23, 24].

Within the Medical realm, both ML and DL have shown potential and have gained attention towards addressing clinical challenges in diagnosis and treatment, offering clinical decision support [25], promising both enhanced accuracy and efficiency [26, 27].

Cancer screening constitutes one of these challenges where the application of AI may be advantageous, as elaborated in the next section.

3.2   How AI Can Help in Cancer Screening

Cancer screening is important for early detection and accurate cancer diagnosis, which will be crucial in determining treatment decisions and patient outcomes. Cancer screening and early diagnosis of tumours heavily rely on Imaging, including X-ray mammography (breast cancer), MRI for brain/prostate cancers, CT (pancreatic and lung cancer), PET (pancreatic cancer), optical imaging for skin, oesophageal, or colorectal cancers, and ultrasound elastography (liver cancer). Manually examining this data has resulted in a bottleneck, due to the big volume and production rate of these data, as well as the time-consuming procedures for manual processing. This raised the need for computerized tools and pipelines that can quantify image characteristics (radiomics) and detect/characterize the lesion, supporting medical experts in their decisions. Benefits of this approach have been found in many cases [28, 29] some of which are discussed below.

Breast cancer screening is crucial for timely treatment In [30], the area under the receiver operating characteristic curve (AUC-ROC) for the AI system was greater than the AUC-ROC for the average radiologist by an absolute margin of 11.5%. However, a systematic review [31] took place to evaluate the reported standalone performances of AI for the interpretation of digital mammography, among 16 studies. Results were positive, for example, pooled AUCs were significantly higher for standalone AI than radiologists in the six reader studies on digital mammography, and stand-alone AI performed as well as or better than radiologists, but results were not conclusive, more studies are needed.

In this context, AI-human synergy is considered in [32]. Specifically, a decision-referral approach for integrating artificial intelligence (AI) into the breast cancer screening pathway is proposed, where AI prediction uncertainty is taken into account, and the assessments with lower certainty are referred to the radiologist, resulting in AI triage normal mammography exams and high sensitivity in cancer detection. Such a screening system leverages the strengths of both the radiologist and AI, demonstrating improvements in sensitivity and specificity beyond both the individual radiologist and the standalone AI system, also allowing for the reduction of workload.

Regarding lung cancer, in the study by Rajpurkar et al. [33], Rajpurkar and team developed a CheXNeXt, a convolutional neural network to classify among 14 different pathologies, including pneumonia, pleural effusion, pulmonary masses, and nodules in frontal-view chest X-rays, and was found to perform well, classifying clinically important abnormalities at a level comparable to practicing radiologists.

In a study by Liu et al. [34], Liu and colleagues assessed the value of AI-assisted lung cancer diagnosis. The AI-assisted diagnostic system for computerized tomography (CT) imaging was found of considerable diagnostic accuracy for lung cancer diagnosis. In addition, many novel markers associated with lung cancer have been identified, including methylated DNA, and exhaled volatile organic compounds, and can be of value if standardized, and can potentially be integrated in future models.

In a study by Spadaccini et al. [35], Spadaccini and colleagues presented AI to support screening based on endoscopy, focusing on colorectal cancer as a significant global health concern. Colonoscopy-based screening is crucial, but as a manual task of endoscopists, it presents a high burden and suboptimal outcomes. AI applications for detection and characterization have demonstrated the potential to enhance adenoma detection and optical diagnosis accuracy. However, further well-designed studies are needed to validate the clinical impact and cost-effectiveness of AI-assisted colonoscopy before its widespread implementation.

Regarding skin cancer risk assessments, mHealth applications have been integrated with deep learning offering this functionality. As an example, in a study by Sangers et al. [36], Sangers and colleagues enabled such a system with a convolutional neural network for the detection of premalignant and malignant skin lesions. When evaluating its diagnostic accuracy, it was found far from perfect, yet promising in empowering patients to self-assess skin lesions before consulting a health care professional.

The cases presented above illustrate the virtue of cancer imaging and AI in screening. Several success stories are identified, while there is still room for improvement. While cancer imaging is of great value, it can be complemented by biomarkers based for example on liquid biopsy technologies, as well as clinical data, favouring the generation of integrative models. In addition, the investigation of the AI-human synergy options and optimal AI-enabled pathways needs further investigation.

4   INCISIVE Case Studies

There are two major results stemming from endeavours of the INCISIVE project: (1) the INCISIVE cancer imaging data repository, a collection of 18,650 imaging studies accompanied with clinical data, and (2) INCISIVE AI Toolbox, a platform facilitating usage of the developed AI services for health care providers (HCPs), data sharing (for data providers, DPs) and AI model development based on imaging repository (for AI researchers). Most of the data collected within INCISIVE relates to diagnostic imaging, facilitating the development of AI screening services, especially for lung (X-ray images comprise 18% of the database) and breast [mammography images (MG) 53% of the database].

AI services developed within INCISIVE have been tailored to the needs of HCPs identified through joint workshops of clinicians from nine hospitals and four European countries. Diagnostic AI services play an important role due to the lack of experts engaged in screening programmes. INCISIVE AI Toolbox comprises 15 AI models integrated as AI services for four cancer types: breast, lung, prostate, and colorectal. These services have been developed based on imaging studies collected through two data collection cycles and later validated through two validation studies: (1) prospective observational study aiming for an objective evaluation of the INCISIVE AI services using additionally collected data, and (2) prospective feasibility study aiming at assessment of user experience and qualitative evaluation of AI services.

4.1   Observational Study

The observation study protocol aims at the evaluation of generalization potentials of INCISIVE AI services using objective performance quality metrics: precision (P, positive predictive value), recall (R, sensitivity), F1-Score (harmonic mean of precision and recall), and the specificity (Sp, true negative rate). It is worth noting that the research question related to performance has been aligned with the type of AI model and metrics used on the development test set to facilitate fast performance comparison and evaluation of the generalization potentials of the AI models developed. Moreover, as more DPs are available, the performance on observational data sets from different DPs has been separately presented to obtain a clear perspective on the potential and maturity of AI services to be applied with stable performance metrics regardless of slight differences in acquisition protocols and image quality metrics.

Sensitivity and specificity indicate as to how much confidence we can put into the INCISIVE output, applicable in certain prioritization models. Diseased individuals predicted as positive are called true positives and non-diseased individuals predicted as negative are called true negatives. Diseased individuals predicted as negative are called false negatives and non-diseased predicted as positive are called false positives. The sensitivity of a model is calculated as the number of diseased that are correctly classified, divided by all diseased individuals. The specificity is calculated as the number of correctly classified non-diagnosed patients divided by all non-diagnosed individuals.

Breast cancer services are tailored for mammography images (MGs), as the most often used modality related to screening and follow-up of breast cancer, supporting an automated MG image analysis. MG-based models developed for the prioritization service, which classifies mammographic images as normal (no lesions detected) or suspicious (lesion detected), have been designed with the aim of fast, automated processing of images obtained during daily clinical routine. All such models have been developed based on the YOLOv5 [37] detection architectures of varying sizes. The training was performed on a combined dataset, using both annotated MG images from open databases and collected by data providers of the INCISIVE consortium. For computational reasons, during training, validation, and testing, all images were proportionally reduced to 640 pixels in height.

Due to the heterogeneity of the available dataset, two types of detection models were developed. In the first type, raw (downscaled and down-sampled) images were presented to the model in the hope that the deep neural architecture would be able to automatically extract features regardless of the image content. In the second type, a custom-made pre-processing procedure was developed to harmonize image appearance and level their dynamic range, ensuring effective intensity range utilization across all the MG images, and finally simplifying the task of feature extraction later performed by the backbone of the YOLO network.

MG prioritization service aims to flag MG image as a high priority in cases when there is an indication of the presence of suspicious lesions. For each MG image labelled as a high priority, the service offers visualization of the areas considered suspicious (MG localization service). The input for these services is a single-sided, single-view mammography image, whereas the output contains a prediction of whether the image contains a lesion or not and the model confidence, This is followed by the visualization supporting the decision, presented in Fig. 1: (left) processed input image with a green/red outline depending on whether a lesion was detected, (centre) processed input image with a bounding box showing that area lead to a positive lesion detection (serving as a decision explanation), and (right) an image showing the original input image along with their properties (acquisition details and size) in comparison with the MG present in INCISIVE dataset based on which the model has been developed.

A total of 686 MG studies were available for evaluation of INCSIVE MG services in the observational study, resulting in 1121 single-sided MG images with the presence of some lesion, and 347 single-sided MG images without any lesion (these were used for evaluation of lesion detection services). The imaging studies come from three INCISIVE DPs: the University of Novi Sad, Serbia (UNS), Hellenic Cancer Society (HCS), Greece and Aristotle University of Thessaloniki (AUTH), Greece. The performance of the prioritization service for two models integrated into the INCISIVE AI toolbox: In-N-n and InOD-y-n (without and with image pre-processing respectively) is presented in Table 1. It could be noticed that on the large and representative datasets (UNS and HCS), the average results (ALL)

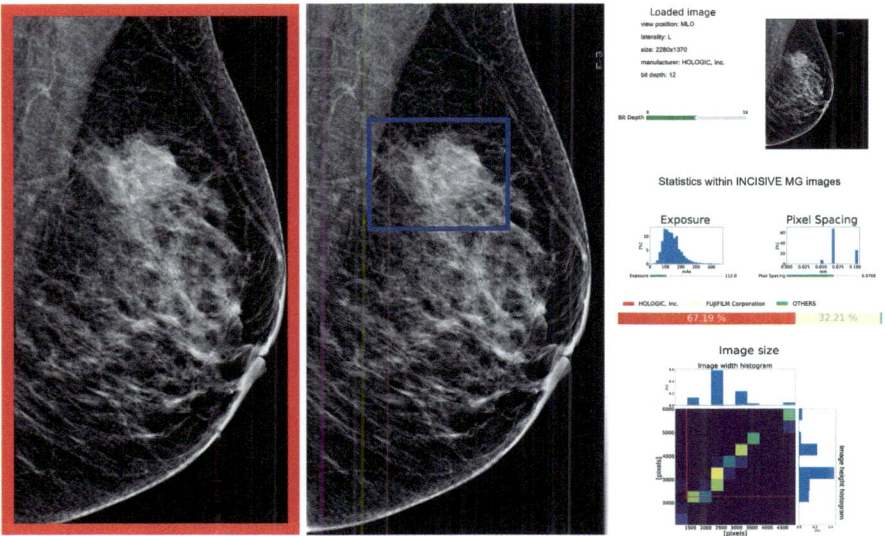

Fig. 1 MG prioritization service output: (left) pre-processed image encircled in red to indicate the presence of a suspicious lesion; (centre) the bounding box indicating the suspicious part of the breast, and (right) the analysed image properties compared to the database of INCISIVE MG images

regardless of pre-processing models perform comparably and slightly better results could be noticed if datasets are more balanced and of higher image quality (UNS, AUTH).

Table 2 presents the results of lesion bounding box detection, i.e., lesion localization, which implies strict pixel correspondence of the annotated and predicted bounding boxes. The observational generalization error is comparable or slightly improved compared to the development test set error. It is worth noting that they are significantly different in size and contain different ratios of data coming from various data providers. During training, it was observed that data coming from different providers tend to be quite distinct and that the trained models tend to perform differently (on average) when evaluated on data coming from different providers. However, our aim here is to provide performance as close as possible to the one that can be achieved for quite a large span of quality levels that can be seen in clinical practise.

Lung cancer services work with X-ray images and CT scans. Chest X-ray classification service has been designed as a prioritization service intended for use in routine daily diagnostics to identify potential abnormal findings (normal/suspicious classification) and specifically targeted at oncological findings. The model training has been done using chest X-rays with oncological, and other pathological and no findings (normal). The image analysis pipeline consists of three consecutive blocks: 1) image pre-processing; 2) lung segmentation using U-NET [38]; and 3) classification using the EfficientNetB2 architecture as a backbone. Both models are designed to achieve high accuracy, preserving computational efficiency. For each DICOM

Table 1 Performance evaluation of two integrated MG prioritization (classification) models: confusion matrices

Model name	Pre-processed	SUBSET	Th = 25%								
			POS	NEG	TP	TN	FP	FN	P	R	F1
In-N-n	NO	ALL	1122	347	753	131	217	367	0.85	0.67	0.75
		AUTH	10	7	8	3	4	2	0.67	0.8	0.73
		UNS	165	75	139	42	33	26	0.81	0.84	0.82
		HCS	945	266	607	169	97	338	0.86	0.64	0.74
InOD-Y-n	YES	ALL	1122	347	647	264	83	447	0.89	0.60	0.72
		AUTH	10	7	9	6	1	1	0.9	0.9	0.9
		UNS	165	75	111	66	9	54	0.93	0.67	0.78
		HCS	945	266	555	191	74	391	0.88	0.59	0.70

The total number of images is 1469 (out of which 347 are patients with no lesions reported). The model's name indicates what type of data has been used in the model development process (*In* INCISIVE, and/or *OD* open data) if the images were pre-processed (*Y* yes, *N* no) and the size of the model (*n* nano)

Table 2 Performance of the lesion localization models integrated in the INCISIVE AI platform, measured on the development test set and the observational data

Model	Data set	Localization		
		P	R	F1
In-N-n	DEVELOPMENT TEST SET	0.554	0.353	0.431
	OBSERVATIONAL DATASET	0.455	0.483	0.468
InOD-Y-n	DEVELOPMENT TEST SET	0.628	0.334	0.436
	OBSERVATIONAL DATASET	0.593	0.41	0.485

Table 3 Summary of performance measures of the trained chest X-ray classification model on different evaluation datasets

Dataset performance measure	VIS (INCISIVE) Threshold = 0.5	AUTH+DISBA+UOA (INCISIVE) Threshold = 0.05	UOA (INCISIVE) Threshold = 0.05
True positive rate (sensitivity)	94.1%	59.2%	61.8%
True negative rate (specificity)	90.6%	85.7%	85.7%
False positive rate	9.4%	14.3%	14.3%
False negative rate	5.9%	40.8%	38.2%
AUC	0.96	0.79	0.82
F1	0.81	0.73	0.74

lung X-ray image input, the service outputs the likelihood of an abnormal finding and the likelihood of an oncological finding. Explainability tools for this service are based on the Local Interpretable Model-agnostic Explanations (LIME) algorithm offering a view of what the model "saw" and concluded to the visualized results.

The model was trained mainly using INCISIVE DP VISARIS (VIS) X-ray images, while in the observational stage, images from multiple DPs [VIS, University of Athens (UoA) Greece, AUTH, DISBA, Italy] have been used to evaluate the generalization performance (Table 3). It can be noticed that the image pre-processing procedure and model itself are fine-tuned to the specific image source (VIS), while the performance on other images, even for the classification thresholds reduced 10x is significantly lower. This calls for a need to involve multiple data in the process of model training to avoid model bias towards certain acquisition equipment and protocols, as in this case.

Lung CT scans are one of the primary diagnostic tools that are utilized in the clinical workflow to inspect the presence of abnormal findings. CT lesion segmentation service can be used in multiple modes: in the prioritization mode, the service scans the CT scan and assigns a low/high priority to the patient depending on whether any findings were identified, in the localization mode, the service identifies the slices of the scan where the model predicted lesions, and in the segmentation mode, it performs annotation of the potential findings. The model architecture that was chosen to implement this service is inspired by ResUnet++ [39]. Several experimentations were performed, mainly focused on model depth, and loss function, as well as testing whether data heterogeneity affects performance. Model training was first been implemented on the open-source NSCLC Radiomics [40] dataset.

During the evaluation in the observational study, 177 new lung CT scans were collected. The prioritization (classification) service was successful in all cases in detecting the scans with lesions as positive, there were no false negative predictions. The results of the localization service, which aims to provide the list of slices where the lesion was segmented, and the segmentation service which identifies all the pixels belonging to a lesion in each scan, are provided in Table 4. The results indicate that despite the correct classification of new scans collected in the observational study, the exact localization and segmentation service show downgraded performance in comparison with the development test set, which probably indicates that there are inherent differences between these datasets and a more robust image harmonization procedure is required.

For prostate cancer, the research team have focused on MRI scans since they are the main diagnostic imaging modality utilized in the clinical workflow. MRI lesion segmentation service performs lesion delineation on T2W Axial View MRI Scan in DICOM format with annotated prostate gland, for which prostate gland segmentation service has been developed. Similarly, to other segmentation services in 3D imaging modalities, MRI prostate lesion segmentation can be used in the prioritization mode, localization mode which extracts the potentially suspicious slices, and the segmentation mode performs annotation of the potential findings.

In the training process, T2W MRI scans from 100 patients were used. This data has been collected by one DP (UoA) within INCISIVE. The dataset split was applied among the patients and not standalone MRI slices. In this way, having slices from a specific patient in both the training and testing set was avoided. 70% of the patients' MRI scans are used for the training set, 20% for the validation set, and 10% for the development test set. For the development of this service U-Net [38] architecture was explored, and the training procedure lasted for 60 epochs.

In the observational study altogether 94 new MRI scans were collected, 44 from UoA, and 50 from another INCISIVE DP Fundacio Clinic Per A La Recerca Biomedica (IDIBAPS). Here we report the performance of both data sets, to present the differences in generalization errors stemming from different acquisition and data quality levels. The prioritization service results, which assign a low/high priority to the examination, are presented in Table 5. The localization and segmentation

Table 4 Evaluation performance of lung CT scan localization and segmentation service—comparison of performance on the development test set (single image source, INCISIVE DP UoA) and performance on the observational datasets collected from UoA and AUTH, INCISIVE DPs

	Localization service		Segmentation service
Dataset	Sensitivity (%)	Specificity (%)	F1-score (%)
DEVELOPMENT TEST SET (UoA)	64.7	94.7	66.2
UoA	50.6	93.5	51.8
AUTH	45.5	94.4	39.9

Table 5 Evaluation performance of Prostate MRI scan prioritization service

Dataset	F1-score (%)
DEVELOPMENT TEST SET (UoA)	100
UoA	88.8
IDIBAPS	65.4

Table 6 Evaluation performance of Prostate MRI scan localization and segmentation service

	Localization service		Segmentation service
Dataset	Sensitivity (%)	Specificity (%)	Sensitivity (%)
DEVELOPMENT TEST SET (UoA)	100	100	87
UoA	95.5	97.3	72.9
IDIBAPS	70.5	96.2	14.3

service results are presented in Table 6, indicating how successful was the model in the prediction of slices where the lesion was present.

As one can observe, the performance of the model on the UoA prospective observational data is well enough, comparing it to its performance on the development test set. The decline in the performance of the model, while it is evaluated on the IDIBAPS dataset, is substantial. Following further examination of this, we assume the following reasons for this behavior: (1) intensity range differs significantly, (2) annotation style which is less strict than in UoA images, inevitably produces additional errors in the segmentation process.

Both the development and evaluation of the models in the setting with multiple data providers, enriched with extensive open data sets, stressed the importance of data quality at the input and relevance of heterogeneous data volumes. The quantitative evaluation of models has indicated that stable and robust model performance is possible only in cases of models developed for image modalities having the largest representation within the INCISIVE repository. In some more demanding tasks, such as disease characterization, the team had to rely on fused imaging and clinical data and extensively analyse and re-evaluate different types of errors. These investigations have contributed set of directions for future developments beyond the project's lifetime.

4.2   Feasibility Study

The feasibility study of the INCISIVE AI toolbox explored the utility of INCISIVE services in cancer screening, diagnosis, and treatment decisions within clinical settings. A rigorous methodology was adopted employing both quantitative and qualitative approaches. Patient participants meeting stringent inclusion criteria were selected as a case. To assess usability, 24 Healthcare professionals (HCPs) were recruited from eight partners in five countries. A total of 1205 cases were assessed over 3 months. Four standardized tools were used to measure usability [41], technology acceptance [42], explainability [43], and trust [44]. Based on the literature recommendations [43–45], trust was measured at two different episodic time points (midterm and post-study). Additionally, a face-to-face interview was conducted with all 24 HCPs to obtain their experiences with using the INCISIVE AI toolbox. A semi-structured interview guide was prepared with 13 questions aimed at assessing aimed at evaluating the user experience, implementation, usability, safety, training, and future perceptions, including advantages, drawbacks, and suggestions for improvement. Quantitative analysis was done with the help of Statistical Package for Social Sciences (SPSS) software. Thematic analysis [46] was done with the qualitative data collected through face-to-face interviews.

Overall, the study results showed (Table 7) relatively positive user experiences. System usefulness and information quality scored moderately. HCPs believed that employing INCISIVE would improve job performance, according to the Technology Acceptance model questionnaire (mean score 4.37). The XAI explanation satisfaction scale reported moderate satisfaction (mean score of 3.54). Trust was also found to be moderate, with a post-study score of 2.96. Despite a little rise in trust between the mid-point and the post-study (mean difference = 0.16), the difference was not statistically significant ($p = 0.090$).

The insightful experiences shared in the qualitative study provided several uses of INCISIVE such as reducing HCPs' workload, helping in simplifying diagnosis, and supporting less experienced radiologists. They also reported that it improves decision-making, serves as a reliable secondary opinion, and enhances trust with rapid diagnosis. The usability of INCISIVE in remote hospitals was also highlighted. The wide applicability of INCISIVE in cancer care stages especially in baseline assessments and diagnosis was highlighted. However, there were concerns about false negatives and the need for more validation studies. The ease of use and user experience were regarded as positive, however, speed in producing the results was suggested. The prior training on the use of INCISIVE and step-by-step explanations in the handbook was considered some of the facilitators in the successful implementation. Insufficient clinical studies, financial scarcity, and resistance from experienced professionals were highlighted as some of the barriers to implementation in clinical settings. The need for retraining algorithms, ensuring high data

Table 7 The results of the quantitative analysis

Tool	Component measured	Mean (95% CI)	SD	Min	Max
Post-study system usability	Overall system usability	2.86 (2.40,3.33)	1.10	1.06	5.00
	System usefulness	2.72 (2.23,3.31)	1.16	1.00	4.83
	Information quality	2.79 (2.30,3.29)	1.17	1.00	4.67
	Interface quality	3.08 (2.55,3.61)	1.24	1.00	5.67
Technology acceptance model	Overall acceptance	4.93 (4.40,5.46)	1.25	2.00	6.75
	Perceived usefulness	4.37 (3.66,5.08)	1.67	1.00	6.67
	Perceived ease of use	5.49 (5.01,5.97)	1.14	2.00	7.00
XAI explanation satisfaction	Explainability	3.54 (3.22,3.86)	0.75	1.88	5.00
Merrit scale	Trust (post)	2.96 (2.57,3.35)	0.92	1.00	4.83
	Trust (mid-point)	3.13 (2.73,3.53)	0.94	1.17	5.00

quality, enhancing the AI output's clarity, and integrating user feedback were suggested as some of the recommendations.

5   Conclusion

AI applications, especially in cancer imaging, have exponentially grown to change the healthcare landscape. The INCISIVE project was a testament to witnessing this change by showcasing its ability to streamline cancer care, especially in cancer screening and diagnosis. The outcomes of the observational and feasibility study have shown great promise even though there were limitations but overall, all these efforts prove that AI has an irevitable role in cancer care

References

1. Bray F, Laversanne M, Weiderpass E, Soerjomataram I. The ever-increasing importance of cancer as a leading cause of premature death worldwide. Cancer. 2021;127(16):3029–30.
2. Bray F, Laversanne M, Sung H, Ferlay J, Siegel RL, Soerjomataram I, et al. Global cancer statistics 2022: GLOBOCAN estimates of incidence and mortality worldwide for 36 cancers in 185 countries. CA Cancer J Clin. 2024;74(3):229–63.
3. Cancer [Internet]. [cited 2023 Aug 1]. https://www.who.int/news-room/fact-sheets/detail/cancer.
4. Hesso I, Kayyali R, Zacharias L, Charalambous A, Lavdaniti M, Stalika E, et al. Cancer care pathways across seven countries in Europe: what are the current obstacles? And how can artificial intelligence help? J Cancer Policy. 2024;39:100457.
5. SAPEA. Improving cancer screening in the European Union. Berlin: SAPEA [Internet]. [cited 2023 Aug 1]. https://sapea.info/topic/cancer-screening/.
6. Jani C, Marshall DC, Singh H, Goodall R, Shalhoub J, Omari OA, et al. Lung cancer mortality in Europe and the USA between 2000 and 2017: an observational analysis. ERJ Open Res. 2021;7(4):00311-2021.
7. Field JK, Dekoning H, Oudkerk M, Anwar S, Mulshine J, Pascorino U, et al. Implementation of lung cancer screening in Europe: challenges and potential solutions: summary of a multidisciplinary roundtable discussion. ESMO Open. 2019;4(5):e000577.
8. Commission E. Communication from the commission to the European Parliament and the Council. eumonitor.eu [Internet]; 2021. https://op.europa.eu/en/publication-detail/-/publication/8dec84ce-66df-11eb-aeb5-01aa75ed71a1.
9. Crosby D, Bhatia S, Brindle KM, Coussens LM, Dive C, Emberton M, et al. Early detection of cancer. Science. 2022;375(6586):eaay9040.
10. Bannister N, Broggio J. Cancer survival by stage at diagnosis for England (experimental statistics): adults diagnosed 2012, 2013 and 2014 and followed up to 2015. Prod Collab Public Health Engl [Internet]. 2016; [cited 2024 Jul 6]. https://backup.ons.gov.uk/wp-content/uploads/sites/3/2016/06/Cancer-survival-by-stage-at-diagnosis-for-England-experimental-statistics-Adults-diagnosed-2012-2013-and-2014-.pdf.
11. Schiffman JD, Fisher PG, Gibbs P. Early detection of cancer: past, present, and future. Am Soc Clin Oncol Educ Book. 2015;35:57–65.
12. Batumalai V, Jameson MG, King O, innovations & … RWT. Cautiously optimistic: a survey of radiation oncology professionals' perceptions of automation in radiotherapy planning. Elsevier [Internet]; 2020. https://www.sciencedirect.com/science/article/pii/S2405632420300263.
13. Khanijahani A, Iezadi S, Dudley S, Policy MGH, et al. Organizational, professional, and patient characteristics associated with artificial intelligence adoption in healthcare: A sys-

tematic review. Elsevier [Internet]; 2022. https://www.sciencedirect.com/science/article/pii/S2211883722000089.

14. Takamatsu M, Yamamoto N, methods HKC, …. Prediction of early colorectal cancer metastasis by machine learning using digital slide images. Elsevier [Internet]; 2019. https://www.sciencedirect.com/science/article/pii/S016926071930197X.

15. Chua IS, Gaziel-Yablowitz M, Korach ZT, Kehl KL, Levitan NA, Yull, et al. Artificial intelligence in oncology: path to implementation. Wiley Online Libr. 2021;10(12):4138–49.

16. Claudio Luchini AP Aldo Scarpa. Artificial intelligence in oncology: current applications and future perspectives. 2021 [cited 2023 Aug 1]. https://www.nature.com/articles/s41416-021-01633-1.

17. Lazic I, Agullo F, Ausso S, Alves B, Barelle C, Berral JL, et al. The holistic perspective of the INCISIVE project—artificial intelligence in screening mammography. Appl Sci Switz. 2022;12(17):8755.

18. Hesso I, Zacharias L, Kayyali R, Charalambous A, Lavdaniti M, Stalika E, Ajami T, Acampa W, Boban J, Nabhani-Gebara S. Artificial intelligence (AI) and machine learning (ML) for optimising cancer imaging: a user experience (UX) study. JMIR Cancer. 2024;10:e52639.

19. Hesso I, Kayyali R, Charalambous A, Lavdaniti M, Stalika E, Lelegianni M, et al. Experiences of cancer survivors in Europe: has anything changed? Can artificial intelligence offer a solution? Front Oncol. 2022;12:888938.

20. Hesso I, Kayyali R, Dolton DR, Joo K, Zacharias L, Charalambous A, et al. Cancer care at the time of the fourth industrial revolution: an insight to healthcare professionals' perspectives on cancer care and artificial intelligence. Radiat Oncol. 2023;18(1):167.

21. Home—incisive project [Internet]. [cited 2023 Aug 1]. https://incisive-project.eu/.

22. Banafa A. 9 narrow AI vs. general AI vs. super AI. 2024 [cited 2024 Jul 17]; https://ieeexplore.ieee.org/abstract/document/10359414/.

23. Sathvika VBT, Anmisha N, Thanmayi V, Suchetha M, Dhas DE, Sehastrajit S, et al. Pipelined structure in the classification of skin lesions based on Alexnet CNN and SVM model with bisectional texture features. IEEE Access [Internet]. 2024; [cited 2024 Jul 17]. https://ieeexplore.ieee.org/abstract/document/10496674/.

24. Das PK, Diya VA, Meher S, Panda R, Abraham A. A systematic review on recent advancements in deep and machine learning based detection and classification of acute lymphoblastic leukemia. IEEE Access. 2022;10:81741–63.

25. Bizzo BC, Almeida RR, Michalski MH, Alkasab TK. Artificial intelligence and clinical decision support for radiologists and referring providers. J Am Coll Radiol. 2019;16(9):1351–6.

26. Yin J, Ngiam KY, Teo HH. Role of artificial intelligence applications in real-life clinical practice: systematic review. J Med Internet Res. 2021;23(4):e25759.

27. Martinez-Millana A, Saez-Saez A, Tornero-Costa R, Azzopardi-Muscat N, Traver V, Novillo-Ortiz D. Artificial intelligence and its impact on the domains of universal health coverage, health emergencies and health promotion: an overview of systematic reviews. Int J Med Inform. 2022;166:104855.

28. Gillies RJ, Schabath MB. Radiomics improves cancer screening and early detection. Cancer Epidemiol Biomarkers Prev. 2020;29(12):2556–67.

29. Chen Z, Lin L, Wu C, Li C, Xu R, Sun Y. Artificial intelligence for assisting cancer diagnosis and treatment in the era of precision medicine. Cancer Commun. 2021;41(11):1100–15.

30. McKinney SM, Sieniek M, Godbole V, Nature JG. International evaluation of an AI system for breast cancer screening. nature.com [Internet]; 2020. https://idp.nature.com/authorize/casa?redirect_uri=https://www.nature.com/articles/s41586-019-1799-6.

31. Yoon JH, Strand F, Baltzer PAT, Conant EF, Gilbert FJ, Lehman CD, et al. Standalone AI for breast cancer detection at screening digital mammography and digital breast Tomosynthesis: a systematic review and meta-analysis. Radiology. 2023;307(5):e222639.

32. Leibig C, Brehmer M, Bunk S, Byng D, Pinker K, Umutlu L. Combining the strengths of radiologists and AI for breast cancer screening: a retrospective analysis. Lancet Digit Health. 2022;4(7):e507–19.

33. Rajpurkar P, Irvin J, Ball RL, Zhu K, Yang B, Mehta H, et al. Deep learning for chest radiograph diagnosis: a retrospective comparison of the CheXNeXt algorithm to practicing radiologists. PLoS Med. 2018;15(11):e1002686.
34. Liu M, Wu J, Wang N, Zhang X, Bai Y, Guo J, et al. The value of artificial intelligence in the diagnosis of lung cancer: a systematic review and meta-analysis. PLoS One. 2023;18(3):e0273445.
35. Spadaccini M, Trova J, Khalaf K, Facciorusso A, Maselli R, Hann A, et al. Artificial Intelligence-assisted colonoscopy and colorectal cancer screening: Where are we going? Dig Liver Dis [Internet]. 2024; [cited 2024 Jul 17]. https://www.sciencedirect.com/science/article/pii/S1590865824002494.
36. Sangers T, Reeder S, van der Vet S, Jhingoer S, Mooyaart A, Siegel DM, et al. Validation of a market-approved artificial intelligence mobile health app for skin cancer screening: a prospective multicenter diagnostic accuracy study. Dermatology. 2022;238(4):649–56.
37. Jocher G. YOLOv5 by ultralytics [Internet]. 2020 [cited 2024 Jul 17]. https://github.com/ultralytics/yolov5.
38. Ronneberger O, Fischer P, Brox T. U-Net: convolutional networks for biomedical image segmentation. In: Navab N, Hornegger J, Wells WM, Frangi AF, editors. Medical image computing and computer-assisted intervention—MICCAI 2015 [Internet]. Cham: Springer; 2015. [cited 2024 Jul 17]. p. 234–241. (Lecture Notes in Computer Science; vol. 9351). http://link.springer.com/10.1007/978-3-319-24574-4_28.
39. Jha D, Smedsrud PH, Riegler MA, Johansen D, De Lange T, Halvorsen P, et al. Resunet++: an advanced architecture for medical image segmentation. In: 2019 IEEE international symposium on multimedia (ISM) [Internet]. IEEE; 2019. [cited 2024 Jul 17]. p. 225–2255. https://ieeexplore.ieee.org/abstract/document/8959021/.
40. Aerts H, Velazquez ER, Leijenaar RT, Parmar C, Grossmann P, Cavalho S, et al. Data from NSCLC-radiomics. Cancer Imaging Arch; 2015.
41. Lewis JR. Psychometric evaluation of the post-study system usability questionnaire: the PSSUQ. Proc Hum Factors Soc Annu Meet. 1992;36(16):1259–60.
42. Davis FD. Perceived usefulness, perceived ease of use, and user acceptance of information technology. MIS Q. 1989;13:319–40.
43. Hoffman RR, Mueller ST, Klein G, Litman J. Metrics for explainable AI: challenges and prospects [Internet]. arXiv; 2019 [cited 2024 May 29]. http://arxiv.org/abs/1812.04608.
44. Merritt SM. Affective processes in human–automation interactions. Hum Factors J Hum Factors Ergon Soc. 2011;53(4):356–70.
45. Siau K, Wang W. Building trust in artificial intelligence, machine learning, and robotics. Cut Bus Technol J. 2018;31(2):47–53.
46. Clarke V, Braun V. Successful qualitative research: a practical guide for beginners. Sage; 2013. p. 1–400.

Design, Development, Piloting, and Evaluation of Smart, Digital Health Applications to Tackle Urgent Cancer Priorities

Antonios Billis, Paraskevas Lagakis, Georgios Petridis,
Panagiotis-Emmanouil Kartsidis, Despoina Mantziari,
Ioannis Poultourtzidis, Sofia Reppou,
and Panagiotis D. Bamidis

1   Introduction

Cancer remains one of the most pressing health challenges of our time, with its incidence dramatically increasing as populations age. In 2012, an estimated 14.1 million new cancer cases and 8.2 million deaths occurred worldwide [1]. The burden of cancer is particularly heavy on older adults, with two thirds of incident cases diagnosed in men and women over the age of 65 [2]. This demographic shift presents unique challenges in cancer care, as older patients often face complex health and social care needs alongside their primary cancer diagnosis [3].

Despite these statistics, current cancer care practices often fall short in addressing the specific needs of older cancer patients. Evidence suggests that older patients remain vastly under-represented in research and are frequently under-treated, leading to inequitable access to care and poorer outcomes [4, 5]. This disparity highlights an urgent need for innovative approaches to cancer care that can address the multifaceted needs of older cancer survivors, including management of comorbidities, frailty, and maintaining quality of life (QoL) [6].

In recent years, smart digital health applications have emerged as promising tools to revolutionize healthcare delivery, particularly in the field of cancer care. These technologies offer the potential to enhance patient monitoring, facilitate personalized interventions, and improve overall quality of care [7]. By leveraging advancements in artificial intelligence (AI), machine learning (ML), and Internet of

A. Billis (✉) · P. Lagakis · G. Petridis · P.-E. Kartsidis · D. Mantziari · I. Poultourtzidis ·
S. Reppou · P. D. Bamidis
School of Medicine, Aristotle University of Thessaloniki, Thessaloniki, Greece
e-mail: ampillis@auth.gr; plagakis@csd.auth.gr; gpetridi@auth.gr; pkartsidis@auth.gr;
mantziad@auth.gr; poultourtzidis@auth.gr; reppou@auth.gr; bamidis@auth.gr

Things (IoT) devices, digital health solutions can provide real-time data collection, analysis, and decision support, thereby enabling more proactive and patient-centered care [8, 9].

The LifeChamps project, funded by the European Union's Horizon 2020 research and innovation program, represents a concerted effort to harness the power of digital health technologies in addressing the urgent priorities in cancer care for older survivors. By integrating various clinical tools and digital technologies, including electronic patient-reported outcome measures (PROMs), electronic health record (EHR) data, wearables, IoT sensors, mHealth apps, Big Data infrastructure and AI-powered analytics, LifeChamps offers a comprehensive approach to geriatric oncology care.

This chapter presents the design, development, piloting, and evaluation of the LifeChamps digital platform, which aims to improve the monitoring, anticipation, and support for complications that can deteriorate the health-related quality of life (HRQoL) of older cancer survivors [10], and also explores the ways that such a platform can address current gaps in clinical practice, promote patient-centered care, and potentially transform the landscape of cancer survivorship care for older adults.

The structure of the current chapter is as follows:

Section 2 outlines the background and motivation that underpins digital care platforms and specifically the LifeChamps initiative toward coordinated, integrated supportive care.

Section 3 presents the importance of patients and healthcare professionals' active involvement in the design and development of such platforms, as well as the way in which this was realized within LifeChamps.

Section 4 gives an overview of the development process and the technical solution of LifeChamps digital care platform, including the AI models.

Section 5 presents the pilot implementation strategy according to the study design and touches upon the evaluation framework employed along with some lessons learnt during the pilot phase of LifeChamps.

Finally, Sect. 6 concludes with main remarks and future directions.

2   Background and Motivation

2.1   Current Challenges in Care of Older Cancer Survivors

The landscape of cancer care, particularly for older adults, is fraught with complex challenges that demand innovative solutions. As the global population ages, healthcare systems face increasing pressure to provide effective, personalized care for older cancer patients who often present with multimorbidity, frailty, and complex psychosocial needs [11].

One of the primary challenges in geriatric oncology is the lack of systematic care and assessment approaches. Traditional tools often fail to adequately assess physiological reserve and predict clinical outcomes in older patients [12]. This can lead to suboptimal treatment decisions, either resulting in under-treatment due to concerns about toxicity or over-treatment, that fails to consider the patient's overall health status and preferences [13].

Moreover, the current healthcare model often struggles to provide comprehensive, continuous monitoring of patients' health status and quality of life outside of clinical settings and during the cancer survivorship stage. This gap in care is particularly pronounced for older cancer survivors, who may experience a range of late effects and psychosocial challenges that significantly impact their daily lives [14].

Another critical issue is the insufficient integration of geriatric assessment into routine oncology practice. Despite evidence supporting its value in risk stratification and treatment planning, comprehensive geriatric assessment is not consistently implemented due to time constraints, lack of geriatric expertise, and logistical challenges [15].

2.2   The Role of Digital Health in Addressing These Challenges

Digital health technologies offer promising solutions to many of these challenges. By leveraging advances in sensor technology, data analytics, and artificial intelligence, digital health applications can provide real-time, continuous monitoring of patients' health status, enabling early detection of complications and more timely interventions [16]. These technologies also have the potential to facilitate more comprehensive and frequent assessments of patients' functional status, symptoms, and quality of life through the use of electronic patient-reported outcome measures (ePROMs) and remote monitoring devices. This can provide clinicians with a more holistic view of the patient's health status, supporting more informed and personalized treatment and care decisions.

Furthermore, digital platforms can enhance communication between patients and healthcare providers, potentially improving care coordination and patient engagement. They can also serve as vehicles for delivering targeted educational content and self-management support, empowering patients to take a more active role in their care [17].

2.3   The Role of AI in Digital Health Interventions

Artificial intelligence (AI) models have shown promising potential in enhancing cancer care, particularly in addressing complex aspects such as quality of life (QoL), mental health issues like anxiety and depression, and specific concerns such as erectile dysfunction in cancer survivors.

In the realm of QoL assessment, AI models have been developed to analyze patient-reported outcomes and sensor data to provide a more comprehensive and nuanced understanding of a patient's well-being. These models can identify patterns and trends in QoL data that may not be timely apparent to clinicians, potentially enabling earlier interventions and more personalized care plans [18, 19].

Anxiety and depression are common comorbidities in cancer patients, particularly in older adults. AI models have been employed to detect early signs of these mental health issues by analyzing various data sources, including patient-reported outcomes, social media activity, and even voice and facial expression analysis. These models can help identify patients at risk of developing anxiety or depression, allowing for timely intervention [20, 21].

Environmental sensors as a data source, quantifying non-static activities, time out of home, sleep quality and nightly routines, were used in a multidimensional frailty model proposal encompassing Activities of Daily Living (ADL), social, and physical dimensions, in a trial described by Bellmunt et al. [18]. In the contemporary healthcare landscape [22–24], an increasing emphasis has been placed on investigating the potential of predictive modeling approaches, for identifying frailty, or a proxy, in older adults, with some emphasizing its importance in geriatric oncology [25, 26].

2.4   Objectives of Digital Health Interventions: The LifeChamps Approach

The LifeChamps project (https://lifechamps.eu/) is dedicated to developing an intelligent and integrated digital care platform tailored specifically for older cancer survivors. This innovative initiative aims to tackle several significant challenges faced by this vulnerable population.

LifeChamps primarily aims to improve patient outcomes and enhance the quality of life for older cancer patients. This goal is achieved through continuous health status monitoring and early detection of adverse events, which can significantly impact a patient's well-being. The platform facilitates personalized care by integrating diverse data sources such as electronic patient-reported outcome measures (ePROMs), wearable devices, and electronic health records, ensuring that care is tailored to the individual needs of each patient.

In addition to personalized care, LifeChamps supports clinical decision-making by providing healthcare professionals with comprehensive, real-time patient data, and predictive analytics. This wealth of information helps healthcare professionals make informed decisions, thereby improving the overall standard of care.

Empowering patients is another critical objective of LifeChamps. The platform offers self-management tools, educational resources, and improved communication channels with care teams, enabling patients to take an active role in managing their health and fostering a sense of control and confidence.

Moreover, LifeChamps contributes to advancing the field of geriatric oncology by generating extensive real-world data sets. This data may inform future research and care practices, paving the way for further innovations in the follow-up of older cancer patients.

Ultimately, LifeChamps envisions to create a more responsive, patient-centered model of care, addressing the complex needs of older cancer survivors to significantly improve their health outcomes and overall quality of life.

3 Design of Digital Health Applications

3.1 The Importance of User-Centered Design and the LifeChamps User-Centered Design Approach

As already mentioned, adopting a user-centered approach and engaging stakeholders throughout the development process is pivotal for enhancing the effectiveness and acceptability of digital health solutions [27]. This approach aligns with the frameworks of user-centered and participatory design, which emphasize incorporating end-users' perspectives into the development lifecycle to ensure that technologies meet their needs and preferences [28]. In the context of the LifeChamps project, actively involving older cancer survivors, caregivers, and healthcare professionals at every stage—from initial needs assessments to co-design sessions and iterative refinements—ensured that the digital solution was both practically relevant and user-friendly. This collaborative process helps developers understand end-users' contexts, challenges, and interactions with technology, allowing them to create solutions that are more likely to be adopted and effectively used in real-world settings [29].

Furthermore, stakeholder engagement through concepts like "co-creation" highlights the benefits of collaborative design processes. Co-creation involves users in the design process, allowing their feedback to shape and refine the product [28, 30]. In LifeChamps, this meant conducting detailed needs assessments, and then validating preliminary designs through co-design sessions and usability testing. This participatory process ensured that the platform was tailored to the specific needs of its users—addressing concerns like ease of use for older adults and seamless integration with existing electronic health records—while fostering a sense of ownership and trust among stakeholders. Such engagement is crucial for overcoming potential barriers to adoption and achieving higher rates of utilization [31]. By integrating these principles into its design strategy, LifeChamps enhanced the platform's relevance and effectiveness, ultimately supporting better patient-centered cancer care and improving health outcomes.

Additionally, LifeChamps successfully built a sustainable community of stakeholders who remained active and engaged throughout the entire project lifecycle. Feeling like co-owners and ambassadors of the project, stakeholders participated with enthusiasm in every activity and remained engaged during the piloting phase. Although the participants varied across different activities, the sense of contributing to a solution designed by and for peers was important, fostering ongoing commitment and support.

From the beginning of the LifeChamps lifecycle, the project research team implemented several activities to identify and categorize relevant stakeholders into primary and secondary end-users of the LifeChamps solution (Fig. 1). This mapping included older cancer patients as primary end-users, followed by healthcare professionals from various disciplines, family and informal caregivers, as well as health and technology providers and policymakers involved in cancer care. Incorporating various perspectives through a multi-stakeholder approach is crucial

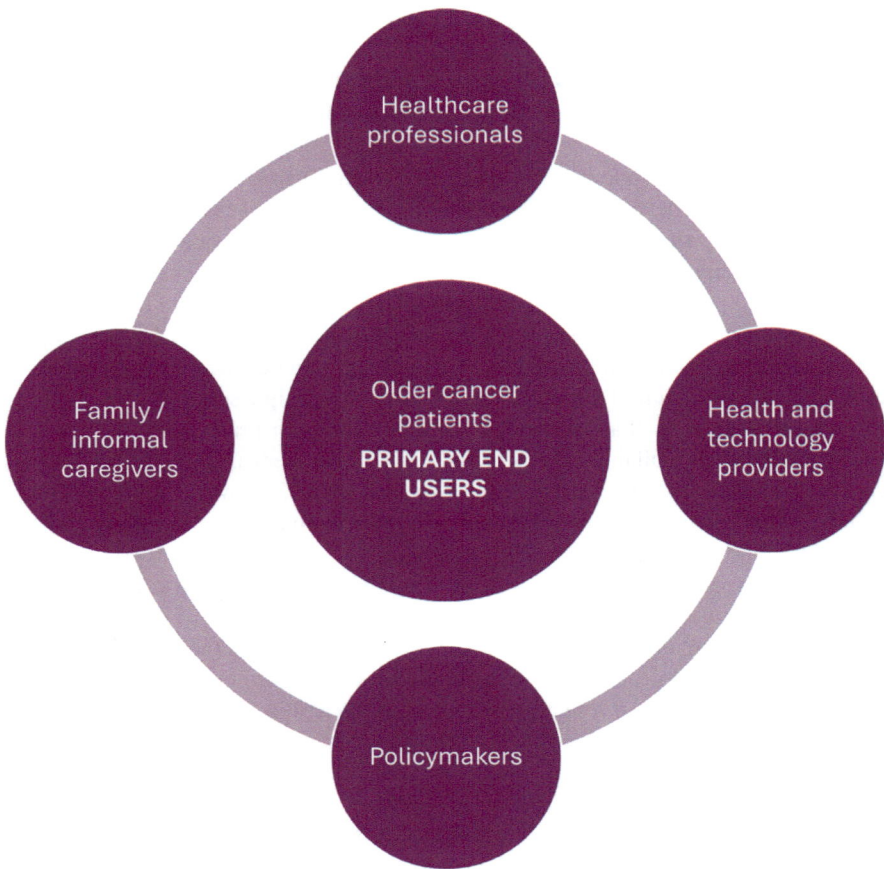

Fig. 1 Mapping of the relevant stakeholder ecosystem

for ensuring that the developing solution is comprehensive, relevant, and effectively addresses the diverse needs of all end-users involved in cancer care.

Stakeholder involvement in LifeChamps can be identified in three main activities during the design and development phases as shown in Fig. 2.

Specifically, recognizing the importance of the different stakeholder perspectives, the multidisciplinary team of experts conducted, just after the mapping activity, a comprehensive needs assessment to understand the challenges faced by older cancer survivors and their caregivers, as well as the limitations of current care practices from the viewpoint of healthcare professionals, and collect requirements and needs to proceed with the development of the solution. To gather user requirements and feedback, LifeChamps employed in-depth interviews with cancer survivors, caregivers, and healthcare professionals, as well as a Delphi study, which provided detailed insights into user experiences and needs. The mixed approach of interviews and group discussions, along with Delphi's online surveys, facilitated a broader

Fig. 2 Co-creation
iteration steps

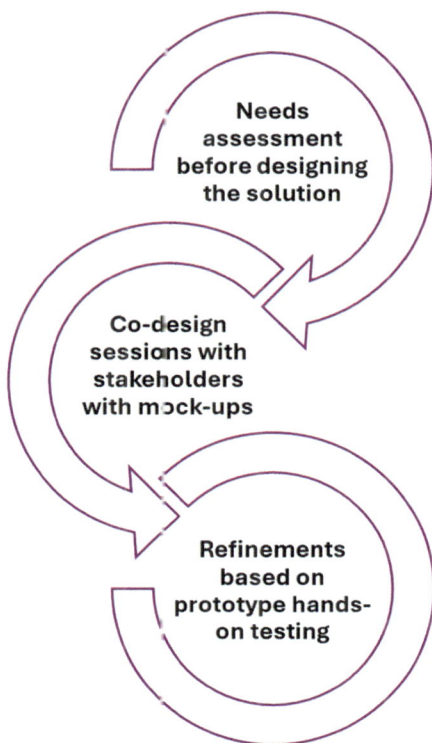

Fig. 3 Participants in
online and onsite
co-creation sessions

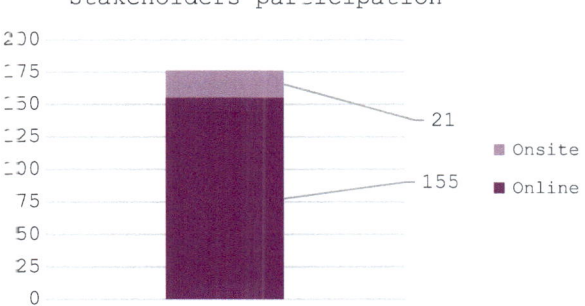

exchange of ideas and experiences, while also reached a wider audience, collecting both qualitative and quantitative data on user preferences. In total, 155 stakeholders participate in the first phase of the project, which due to COVID-19 took place online with success. During the second phase of the project, a new round of co-validation sessions took place. With COVID-19 restrictions lifted, onsite meetings were preferred for this phase. with 21 stakeholders participating (see Fig. 3).

Based on the collected needs, the project team started the development of preliminary versions of the solution components, which were validated by stakeholders during a series of co-design sessions. In those sessions, stakeholders (i.e., cancer survivors, caregivers and healthcare professionals) were actively engaged to review and provide feedback on early mock-ups of the solution. These sessions were crucial in gathering further insights and improvements from end-users, ensuring that the design was user-friendly and aligned with their needs and expectations.

The entire design process was iterative, involving multiple rounds of refinements, based on continuous feedback from all the involved stakeholders. This iterative design ensured that the digital platform evolved to better meet the needs of its end-users, with a special focus on cancer patients and healthcare professionals. In particular, a series of co-validation workshops and prototype testing sessions were organized [10]. The co-validation workshops engaged stakeholders in the final designing phase, where they had the opportunity to provide valuable input and last remarks on features, user interface, and functionality, in view of solution's finalization and launching. Additionally, usability testing sessions with early prototypes offered practical insights into how users interacted with the platform, highlighting areas for improvement, before the real-life piloting phase.

Co-creation was not limited to the various end-user applications or tools integrated into the LifeChamps platform. Clinicians-in-the-loop paradigm was adopted, since healthcare experts were involved in the design of the AI-driven clinical predictive models indicating the necessary inputs and outputs of the models, as well in the iterative co-creation sessions, called "data rodeos" workshops, where they co-created with the LifeChamps data science team the clinically relevant process indicators for geriatric oncological care and QoL, facilitated continuous improvement and refinement of the LifeChamps solution. This approach not only ensured the dashboard's relevance and usability, but also played a pivotal role in integrating technology into clinical practice and letting clinicians better understand the data collected outside the clinical environment.

This participatory approach ensured that the LifeChamps platform was carefully tailored to meet the specific needs and preferences of its intended users. By involving stakeholders throughout the design process, the project significantly increased the likelihood of the platform's acceptability and effectiveness in real-world settings. Indeed, the stakeholder engagement process for the LifeChamps digital platform revealed several critical requirements from various perspectives, shaping the platform's design and functionality. From the patient perspective, it became clear that the platform needed an easy-to-use interface suitable for older adults with varying levels of technology literacy. Healthcare professionals had their own set of requirements. They needed a comprehensive patient monitoring dashboard and seamless integration with existing electronic health record systems. The stakeholder involvement process also uncovered potential barriers to adoption, such as concerns about technology use among older adults and the necessity for adequate training and support for both patients and healthcare professionals. These insights were crucial in shaping the design and functionality of the LifeChamps platform, ensuring it was both technologically sophisticated and deeply attuned to the everyday experiences of its users.

4   Development Process

4.1   Agile Development Methodology

The LifeChamps project adopted an agile development methodology [32] to ensure flexibility, rapid iteration, and continuous improvement throughout the development process (Fig. 4). This approach was particularly well-suited to the complex and evolving nature of the project, both in terms of coordinating the technical work of a medium-sized development team and potential blockers/integration issues, as well as in terms of adjusting to the limitations that came up during the Covid-19 period and had a major impact in the timeline of the technical work. Having an agile framework to work with, helped the team be transparent with issues and progress, adapt and discuss blockers early on, and come up with solutions as a group. This agile framework involved not only the technical partners but also the clinical ones, where their input and expertise were deemed crucial. Technical and clinical partners worked hand in hand at several steps of the development lifecycle, e.g., in the decision of the selected IoT devices, since it was crucial to integrate devices, that from one hand could provide all the information and variables that were important for the clinical partners, while they also had to cover certain technical specifications.

The development process was organized into 2-month sprints, aligning with the integration plan. Each sprint involved several key phases:

– Planning: The team identified priorities and set specific goals for the sprint, based on stakeholder feedback and technical requirements.

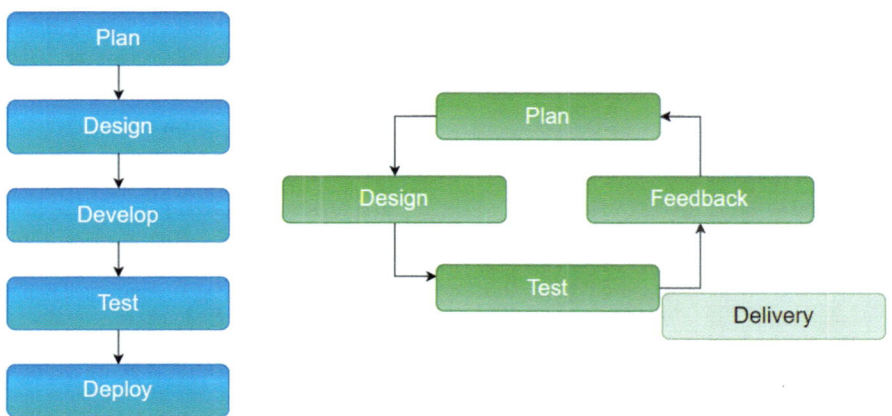

Fig. 4 Traditional vs agile development methodology

- Design: User interface and experience designers worked on refining the platform's look and feel, incorporating insights from user testing and stakeholder input.
- Development: Engineers and developers implemented new features and refined existing ones, focusing on both front-end and back-end components of the system.
- Testing: Rigorous testing was conducted throughout the sprint to identify and address any bugs or usability issues.
- Retrospective: At the end of each sprint, the team (including both technical and clinical experts where relevant) collectively evaluated the completion of sprint goals and identified areas for improvement.

The development process also involved extensive testing to ensure the robustness of the entire solution. Three iterative rounds of testing were conducted, resulting in the tracking and fixing of 210 issues related to the core platform and approximately 800 language and user experience issues in the mobile application.

This iterative approach allowed for continual refinement of the LifeChamps platform, ensuring that it remained aligned with user needs and technological advancements.

4.2   LifeChamps Digital Care Platform

The LifeChamps digital care solution was designed to support the complex requirements of a comprehensive digital health platform for cancer care [33]. The backbone of the solution consists of two major components: the Cloud Platform and the Edge (see Fig. 5).

The Cloud Platform houses various services, including end-user applications, computational models, and business logic. It incorporates a Data Warehouse for

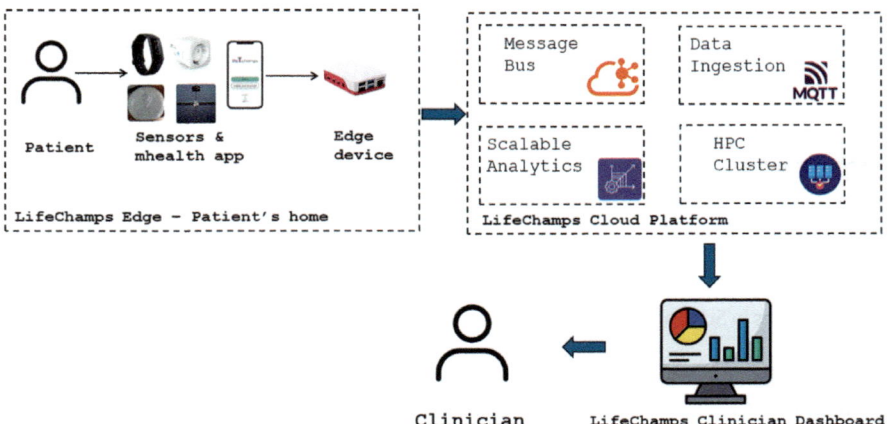

Fig. 5 LifeChamps AI suite

secure storage of data gathered from multiple sources. Key components of the Cloud Platform include:

- Message Bus: Powered by Apache Kafka, facilitating communication between services through dynamically defined topics.
- Data Ingestion: Utilizing MQTT brokers and Apache Flink for real-time data processing and transformation.
- Scalable Analytics Engine: Implementing AI, ML, and deep learning predictive models for health status monitoring and quality-of-life improvement.
- High-Performance Infrastructure (HPC): Part of the cloud platform is also the HPC infrastructure. This part of the platform enables the rapid training of AI models on vast amount of data that builds toward the robustness of the platform.

The Edge component is installed in patients' homes and streams data to the LifeChamps Platform. It includes various sensors and IoT devices that collect patient data and send them to an Edge device—a Raspberry Pi. The Edge device acts as a hub for collecting data and deploying relevant services, such as the Edge Analytics Engine for pre-processing and arbitrary computations.

Regarding the various data sources that are integrated into the platform, these include:

- A Wearable device: A Fitbit Charge 4 wristband for continuous monitoring of physical activity, heart rate, and sleep patterns.
- A Smart Weight scale: Withings Body+ for tracking weight and body composition.
- Ambient home sensors: MySphera LOCS sensors, a set of infrared motion sensors, for passive monitoring of patients' daily in-home ambulation.
- Smart plug: A smart plug, specifically the Teckin SP22, was employed to monitor the television's power status, recording on/off transitions every 5 min. This served as a proxy to one of the participants' Activities of Daily Living (ADLs), offering insights into sedentary and leisure activities.
- Mobile application (mHealth application): A smartphone app for quality-of-life assessment and patient self-management.

4.3   LifeChamps AI Suite

The LifeChamps project seeks to harness the power of AI to significantly enhance the care of older cancer survivors. This innovative initiative focuses on several key areas to achieve its goals.

Firstly, LifeChamps employs AI-based clinical monitoring algorithms for predictive modeling. These algorithms are designed to foresee and prevent disorders, morbidities, or QoL decline related to cancer treatment at an early stage. By analyzing data from multiple sources—such as patient-reported outcomes, wearable devices, and electronic health records—the models can identify potential issues before they become severe, enabling timely interventions.

Personalized risk assessment is another crucial aspect of the project. AI models are developed to stratify patients based on their risk profiles, with a particular emphasis on frailty and quality-of-life subtypes. This stratification allows healthcare providers to tailor interventions and follow-up care to meet each patient's specific needs and risk factors, ensuring a more individualized approach to treatment.

Two models were successfully produced during the project's lifetime. The first model was trained to predict the frailty status of patients, while the second model predicted the presence of mental health issues (i.e., anxiety and/or depression). Both models demonstrated good levels of accuracy. The development of these models involved overcoming several challenges due to the nature of the study and the data. Data completeness and quality were evaluated before proceeding with pre-processing and digital biomarker extraction. The varying levels of engagement required from patients to collect data from different sensors resulted in significant variations in data quality and completeness. Additionally, differences in data granularity from various sensors presented another challenge. To address these issues, a comprehensive pipeline was established for data ingestion, pre-processing, and quality control. Features were homogenized within a common timeframe, and the models were re-trained at specific intervals.

For healthcare professionals, the LifeChamps dashboard integrates AI-driven insights to support clinical decision-making. Through processing complex, multimodal data to deliver actionable information, LifeChamps aims at improving the efficiency and effectiveness of care delivery. This support is invaluable in helping clinicians make informed decisions based on comprehensive visualizations of patient daily, continuous, multi-source data, that otherwise would not be possible to collect and analyze.

Furthermore, the AI models in LifeChamps are designed for continuous learning and improvement. They continuously learn from new data, enhancing their accuracy and relevance over time. This adaptive approach ensures that the models remain up-to-date and effective as more patient data is collected and analyzed. Toward this continuous improvement, the clinician in the loop paradigm mentioned earlier, once again plays an important role. Clinicians have the ability to rate a prediction made by the models through their dedicated dashboard, based on a review of the data that accompany each prediction as part of LifeChamps' explainable AI. These ratings, along with any natural language comment that is given with them, help the models correct their mistakes and stay relevant.

The project also focuses on personalized interventions. By analyzing individual patient data and comparing it with larger population datasets, the AI models in LifeChamps can aid toward more tailored interventions. These might include lifestyle modifications, all aimed at enhancing patient outcomes.

Through these AI applications, LifeChamps aims to create a more responsive, personalized, and effective care model for older cancer survivors. The project acknowledges the transformative potential of AI in cancer care, while also recognizing the necessity of integrating these technological advances with human expertise and compassionate care.

5   Pilot Implementation

5.1   Pilot Study Design

The LifeChamps project implemented a comprehensive pilot study to evaluate the feasibility, usability, acceptability and effectiveness of the digital platform in real-world settings. The pilot study implemented a mixed-methods, multi-centered exploratory design, involving four study sites across Europe: Greece, Spain, Sweden, and the United Kingdom.

The feasibility study adopted a single-group, pre-post design to allow for data collection before, during, and after the deployment of the LifeChamps platform [34]. This design enables better attribution of changes in measured outcomes to the intervention. The study was structured in three phases:

1. Pre-deployment phase: Collection of baseline data using endpoint patient-reported outcome measures (PROMs).
2. Deployment phase: A 12-week period during which participants used the LifeChamps platform, including the smartphone app and IoT sensors.
3. Post-deployment phase: Collection of endpoint PROMs and additional data on the Global Rating of Change Scale, followed by an evaluation process to assess acceptability, usability, and perceived impact of the platform. Clinicians utilized and evaluated the dashboard to monitor patients' progress during this phase of the study.

Participant selection criteria were carefully defined to achieve a representative sample of older cancer survivors. The study recruited 121 patients and 36 healthcare professionals across the four sites within 7 months. Inclusion criteria for patients encompassed individuals aged 65 and above, diagnosed with breast cancer, prostate cancer, or melanoma, who had completed primary treatment within specified timeframes.

To assess the platform's performance and its influence on cancer care, the LifeChamps project established a comprehensive evaluation framework (Fig. 6) encompassing several key domains:

- **Feasibility**: Metrics included recruitment rates, retention rates, and adherence to the study protocol to determine if the platform could be successfully implemented in real-world clinical and non-clinical settings.
- **Usability**: Focused on the ease of use and user experience of both the patient-facing app and the clinician dashboard. Factors such as learnability, efficiency, memorability, and user satisfaction were thoroughly assessed.

Fig. 6 LifeChamps
evaluation framework

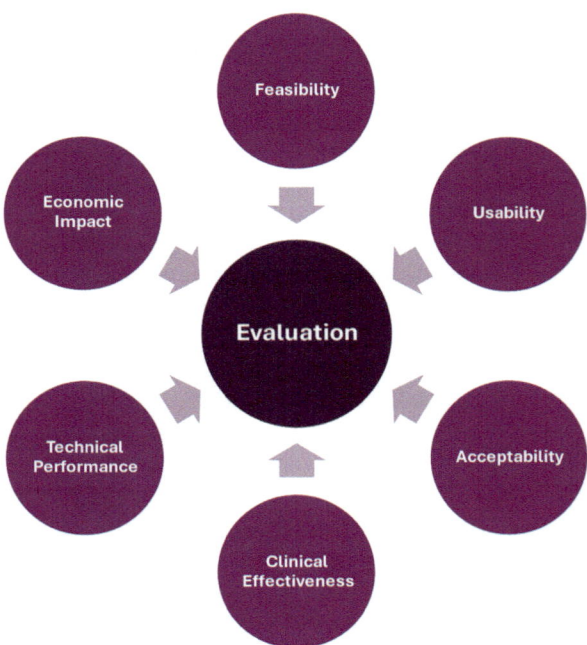

- **Acceptability**: Evaluated the willingness of patients and healthcare profession-als to incorporate the LifeChamps platform into routine care, including perceived usefulness, integration into existing workflows, and overall satisfaction.
- **Clinical Effectiveness**: Assessed by examining changes in quality-of-life mea-sures, symptom management, and healthcare utilization to determine the impact on patient outcomes and clinical decision-making.
- **Technical Performance**: Measured the reliability, responsiveness, and accuracy of the platform's components, including data collection from sensors, data pro-cessing, and the performance of predictive models.
- **Economic Impact**: Provided a preliminary analysis of the platform's cost-effectiveness and its influence on healthcare resource utilization.

To evaluate these domains, the LifeChamps project employed a variety of patient-centered metrics and assessment tools. Patient-Reported Outcome Measures (PROMs) such as the European Quality of Life Scale (EQ-5D-5L), Functional Assessment of Cancer Therapy (FACT-G7), EORTC Quality of Life Utility Measure—Core 10 Dimensions (QLU-C10D), and the Tilburg Frailty Indicator (TFI) were used to assess changes in health status and quality of life.

The Global Rating of Change Scale (GROC) was utilized to detect changes in well-being from the patient's perspective. The System Usability Scale (SUS) and the Mobile App Rating Scale (MARS) were applied to evaluate the usability of the clinician dashboard and the mhealth application for patients, respectively.

The Technology Acceptance Model (TAM) Questionnaire gauged user acceptance and perceived usefulness of the platform. Qualitative interviews with patients and healthcare professionals provided in-depth insights into their experiences. Usage analytics tracked app usage frequency and duration, completion rates of PROMs, and engagement with educational content.

The evaluation process was conducted in phases, starting with baseline assessments before deployment, followed by ongoing monitoring during the intervention period, and concluding with post-intervention assessments. This phased approach allowed for the detection of changes over time and the assessment of both short-term and long-term impacts of the LifeChamps platform.

Through this comprehensive evaluation framework, the LifeChamps project gathered robust evidence on the feasibility, acceptability, usability and potential effectiveness of its digital platform in enhancing cancer care for older adults. The findings from this evaluation will not only guide future refinements of the LifeChamps platform but also contribute to a broader understanding of how digital health interventions can be effectively implemented and evaluated in geriatric oncology care.

5.2   Implementation Strategy

The implementation of the LifeChamps platform in the pilot study followed a structured approach to ensure smooth deployment and maximize older cancer survivors' and healthcare professionals' engagement. Key steps in the implementation strategy included:

Technology Installation and Activation: Each participant's home was equipped with the LifeChamps edge device (Raspberry Pi), wearable devices (Fitbit Charge 4), smart scales (Withings Body+), and ambient home sensors. Pre-generated and pseudonymized user accounts were provided for the mHealth application and the associated third-party services of the above devices and sensors to protect the personal data of the participants.

Participant Training Comprehensive training sessions were conducted for both patients and healthcare professionals. Patients received guidance on using the smartphone app, and the smart devices. Healthcare professionals were trained on utilizing the clinician dashboard and interpreting the data presented.

Support Process: A two-tiered support system was established to address issues effectively. The first level of support was managed by research assistants at each pilot site, who either resolved problems directly or acted as intermediaries between patients and technical partners, if the issue required further assistance. The second level of support involved technical partners who specialized in the specific devices or components of the platform.

Data Collection: Throughout the 12-week deployment phase, data was continuously collected from various sources, including wearable devices, ambient home sensors, patient-reported outcomes via the smartphone app, and clinician inputs through the dashboard.

Monitoring and Feedback: Collected data was checked daily to recognize and address any potential technical issues. In such case, issues were resolved by participants with the guidance of researchers or home visits were scheduled when more serious technical issues needed to be addressed. Patients were instructed to contact the researcher at any time to discuss any issues or concerns. Other than that, no contact was initiated from the researchers' side, to ensure that the feasibility results were as accurate as possible in regard to the usage of the technology.

The implementation strategy also included contingency plans for addressing technical issues, ensuring data privacy and security, and managing withdrawals from the study. Special consideration was given to the needs of the participants who might have limited experience with digital technologies, with additional support provided as needed.

By carefully designing the pilot study and implementing a comprehensive strategy, the LifeChamps project aimed to gather robust data on the platform's performance, user acceptance, and potential impact on cancer care for older adults. This approach allows for a thorough evaluation of the platform's feasibility and effectiveness in real-world clinical settings, providing valuable insights for future refinement and potential wider implementation.

5.3   Preliminary Results and Lessons Learnt

The LifeChamps platform usage by the population of interest (cancer survivors over the age of 65) is feasible in operational terms, as it can collect real-time data from a wide range of sources in challenging, real-life settings, create and deliver predictions based on the collected data for the risk of frailty to the participating HCPs. Additionally, the Real-Life pilot was feasible in terms of recruitment across all pilots, requiring 210 days to exceed the target number of 120, as well as in achieving a drop-out rate of less than 7%. Expanding on the reasons for not enrolling or withdrawing, the most prevalent replies were that of the platform not being compatible with iPhones, the necessity to not move to a vacation house or travel for long periods and mild technophobia, either by the participants or family members living in the same house.

Overall, the platform was adopted in their daily lives by the participants, even though the degrees of adoption were uneven between the devices and the mHealth app with the overall feedback regarding acceptance and usability being positive, with minimal security concerns. Patients perceived, on average, the app useful and easy to use and would recommend it to their peers. Furthermore, the usability of the app was classified, on average, as "Good," according to the SUS score. Interestingly, an expected patient disengagement from the use of smart devices was only observed with the smartwatch with a reduction of 15% per month, while the smart scale adherence to weekly usage receded only by 5.5% over 3 months.

Regarding the HCP's dashboard, the feedback from the HCPs was considered as negative, with an average rating of "Poor" for its usability, according to the SUS score. However, although the replies were not as positive as the patients, yet they reported positively about the acceptability, feasibility, the care management efficiency, and they were happy with the information presented in the LifeChamps dashboard. Assumption regarding this contradictory finding was that the training received and the time for using the dashboard were very limited, due to the tight schedule of the healthcare professionals.

On the technical side of the study, numerous technical issues were identified, which was expected as the diversity of devices, house layouts and Wi-Fi routers introduced unforeseen incompatibilities. Ambient home sensors proved challenging to install to prevent overlapping events, especially within the Raspberry Pi's limited Bluetooth range. The LifeChamps mHealth app encountered instances of user account logouts and difficulties in establishing connection with the edge device. While comparing these technical issues to similar studies is challenging due to limited reporting, it is acknowledged that addressing these issues is crucial for enhancing the acceptance and engagement of home-based digital health systems [35]. Examples of the impact that technical issues can have to a study can be found in Lee et al. [36] where a feasibility study had to be discontinued, or in Lau et al. [37] where 9 out of 19 older adult participants completed the study with technical and complexity issues being reportedly one of the main reasons. In LifeChamps, the absence of withdrawals due to technical issues, and the overall low drop-out rate, may be attributed to the significant allocation of resources in identifying and solving technical issues and communicating with the participants, which was to be expected according to the experience of other similar studies.

6   Conclusion and Future Directions

The LifeChamps project represents a significant advancement in addressing the complex care needs of older cancer survivors through digital health technologies. Its development and evaluation have important implications for the field of cancer care. By integrating digital solutions, the project highlights the potential to bridge existing gaps in geriatric oncology care. The combination of continuous monitoring through wearable devices and home sensors with regular patient-reported outcomes offers a more comprehensive view of patients' health status when compared to the traditional episodic care models. This approach enables earlier detection of deteriorating conditions and allows for more timely interventions, potentially reducing hospitalizations and improving the quality of life for older cancer survivors.

The incorporation of AI-driven predictive models in LifeChamps demonstrates the power of data analytics in personalizing cancer care. These models, which analyze diverse data streams to predict risks and drive personalized and timely interventions, have the potential to transform clinical decision-making. By providing clinicians with actionable insights based on real-time patient data, LifeChamps supports a more proactive and personalized approach to care, aligning with the growing emphasis on precision medicine in oncology.

Moreover, the project's focus on user-centered design and stakeholder engagement throughout the development process offers valuable lessons for future digital health initiatives. The iterative approach to refining the platform based on user feedback ensures that the resulting solution is not only technologically advanced but also practical and acceptable to both patients and healthcare providers. This user-centric approach is crucial for the successful implementation and adoption of digital health technologies in real-world clinical settings.

The LifeChamps platform also addresses the often-overlooked psychosocial aspects of cancer survivorship. By incorporating tools for monitoring mental health and quality of life, and providing educational resources and self-management support, the platform takes a holistic approach to patient care. This comprehensive care model could potentially lead to improved patient outcomes and increased patient satisfaction.

The scalability and broader adoption of the LifeChamps platform depend on several factors. The modular architecture of the system, which allows for integration with existing healthcare IT infrastructure, enhances its potential for widespread implementation. However, successful scaling will require addressing challenges such as interoperability with diverse electronic health record systems and ensuring data security and privacy compliance across different jurisdictions.

The project's multinational approach, involving pilot sites across different European countries, provides valuable insights into the adaptability of the platform to various healthcare contexts. This cross-cultural validation enhances the potential for broader international adoption, although further studies may be needed to assess its applicability in significantly different healthcare systems and cultural contexts.

The cost-effectiveness of the LifeChamps solution is a crucial factor in its potential for large-scale adoption and economic sustainability. While the initial implementation may require significant investment in technology and training, the potential long-term benefits in terms of improved patient outcomes and reduced healthcare utilization could make it an attractive option for healthcare systems struggling with the growing burden of cancer care in aging populations.

Adoption of the LifeChamps platform may also be influenced by healthcare policy and reimbursement structures. The shift toward value-based care models in many healthcare systems could create favorable conditions for the adoption of comprehensive digital health solutions like LifeChamps, which aim to improve outcomes and efficiency of care delivery.

6.1   Future Directions

As digital health continues to evolve, several key areas warrant further exploration to build upon the foundations laid by the LifeChamps project.

Future research should focus on assessing the long-term impact of the LifeChamps platform on patient outcomes, healthcare utilization, and cost-effectiveness.

Longitudinal studies will be crucial in determining the sustained benefits of such digital interventions in geriatric oncology care. Furthermore, while the current project focused on older adults with specific cancer types, future work should explore the applicability and adaptability of the LifeChamps approach to a broader range of cancer types and patient populations, including those with multiple comorbidities.

LifeChamps utilized a selection of IoT devices based on a comprehensive analysis of their features with the help of clinical experts. As new sensor technologies continue to develop though, ongoing research should investigate their integration into platforms like LifeChamps to further enhance monitoring capabilities and their easier adaptation from patients, who already use such kind of devices. This also means that efforts should be made to establish standards for data integration and interoperability.

Finally, as digital health solutions become more prevalent, continued attention must be paid to ethical considerations, data privacy, and security. Future research should explore more the robustness of such frameworks for protecting patient data while maximizing the benefits of data sharing for improved care and research.

In conclusion, the LifeChamps project has demonstrated the potential of integrated digital health solutions to enhance care for older cancer survivors. By combining user-centered design, advanced technologies, and a holistic approach to patient care, it provides a model for future innovations in geriatric oncology. As healthcare systems worldwide struggle with the challenges of aging populations and increasing cancer prevalence, initiatives like LifeChamps offer a promising path toward more personalized, efficient, and effective cancer care for older adults.

References

1. Ferlay J, Soerjomataram I, Ervik M, Dikshit R, Eser S, Mathers C, Rebelo M, Parkin DM, Forman D, Bray F. GLOBOCAN 2012: Estimated Cancer Incidence, Mortality and Prevalence Worldwide in 2012 v1.0 [Internet]. [cited 2024 Jul 22]. https://publications.iarc.fr/Databases/Iarc-Cancerbases/GLOBOCAN-2012-Estimated-Cancer-Incidence-Mortality-And-Prevalence-Worldwide-In-2012-V1.0-2012.
2. Swaminathan D, Swaminathan V. Geriatric oncology: problems with under-treatment within this population. Cancer Biol Med. 2015;12(4):275–83.
3. Chen RC, Royce TJ, Extermann M, Reeve BB. Impact of age and comorbidity on treatment and outcomes in elderly cancer patients. Semin Radiat Oncol. 2012;22(4):265–71.
4. Dharmarajan KV, Presley CJ, Wyld L. Care disparities across the health care continuum for older adults: lessons from multidisciplinary perspectives. Am Soc Clin Oncol Educ Book. 2021;41:1–10.
5. Sedrak MS, Freedman RA, Cohen HJ, Muss HB, Jatoi A, Klepin HD, et al. Older adult participation in cancer clinical trials: a systematic review of barriers and interventions. CA Cancer J Clin. 2021;71(1):78–92.
6. Extermann M, Brain E, Canin B, Cherian MN, Cheung KL, de Glas N, et al. Priorities for the global advancement of care for older adults with cancer: an update of the International Society of Geriatric Oncology Priorities Initiative. Lancet Oncol. 2021 22(1):e29–36.
7. Dicker AP, Jim HSL. Intersection of digital health and oncology. JCO Clin Cancer Inform. 2018;2:1–4.

8. Warrington L, Absolom K, Conner M, Kellar I, Clayton B, Ayres M, et al. Electronic systems for patients to report and manage side effects of cancer treatment: systematic review. J Med Internet Res. 2019;21(1):e10875.
9. Aghdam ZN, Rahmani AM, Hosseinzadeh M. The role of the Internet of things in healthcare: future trends and challenges. Comput Methods Prog Biomed. 2021;199:105903.
10. Marshall-McKenna R, Kotronoulas G, Kokoroskos E, Granados AG, Papachristou P, Papachristou N, et al. A multinational investigation of healthcare needs, preferences, and expectations in supportive cancer care: co-creating the LifeChamps digital platform. J Cancer Surviv. 2023;17(4):1094–110.
11. Dambha-Miller H, Simpson G, Hobson L, Olaniyan D, Hodgson S, Roderick P, et al. Integrating primary care and social services for older adults with multimorbidity: a qualitative study. Br J Gen Pract. 2021;71(711):e753–61.
12. Audisio RA, van Leeuwen B. When reporting on older patients with cancer, frailty information is needed. Ann Surg Oncol. 2011;18(1):4–5.
13. Le Saux O, Falandry C. Is there an age threshold for holding off on testing novel therapies? Curr Oncol Rep. 2018;20(1):6.
14. Tremblay D, Prady C, Bilodeau K, Touati N, Chouinard MC, Fortin M, et al. Optimizing clinical and organizational practice in cancer survivor transitions between specialized oncology and primary care teams: a realist evaluation of multiple case studies. BMC Health Serv Res. 2017;17(1):834.
15. Wildiers H, Heeren P, Puts M, Topinkova E, Janssen-Heijnen MLG, Extermann M, et al. International Society of Geriatric Oncology consensus on geriatric assessment in older patients with cancer. JCO. 2014;32(24):2595–603.
16. Fallahzadeh R, Rokni SA, Ghasemzadeh H, Soto-Perez-de-Celis E, Shahrokni A. Digital health for geriatric oncology. JCO Clin Cancer Inform. 2018;2:1–12.
17. Fitzpatrick PJ. Improving health literacy using the power of digital communications to achieve better health outcomes for patients and practitioners. Front Digit Health. 2023;5:1264780.
18. Bellmunt J, Mokhtari M, Abdulzarak B, Aloulou H, Kodyš M. Experimental frailty model towards an adaptable service delivery for aging people. 2016 21st International conference on engineering of complex computer systems (ICECCS) [Internet]. 2016 [cited 2024 Jul 26]. p. 227–30. https://ieeexplore.ieee.org/document/7816593.
19. Brodie MA, Wang K, Delbaere K, Persiani M, Lovell NH, Redmond SJ, et al. New methods to monitor stair ascents using a wearable pendant device reveal how behavior, fear, and frailty influence falls in octogenarians. IEEE Trans Biomed Eng. 2015;62(11):2595–601.
20. Wahle F, Kowatsch T, Fleisch E, Rufer M, Weidt S. Mobile sensing and support for people with depression: a pilot trial in the wild. JMIR Mhealth Uhealth. 2016;4(3):e111.
21. Pedrelli P, Fedor S, Ghandeharioun A, Howe E, Ionescu DF, Bhathena D, et al. Monitoring changes in depression severity using wearable and mobile sensors. Front Psychiatry [Internet]. 2020 Dec 18 [cited 2024 Apr 22];11. https://www.frontiersin.org/journals/psychiatry/articles/10.3389/fpsyt.2020.584711/full.
22. Wu Y, Jia M, Xiang C, Fang Y. Latent trajectories of frailty and risk prediction models among geriatric community dwellers: an interpretable machine learning perspective. BMC Geriatr. 2022;22:900.
23. Silva J, Sousa I, Cardoso JS. Fusion of clinical, self-reported, and multisensor data for predicting falls. IEEE J Biomed Health Inform. 2020;24(1):50–6.
24. Tang YT, Romero-Ortuno R. Using explainable AI (XAI) for the prediction of falls in the older population. Algorithms. 2022;15(10):353.
25. Jespersen E, Winther SB, Minet LR, Möller S, Pfeiffer P. Frailty screening for predicting rapid functional decline, rapid progressive disease, and shorter overall survival in older patients with gastrointestinal cancer receiving palliative chemotherapy—a prospective, clinical study. J Geriatr Oncol. 2021;12(4):578–84.
26. Massaad E, Williams N, Hadzipasic M, Patel SS, Fourman MS, Kiapour A, et al. Performance assessment of the metastatic spinal tumor frailty index using machine learning algorithms:

limitations and future directions. 2021 May 1 [cited 2024 Jul 29]; https://thejns.org/focus/view/journals/neurosurg-focus/50/5/article-pE5.xml.

27. Vennik FD, van de Bovenkamp HM, Putters K, Grit KJ. Co-production in healthcare: rhetoric and practice. Int Rev Adm Sci. 2016;82(1):150–68.

28. Duque E, Fonseca G, Vieira H, Gontijo G, Ishitani L. A systematic literature review on user centered design and participatory design with older people. In: Proceedings of the 18th Brazilian symposium on human factors in computing systems [Internet]. New York: Association for Computing Machinery; 2019 [cited 2024 Jul 27]. p. 1–11. (IHC'19). doi:https://doi.org/10.1145/3357155.3358471.

29. Tessarolo F, Nollo G, Conotter V, Onorati G, Konstantinidis E, Petsani D, et al. User-centered co-design and AGILE methodology for developing ambient assisting technologies: study plan and methodological framework of the CAPTAIN project. 2019 p. 283–6.

30. Kushniruk A, Nøhr C. Participatory design, user involvement and health IT evaluation. Stud Health Technol Inform. 2016;222:139–51.

31. Mantziari D, Konstantinidis E, Petsani D, Kyriakidis N, Zilidou V, Sidiropoulos E, et al. ThessAHALL—a life-long learning programme for the social inclusion of "Early-Stage" older adult researchers. In: Deserti A, Real M, Schmittinger F, editors. Co-creation for responsible research and innovation. Springer series in design and innovation, vol. 15. Cham: Springer; 2022. p. 89–97. https://doi.org/10.1007/978-3-030-78733-2_9.

32. Cockburn A, Highsmith J. Agile software development, the people factor. Computer. 2001;34(11):131–3.

33. Billis A, Lagakis P, Petridis G, Dimitriadis I, Gounaris A, Vakali A, et al. Enable care of older cancer survivors with digital health technologies: the LifeChamps project. 2023 IEEE 19th international conference on body sensor networks (BSN) [Internet]. 2023 [cited 2024 Jun 10]. p. 1–4. https://ieeexplore.ieee.org/document/10331429.

34. Papachristou N, Kartsidis P, Anagnostopoulou A, Marshall-McKenna R, Kotronoulas G, Collantes G, et al. A smart digital health platform to enable monitoring of quality of life and frailty in older patients with cancer: a mixed-methods, feasibility study protocol. Semin Oncol Nurs. 2023;39(3):151437.

35. Cho Y, Zhang H, Harris MR, Gong Y, Smith EL, Jiang Y. Acceptance and use of home-based electronic symptom self-reporting systems in patients with cancer: systematic review. J Med Internet Res. 2021;23(3):e24638.

36. Lee A, Sandvei M, Asmussen HC, Skougaard M, Macdonald J, Zavada J, et al. The development of complex digital health solutions: formative evaluation combining different methodologies. JMIR Res Protocols. 2018;7(7):e9521.

37. Lau AY, Piper K, Bokor D, Martin P, Lau VS, Coiera E. Challenges during implementation of a patient-facing mobile app for surgical rehabilitation: feasibility study. JMIR Hum Factors. 2017;4(4):e8096.

Training Needs and Programs to Empower Patient and Healthcare Professionals Adopting Telehealth Applications

Despoina Mantziari, Christina Plomariti, Antonios Billis, and Panagiotis D. Bamidis

1   Introduction

Telehealth, which involves delivering healthcare services through digital and tele-communication technologies, has profoundly transformed the healthcare landscape, particularly in the wake of the COVID-19 pandemic [1, 2]. As the adoption of tele-health services continues to grow, thorough training for both healthcare profession-als and patients is crucial. Effective training enables both groups to use telehealth technologies proficiently, thereby improving care delivery, enhancing patient out-comes and care quality, and expanding healthcare accessibility. By addressing train-ing needs and developing effective programs, the potential of telehealth technologies can be maximized, and the overall quality and accessibility of healthcare services can be improved [3]. This chapter explores the training requirements for healthcare professionals and patients in telehealth, highlighting the importance of these educa-tional initiatives and examining the common challenges and opportunities associ-ated with their successful implementation. Additionally, this chapter delves into the essentials of training programs and existing initiatives aimed at empowering both patients and healthcare professionals in adopting telehealth applications.

The COVID-19 pandemic rapidly transformed healthcare delivery, requiring a rigorous shift to telehealth due to social distancing measures. This transition to digi-tal health environments ensured continuous patient care, minimized the exposure of the healthcare workforce and patients, and promoted the use of remote consulta-tions. As a result, telehealth has become increasingly essential to healthcare deliv-ery [4, 5].

Although telemedicine is not a new concept, advancements in information and communication technology have greatly accelerated its widespread adoption in

D. Mantziari (✉) · C. Plomariti · A. Billis · P. D. Bamidis
School of Medicine, Aristotle University of Thessaloniki, Thessaloniki, Greece
e-mail: mantziad@auth.gr; cplomari@auth.gr; ampillis@auth.gr; bamidis@auth.gr

healthcare systems globally. Prior to the COVID-19 pandemic, telehealth was a relatively minor component of overall care, representing less than 2% of healthcare services worldwide in early 2020 [6]. However, recognizing its critical potential, many healthcare organizations quickly adopted and expanded telehealth services even before the pandemic became widespread [6].

The pandemic underscored the critical need for reducing in-person visits while maintaining access to essential health services, propelling telehealth into the global spotlight. Telehealth has addressed chronic shortages of healthcare providers and promoted more equitable access to care, aligning with the Sustainable Development Goal of universal health coverage by providing high-quality, safe, and cost-effective services [7]. This is particularly beneficial for individuals in remote areas, vulnerable populations, and elderly patients with chronic conditions. Additionally, it enhances communication among healthcare professionals and care team members, improving patient care coordination and quality [8, 9]. However, despite its advantages, telehealth cannot always fully replace in-person consultations, and each case must be evaluated individually.

The recent experience highlighted the importance of further developing and diversifying telemedicine services for the post-pandemic era [10]. Moving forward, telehealth is expected to enhance even more healthcare access and equity, decrease the need for patient travel, and improve cost and time effectiveness of the provided healthcare services to underserved populations.

To fully realize these advancements, it is essential to prioritize ongoing training and upskilling of the healthcare workforce as well as patient education [11–13]. According to the World Health Organization, telemedicine involves not only providing health services but also facilitating the continuing education of health professionals [7]. This ongoing education is crucial to ensure that both healthcare providers and patients are well-prepared to adapt to and make the most of evolving telehealth technologies. By investing in comprehensive training programs, the effective use of telehealth can be better supported, ultimately leading to enhanced quality and accessibility of care [9].

1.1   Importance of Receiving Training for Telehealth

Adequate training in telehealth is pivotal for enhancing healthcare delivery and expanding accessibility. It prepares healthcare professionals to effectively utilize telehealth technologies, improving their capability to provide high-quality care and accurately manage patient needs [14]. Concurrently, proper training empowers patients to confidently use telehealth solutions, boosting their digital health literacy, engagement, and satisfaction with remote care [15]. Training also ensures a shared understanding between patients and healthcare providers regarding compliance with legal and ethical standards, security of sensitive information, and maintaining trust in the healthcare system [9].

1.1.1   Enhancing Quality of Care

Training equips healthcare professionals with the necessary skills to deliver high-quality care through telehealth platforms. It enables them to conduct thorough assessments, make accurate diagnoses, deliver appropriate treatments, and monitor patients effectively. For patients, proper training facilitates accurate reporting of symptoms and concerns, equal to traditional in-person consultations. This mutual proficiency helps reduce miscommunication and misdiagnosis, leading to better health outcomes [9, 16].

1.1.2   Improving Patient Outcomes

Effective telehealth training significantly improves patient outcomes. Clinicians who are skilled in using telehealth tools can closely monitor patients and intervene promptly, especially in managing chronic conditions. This capability reduces hospital readmissions and complications. Similarly, well-trained patients are better equipped to adhere to treatment plans, report issues early, and maintain consistent communication with healthcare providers, all of which are essential for achieving optimal health outcomes [15, 17].

1.1.3   Increasing Healthcare Accessibility

Telehealth has the potential to bridge geographical gaps, making healthcare more accessible to individuals in remote or underserved areas. Training empowers both healthcare professionals and patients to leverage telehealth effectively, facilitating timely and efficient healthcare delivery regardless of location. For professionals, this means extending their reach to patients who might otherwise lack access to medical services. Additionally, the frequent and seamless use of telehealth services enables clinicians to collaborate with peers from various regions and countries, enhancing care through shared expertise. For patients, training provides the knowledge and confidence to use telehealth platforms effectively, reducing the need for long-distance travel for care [18].

1.1.4   Increasing Patient Engagement and Satisfaction

When patients feel comfortable and confident in using telehealth technologies, they are more likely to engage proactively in their healthcare. This increased engagement leads to higher satisfaction rates, better adherence to treatment plans, and improved health management and monitoring through tailored interventions and self-care tools. Educated patients are empowered to actively participate in their health care, ask informed questions, and communicate more effectively with their healthcare providers. This proactive approach fosters a collaborative relationship with clinicians, enhancing the overall healthcare experience [19].

1.1.5   Ensuring Compliance and Security

Training is also crucial for understanding and adhering to legal and ethical standards in telehealth. It helps both healthcare professionals and patients recognize the importance of safeguarding sensitive health and personal information, ensuring secure telehealth interactions [18]. Clinicians trained in telehealth are better equipped to comply with regulations such as the EU GDPR and other national or regional laws, protecting patient data. On the other hand, patients gain knowledge about using telehealth platforms safely, understanding potential security risks, and how their data is protected [20].

Comprehensive telehealth training is crucial for optimizing healthcare delivery by equipping both healthcare professionals and patients with the required skills and competencies to effectively utilize remote technologies [12]. Training empowers healthcare professionals to enhance care quality and manage patient health needs with precision, while boosting patients' confidence and engagement, which improves adherence to treatment plans and health outcomes [19]. While existing training programs provide a solid starting point for meeting patients and professionals' training needs, further exploration and enhancement of these initiatives are necessary to fully unlock the potential of telehealth [11]. Expanding and refining training efforts will help both healthcare professionals and patients better adapt to evolving technologies and maximize the benefits of remote care.

2   Current Landscape of Telehealth Training Programs

Existing telehealth training programs encompass a broad spectrum of approaches aimed at equipping both patients and healthcare professionals with the requisite skills and knowledge for effective use of remote and digital healthcare technologies. As telehealth has advanced, these training programs have evolved to accommodate the diverse needs and contexts of different users [1, 21]. The current section provides a brief overview of the range of current training programs, highlighting various methods and structures employed to address specific user requirements. Examining these programs highlights how the adaptation and refinement of training methods have been essential in improving telehealth proficiency and optimizing remote care technologies. However, identifying and addressing ongoing training needs is crucial for further enhancing these efforts and ensuring the continued effectiveness and evolution of telehealth practices.

2.1   Evolution and Integration of Telehealth Training Programs

Telehealth training programs have been developed by a range of institutions, including hospitals, universities, and specialized training organizations. These programs aim to bridge the knowledge gap and ensure the seamless adoption of telehealth services. Although the concept of telehealth and the technological readiness existed before the COVID-19 pandemic, its integration into everyday healthcare has often been abrupt and unplanned [22]. The pandemic necessitated an immediate and widespread shift to telehealth to address urgent healthcare needs. This rapid transition frequently occurred without substantial preparation or training for both healthcare professionals and patients [21]. Consequently, this situation highlighted and amplified the need for comprehensive training programs.

Early telehealth training initiatives were often fragmented and ad hoc, focusing on basic technological training and troubleshooting. However, as the demand for telehealth grew during the pandemic, more comprehensive and structured training programs emerged [12]. These programs now cover a broad spectrum of competencies, from technical skills to clinical decision-making and doctor-to-patient communication. The need for training has become so apparent that telehealth training has been integrated into medical school curricula and incorporated into professional development seminars and continuing education courses for healthcare professionals [12, 22]. Similarly, preparing patients to effectively engage with telehealth services has become a critical focus. Some programs target not only patients but also their family members and informal caregivers, recognizing their crucial role in effective health management [23, 24]. Many programs are also structured around managing specific chronic conditions, such as cancer, dementia, or cardiovascular diseases. These programs train patients, caregivers, and healthcare professionals in specialized technologies and supportive tools tailored to the management of these particular diseases [25].

2.2   Approaches to Telehealth Training Delivery

The diverse needs of healthcare professionals and patients require varied training delivery methods and methodological approaches in telehealth education [3, 12]. To address these needs effectively, several primary types of training programs have been developed, each with unique features and benefits.

2.2.1   Online Courses

Online courses are among the most prevalent forms of telehealth training, often delivered as self-paced programs or Massive Open Online Courses (MOOCs). These courses offer flexibility and accessibility, allowing participants to learn at their own pace. They typically include a series of modules covering various aspects of telehealth, such as technology familiarization, system navigation, online patient engagement and communication, and privacy regulations. Online courses are typically rich in multimedia content, incorporating videos, interactive quizzes for self-evaluation, and discussion forums to enhance learning and retention.

2.2.2   Workshops

Workshops provide an interactive and hands-on approach to telehealth training. These sessions are usually conducted in-person or virtually and are designed to foster practical skills through real-time demonstrations and group activities. Workshops are particularly effective for training healthcare professionals on the use of telehealth equipment and software, as they allow for immediate feedback and troubleshooting. Regarding patient education, workshops offer opportunities for patients to engage with eHealth tools and applications, either with guides support or independently, enhancing their confidence and trust in remote care and self-management health technologies. Additionally, these interactive sessions foster peer-learning, as well as collaboration between healthcare professionals and patients, which is essential for building confidence and competence in telehealth practices.

2.2.3 Simulations

Simulations offer a high-fidelity training environment where participants can practice telehealth scenarios in a controlled setting. These simulations often use standardized patients (i.e. actors trained to portray patient cases) or advanced computer simulations to imitate real-life telehealth consultations (i.e. virtual patient scenarios). This method helps develop critical thinking, decision-making, and communication skills. Simulations are valuable for both initial training and ongoing professional development, offering a safe space to make errors without risking patient safety. Their importance is evident in routine clinical settings and during crises like pandemics. Simulations also offer flexible, accessible learning experiences, even through smartphone applications, democratizing medical education. They foster experiential learning and critical thinking, equipping professionals with essential clinical skills. Additionally, simulations aid in patient education, supporting self-management and informed decision-making amidst abundant online resources.

2.2.4 Webinars and Tutorials

Webinars and tutorials are popular for their convenience and ability to reach a wide audience. These sessions are typically short and informative, including focused presentations on specific topics related to telehealth, such as regulatory updates, best practices in telehealth etiquette, or new technological advancements. Webinars often feature expert speakers and include Q&A sessions, allowing participants to engage directly with the presenters. Tutorials, on the other hand, are usually prerecorded and can be accessed on-demand, offering step-by-step instructions on various telehealth tasks.

The existing array of telehealth training programs demonstrates a rich variety of approaches tailored to meet the diverse needs of both patients and healthcare professionals. These programs utilize online courses, workshops, simulations, and webinars to deliver comprehensive education on the effective use of telehealth technologies. The diverse approaches employed ensure that users can engage with telehealth in a way that aligns with individual needs and specific contexts. By continually assessing and adapting training programs, the healthcare sector can ensure that both professionals and patients are equipped with the knowledge and skills necessary to optimize remote care and improve health outcomes.

3   Identifying Training Needs

Identifying training needs for telehealth involves a multi-faceted approach, though quite important for mapping the current landscape, beginning with a comprehensive analysis of existing practices and literature. This includes a thorough review of current research and reports to identify the common challenges and requirements faced by both patients and healthcare professionals in telehealth environments. This exploration helps pinpoint key areas where focused training is necessary, such as technology use, health literacy, and virtual communication.

Following the review, a needs assessment, through various methods, including surveys, expert consultations, and stakeholder interviews, is also crucial. This assessment provides insights into the specific challenges and needs of users, co-validating the review results and informing the development of targeted training programs [3, 24]. By addressing these needs, the approach ensures that both patients and professionals receive tailored training materials and support, enabling them to their effective upskilling and the successful utilization of telehealth technologies. This targeted support enhances user proficiency and confidence [16, 23].

The recent state-of-the-art analysis from the eCAN Joint Action,[1] an EU-funded initiative focused on enhancing eHealth for cancer patients, illustrates this process. It has identified critical training needs and knowledge gaps for patients, caregivers, and healthcare professionals. Although the eCAN project specifically addresses cancer-related telehealth, its findings underscore broader telehealth empowerment, emphasizing the general training needs and knowledge gaps essential for optimizing telehealth adoption and effectiveness across various medical contexts.

Specifically, the identified training requirements can be broadly categorized into six key areas, encompassing both patients and healthcare professionals. Although the context in which these needs are applied may differ, the fundamental areas of (a) digital literacy, (b) health literacy, (c) communication skills, (d) empathy and trust, (e) ethical and security considerations, and (f) equal access to care are relevant to both groups (Fig. 1). Understanding and addressing these categories of needs is essential for optimizing the benefits of telehealth training and ensuring that all stakeholders can engage with these digital and remote health technologies confidently and effectively.

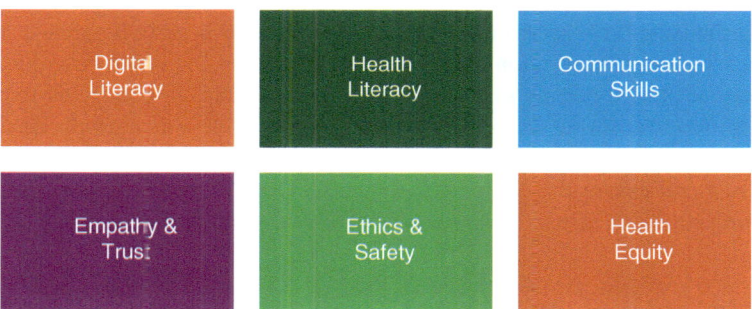

Fig. 1 Key areas of training requirements for telehealth (patients and healthcare professionals)

---

[1] https://ecanja.eu/

3.1   Digital Literacy

For both patients and healthcare professionals, digital literacy is a cornerstone of successful telehealth interactions. Patients and caregivers require training to effectively use telehealth technologies, prepare for virtual appointments, and troubleshoot basic technical issues. This ensures that technical barriers do not impede access to care, allowing patients to navigate telehealth platforms with confidence [26]. Similarly, healthcare professionals need to master telehealth platforms, handle technical problems, and integrate these technologies into their daily workflows. Proficiency in digital literacy helps maintain seamless interactions with patients, thereby enhancing the overall telehealth experience [27].

3.2   Health Literacy

Health literacy training is vital for understanding health conditions and treatment options, and it plays a critical role for both patients and healthcare professionals. Patients and their caregivers benefit from education that helps them understand their health conditions, available treatments, and how to engage with telehealth resources. This knowledge supports informed decision-making and active participation in their care [26, 28]. Healthcare professionals, on the other hand, must adapt their clinical practices to accommodate telehealth, including the integration of hybrid care models that combine in-person and virtual interactions. Training in health literacy equips both groups with the tools needed to navigate the complexities of telehealth effectively [22].

3.3   Communication Skills

Effective communication is pivotal in telehealth, where interactions mostly occur without the benefit of face-to-face engagement. Patients need to be trained in clear and consistent communication with healthcare providers, including providing accurate feedback and reporting symptoms. This training helps in conveying important information and ensuring that care is appropriately tailored to their needs. Healthcare professionals must also develop skills in transparent, empathetic communication to build trust and ensure that patients feel heard and understood. Emphasizing clear communication in a virtual setting is crucial, as non-verbal cues are often limited.

3.4   Empathy and Trust

Empathy and trust are fundamental to successful telehealth interactions. Patients should be educated on actively engaging in their care and understanding their personalized treatment plans, while also learning how to build and maintain trust in a virtual environment. Trust is a crucial component of effective telehealth interactions, and patients need to be aware of how to establish a trusting relationship with their healthcare providers even when not meeting in person. This includes understanding the roles and responsibilities of their healthcare team, actively participating in their care, and feeling confident in the security and confidentiality of their telehealth sessions [29]. Empowering patients with this knowledge fosters a collaborative relationship and enhances the overall effectiveness of telehealth services [24]. For healthcare professionals, training should focus on building rapport and personalizing care to maintain trust in a virtual environment. Empathy is a key factor in patient satisfaction and adherence to treatment plans, making it an essential component of training programs for both patients and healthcare providers [12, 21].

3.5 Ethical and Security Considerations

Understanding and addressing ethical and security concerns is critical for maintaining the integrity of telehealth services. Patients need to be informed about data privacy practices and potential security threats to protect their personal health information. Healthcare professionals must receive ongoing education on privacy regulations, ethical conduct, and strategies to ensure confidentiality in telehealth interactions. Comprehensive training in ethical and security considerations helps safeguard sensitive information and upholds the trust in telehealth services [16, 30].

3.6 Equal Access to Care

Ensuring equitable access to telehealth services is a vital aspect of training. Patients must be trained on how to effectively access telehealth services, especially those from underserved or special populations. Healthcare professionals should be equipped to address disparities in access and ensure that telehealth services are culturally sensitive and inclusive. Training programs should focus on overcoming barriers to access and promoting equality in telehealth care, ensuring that all patients receive the benefits of remote health services [28].

Overall, identifying and addressing training needs in telehealth is essential for preparing both patients and healthcare professionals to effectively use telehealth technologies. By analyzing current practices, conducting needs assessments, and focusing on key areas such as digital literacy, health literacy, communication skills, empathy and trust, ethical considerations, and equal access to care, the training reveals both opportunities and challenges. Tailoring training programs to these needs enhances user proficiency and confidence, contributing to improved healthcare outcomes and equitable access to telehealth services. This approach not only addresses existing gaps but also helps in optimizing the integration and effectiveness of telehealth across various medical contexts.

4   Challenges and Opportunities in Training for Telehealth

As healthcare systems increasingly integrate telehealth into their service delivery models, both the training needs and the practical application of this technology reveal a spectrum of opportunities and challenges. The identified training needs for both patients and healthcare professionals highlight the critical areas where telehealth can transform care but also where obstacles must be addressed. Effective training is essential to leverage the potential benefits of telehealth while navigating its inherent difficulties. Understanding these challenges and opportunities is necessary for optimizing telehealth practices and ensuring successful implementation in the evolving landscape of healthcare [31].

4.1   Challenges in Telehealth Training

Telehealth has brought about significant advancements in healthcare delivery, but it also presents several challenges, particularly for patients and healthcare professionals.

Telehealth training programs, designed to enhance the proficiency of both patients and healthcare professionals, can face several significant challenges. For patients, one major obstacle is the diverse range of technological literacy. Patients with limited experience using digital devices or unfamiliarity with telehealth platforms may struggle to engage effectively with the training [32]. This issue is compounded for older adults or those with disabilities who might face additional barriers. Ensuring that training is accessible, user-friendly, and tailored to varying levels of technological competence is crucial, yet often difficult to achieve [33].

Healthcare professionals also encounter distinct challenges during telehealth training. The shift from in-person consultations to virtual interactions requires them to adapt not only to new technologies but also to new modes of communication and care delivery [31]. Training must address the nuances of conducting consultations through screens, which can differ significantly from face-to-face interactions. Professionals need to be adept at using telehealth tools while maintaining high standards of care, managing patient data securely, and effectively communicating in a digital environment [22]. This demands a comprehensive approach to training that encompasses both technical skills and patient management strategies.

Moreover, the integration of telehealth training into existing workflows presents its own set of difficulties. For both patients and healthcare providers, balancing telehealth training with ongoing responsibilities can be challenging. Scheduling conflicts, limited time for training sessions, and the need for ongoing support can impede the effectiveness of training programs [31]. Addressing these issues requires careful planning and support systems to ensure that the training is not only delivered effectively but also adopted seamlessly into routine practice.

4.2   Opportunities in Telehealth Training

Telehealth training, while presenting its own set of challenges, also opens up a wealth of opportunities for improving patient and healthcare professional experiences. For patients, telehealth training can empower them to engage more actively in their healthcare. Through effective training programs, patients can learn to navigate digital platforms, access their medical records, and participate in virtual consultations with greater ease. This empowerment not only improves patient satisfaction but also promotes better adherence to treatment plans and follow-up care. By becoming proficient in telehealth, patients gain greater flexibility and access to healthcare services that might otherwise be limited by geographical or logistical constraints [34].

Healthcare professionals also stand to benefit significantly from telehealth training. The shift to virtual consultations can lead to enhanced efficiency and increased reach of healthcare services. Training programs can equip providers with the skills to manage multiple patients simultaneously, leverage digital tools for better patient tracking, and utilize data analytics to improve care outcomes. Furthermore, telehealth training fosters a culture of continuous learning and adaptation, which is crucial in an ever-evolving medical landscape [31]. This proficiency can also reduce the strain on healthcare facilities by allowing for more streamlined and effective patient management.

Additionally, telehealth training can foster greater collaboration and knowledge sharing among healthcare professionals [3]. Virtual platforms can facilitate networking opportunities and the exchange of best practices across different regions and specialties. This can lead to the development of innovative approaches to patient care and an overall enhancement in the quality of healthcare services. By embracing these opportunities, both patients and healthcare professionals can experience a more integrated and effective healthcare system, leveraging the full potential of telehealth technology to improve health outcomes and operational efficiency.

5   Designing a Training Program

A well-structured telehealth training program must encompass several key components, including curriculum design and content, methods of delivery, customization for various user groups and demographics, and mechanisms for continuous feedback and improvement [17]. To achieve these objectives effectively, it is crucial to engage all relevant stakeholders—patients, caregivers, and healthcare professionals—through participatory design approaches. By involving these groups even from the early stages of the development process, the training program can be finely tuned to address users' specific needs and preferences, ensuring that the content is relevant and the delivery methods are appropriate for diverse audiences.

Incorporating input from stakeholders helps to create a more user-centered training experience, which enhances engagement and fosters higher levels of satisfaction among participants. This collaborative approach ensures that the training materials are tailored to users' needs, leading to increased rates of consensus and successful completion. Additionally, ongoing feedback from participants allows for the continuous refinement of the program, addressing any emerging challenges or gaps in knowledge. This iterative process not only improves the overall effectiveness of the training but also supports the development of a more adaptable and resilient telehealth infrastructure.

5.1   Curriculum Design and Content

The foundation of an effective telehealth training program is its curriculum design and content. This starts with a thorough needs assessment and gap analysis to identify stakeholders' specific requirements. The content must be practical, relevant, and accessible, incorporating real-world scenarios and examples to illustrate the application of new skills in telehealth settings. Interactive elements, such as simulations and role-playing exercises, can enhance learning by offering hands-on experience with telehealth platforms [12]. Additionally, modules on troubleshooting common technical issues and adhering to ethical and privacy standards are crucial for preparing users to handle various challenges in telehealth interactions [11] [also refer to chapter "Digital Literacy and Preparedness of Healthcare Professionals: The TRANSiTION Project".

5.2   Methods of Delivery

The methods of delivery for telehealth training should be diverse to accommodate different learning styles and accessibility needs. A blended learning approach, combining online resources with in-person or virtual workshops, can be highly effective. As previously mentioned, online modules and webinars offer flexibility, allowing learners to access materials at their own pace with video tutorials, interactive quizzes, and downloadable guides. In-person or live virtual workshops complement online learning by providing hands-on practice, real-time feedback, and interactive discussions. Incorporating peer-learning opportunities can foster a collaborative environment and enhance the training experience [3].

5.3   Customization for Different Demographics

Customization is a critical component of telehealth training, as different demographics may have varying needs and challenges. For patients and caregivers, training programs should be tailored to address factors such as age, technological proficiency, and health literacy levels [8]. For instance, older adults might benefit from simplified instructions and additional support for using telehealth technologies, while caregivers may require guidance on how to assist patients with telehealth interactions effectively. Healthcare professionals also have diverse training needs based on their roles and specialties. Customizing training for different healthcare professionals—such as primary care providers, specialists, and support staff—ensures that the curriculum is relevant to their specific responsibilities and challenges [3]. This targeted approach helps to address the unique aspects of each role and facilitates the development of skills that are directly applicable to their day-to-day telehealth practice.

5.4   Continuous Feedback and Improvement Mechanisms

To maintain the effectiveness of the training program, continuous feedback and improvement mechanisms are essential. This involves gathering input from participants through surveys, interviews, and focus groups to gain insights into the program's strengths and areas for enhancement. Incorporating this feedback into program updates refines the curriculum and delivery methods, ensuring ongoing relevance and effectiveness. Additionally, tracking trainees' progress and performance helps identify where additional support may be needed. Regular evaluation and adaptation of the training program are crucial for addressing emerging challenges and integrating new developments in telehealth technology and practices [2].

Ultimately, a well-designed and responsive training program can significantly impact the effectiveness of telehealth services. By aligning the training with the needs and expectations of patients, caregivers, and healthcare professionals, organizations can ensure that all parties are well-prepared to utilize telehealth technologies efficiently. This approach promotes better user adoption, enhances the quality of virtual care, and contributes to the overall success of telehealth initiatives.

6   Case Studies of e-Training Programs

6.1   Erasmus+ e-Training Programs for Individuals' Capacity Building

Several e-Training Programs under the Erasmus+ EU funding framework focus on capacity building for healthcare professionals and targeted population groups, including chronic patients, older adults, people at risk, and informal caregivers. The aim is to enhance the competences, skills, and attitudes of these populations toward digital health literacy and telehealth adoption. These programs empower individuals for effective self-management of their conditions using assistive technologies and online resources. The training components often include an open-access e-Training platform and a designed curriculum that covers thematic areas for increasing awareness and training skills related to specific health conditions [35–37].

6.1.1   Program and Curriculum Design

These e-Training programs are developed using the participatory design methodology. This approach involves identifying the needs and requirements of the targeted populations and extending to the selection and development of content delivery. The co-created curriculum includes several educational modules tailored to the needs of the primary end-users (i.e., older adults, persons with chronic diseases, and so on), as well as healthcare professionals and informal caregivers. The training materials include practical tips on using technology to assist in everyday living routines, particularly for older adults and chronic patients, as well as training materials to upskill the healthcare workforce and informal caregivers experienced in caring the targeted individuals [38]. Each thematic module features experiential learning, practical interactive group activities, face-to-face and online informative sessions, digital libraries of tools and technology resources for real-life experimentation, and guidelines for trainers to facilitate the training effectively (Fig. 2) [36, 37].

6.1.2 Main Outcomes

The main outcomes of these e-Training programs include increased awareness and skills in using mHealth solutions among the targeted populations. Multinational evaluation studies demonstrated the effectiveness of these programs in enhancing competencies for health self-management using digital tools. Primary end-users reported significant improvements in managing their health conditions with digital health technologies. On the other hand, healthcare professionals and informal caregivers reported overall positive impacts from the e-Training programs, including enhanced technology knowledge and better support for individuals [36, 37].

6.1.3 Lessons Learned

Several key lessons emerged from implementing these e-Training programs. The co-creation approach proved highly effective in customizing the programs to the specific needs of the targeted populations. Despite the positive initial outcomes, evaluations highlighted the need for ongoing improvements to the training tools. Future efforts should aim to extend training periods and involve larger participant groups to offer more comprehensive instruction and collect broader feedback [35, 37, 38]. Incorporating self-evaluation of both acquired knowledge and the training programs themselves is crucial for ensuring continuous improvement and relevance. Key recommendations include enhancing the e-Training platforms for better user experience and accessibility, and refining digital resources, especially interactive tools and gamified components of the training delivery, i.e., serious games to improve their effectiveness in building user confidence and engagement [37].

Table 1 summarizes the mHealth-AD (https://mhealth-ad.eu/), AD-Autonomy (http://ad-autonomy.eu/), and ERMAT (https://erasmus-ermat.eu/platform/el/)

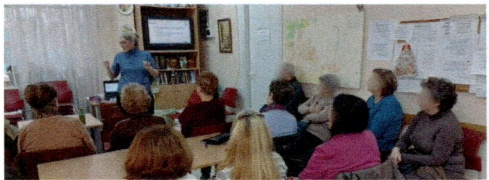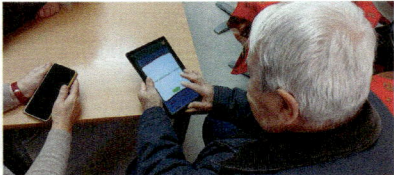

Fig. 2 Shots from E+ Training Programs to enhance digital health literacy (group sessions and experiential activities)

Table 1 Overview of the AD-AUTONOMY, ERMAT, mHealth-AD e-Training Programs

	AD-AUTONOMY	ERMAT	mHEALTH-AD
Primary targeted population	Older adults (over 65 years old) with early/mild dementia, mild cognitive impairment (MCI), initial stages of Alzheimer's disease	Older adults (over 65 years old) with reduced mobility	Older adults (over 65 years old) with early/mild dementia, mild cognitive impairment (MCI)
Other stakeholder groups	Informal caregivers, healthcare professionals from various disciplines	Informal caregivers, healthcare professionals from various disciplines	–
e-Training program (main components)	Open-access online platform, learning materials (handbook and reading resources), Experiential Learning (Hands-On) activities, train-the-trainers handbook	Open-access online platform, learning materials (handbook and reading resources), practical (hands-on) activities, train-the-trainers handbook	Open-access online platform, serious games, learning materials (handbook and reading resources), mHealth tools repository, train-the-trainers handbook
Mult-national study (Pilot Countries)	Greece, Slovenia, Spain, Turkey, UK	Croatia, Germany, Greece, Romania, Slovenia, Spain	Germany, Greece, Slovenia, Spain, Turkey
Number of participants in the study (per stakeholder group)	54 older adults with early/mild Dementia, mild cognitive impairment (MCI), 64 informal caregivers, 49 healthcare professionals	50 older adults with reduced mobility, 40 informal caregivers, 54 healthcare professionals	94 older adults with early/mild dementia, mild cognitive impairment (MCI)

e-Training Programs, funded by the Erasmus+ EU framework. The three initiatives represent significant steps toward integrating digital health solutions into the care and management of various conditions. These programs emphasize the importance of accessible, practical training for both the targeted populations and their caregivers, as well as healthcare professionals, ensuring that the benefits of digital health technologies are widely realized.

6.2　Designing the eCAN Training Program for Telemedicine in Cancer Care

The eCAN Joint Action (JA), funded by the European Union's HaDEA represents a transformative effort to reduce cancer care disparities within the European Union through the integration of telehealth and remote monitoring into healthcare systems. This initiative aims to bridge gaps in cancer care, especially during cross-border emergencies and health crises such as the COVID-19 pandemic. Central to this mission is a comprehensive training program designed to empower healthcare professionals, patients, and caregivers in utilizing telehealth technologies effectively. The following sections provide an in-depth overview of the training program's design, its outcomes, and the lessons learned from its development and implementation.

6.2.1 Program and Curriculum Design

The eCAN training program is designed as a self-paced online course, allowing participants to engage with the material over a flexible timeframe of 1 week. This format ensures that learners can progress at their own pace while adhering to a structured educational approach. The curriculum is organized into five modules, each addressing different aspects of telemedicine and remote care (Fig. 3). Notably, Modules 2, 3, and 4 are tailored to different stakeholder groups, including patients, caregivers, and healthcare professionals, ensuring that the content is relevant and applicable to each audience.

Module 1, "Introduction to Telehealth/Telecare" serves as the foundation of the program, providing all participants with an understanding of telehealth basics. It covers the definition, types, and technologies of telehealth services, such as real-time consultations and remote monitoring. This module includes a core presentation, comprehensive reading, and an interactive quiz to reinforce learning and self-assessment.

Module 2, "Building Trust in Telehealth" is divided into two parts: A) for patients and caregivers and B) for healthcare professionals. This module focuses on building and maintaining trust, as well as effective communication strategies in telehealth interactions. It is split in two parts, since it approaches effective communication, empathy, trust and reliability from either a patient and caregiver or a healthcare professional perspective. Both parts utilize case studies, reading materials, and simulated scenarios to practice trust-building strategies.

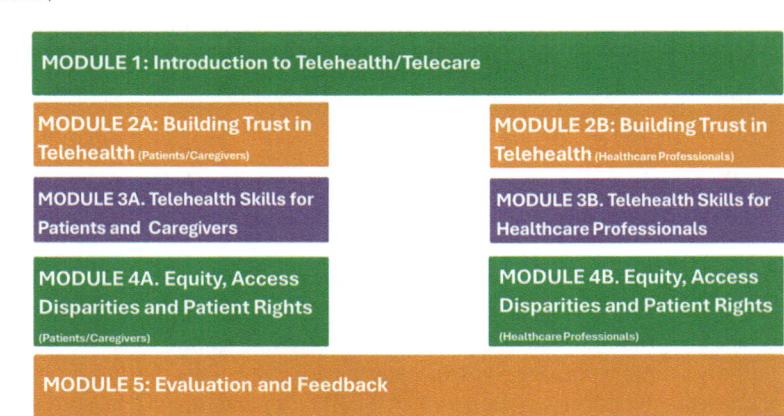

Fig. 3 Overview of the eCan Training Program Curriculum

Module 3, emphasizing "Telehealth Skills," is also divided into two parts, one for patients and caregivers and one for healthcare professionals. Materials developed for patients and caregivers equip them with practical and digital skills for using telehealth platforms, including setting up technology and preparing for appointments. Materials for healthcare professionals provide them with more advanced digital skills to effectively manage telehealth consultations, set-up a virtual appointment and address technical issues. Each part features tutorials, checklists, and interactive simulations, with the use of virtual patient scenarios to enhance practical knowledge and confidence.

Module 4, regarding "Equity, Access Disparities and Patient Rights in Telehealth" is similarly divided in two parts—one for patients and caregivers and one for healthcare professional. Both of them focus on telehealth as a driver for health equity, also promoting a common understanding of patient and clinicians' rights and responsibilities, as well as privacy, and advocacy within the telehealth context. This module includes lectures, detailed reading materials, and simulated scenarios to practice knowledge application and empower both clinicians and patients.

Finally, **Module 5 comprises the "Evaluation and Feedback,"** concluding the training program by assessing its effectiveness and gathering participant feedback. This module uses an online survey to evaluate the training content, delivery, and overall satisfaction and participants readiness to adopt telehealth, providing valuable insights for continuous improvement.

6.2.2   Methodological Approach

The curriculum design for the eCAN training program was meticulously shaped by an initial thorough needs assessment and gap analysis, combined with a review of existing literature and best practices. This comprehensive process identified the specific needs of various stakeholder groups, ensuring that the curriculum effectively addresses these needs. The integration of feedback from a co-validation workshop with technology experts, healthcare providers, and patient representatives further refined the curriculum, enhancing its relevance and applicability.

The rigorous approach to developing the eCAN training program ensured that the curriculum was not only tailored to the distinct needs of each stakeholder group but also actionable and impactful. By integrating insights from a thorough needs assessment, gap analysis, and literature review, the program effectively addressed real-world challenges and advanced telehealth practices in cancer care. The iterative refinement process, bolstered by feedback from a co-validation workshop with technology experts, healthcare providers, and patient representatives, confirmed that the curriculum is both practical and directly aligned with the needs of its intended audience. This comprehensive and adaptive approach has been crucial in creating relevant and effective content, demonstrating the importance of aligning training programs with stakeholder-specific needs and practical feedback.

Table 2 highlights that while all stakeholder groups share similar thematic needs, the intensity of these needs varies, which informed the tailored design of the curriculum to address each group's specific requirements effectively.

Table 2 Identified training needs and weighted interest per eCan stakeholder group

	Patients	Caregivers	Healthcare professionals
Knowledge and Understanding of Telehealth	XXX	XXX	X
Building Trust in Telehealth	XXX	XXX	XX
Telehealth (Digital) Skills	XXX	XXX	XX
Effective Communication and Empathy	XX	X	XXX
Security, Safety and Rights	XXX	X	XXX

Moreover, the flexibility of the self-paced learning format has been beneficial, allowing participants to engage with the material at their own pace. However, it requires careful structuring to ensure that participants remained on track and achieved the learning objectives. Moreover, incorporating interactive elements such as simulations and quizzes is essential for bridging the gap between theoretical knowledge and practical application. These components enhance the overall effectiveness of the training and helped participants apply what they had learned in real-world scenarios.

Finally, the dedicated module for feedback collection from participants has been invaluable for continuous improvement. The training program's ability to adapt based on user feedback ensures that it remains relevant and effective in meeting the evolving needs of its users.

7   Future Directions in Telehealth Training

The future of telehealth training is poised for significant enhancement through advancements in technology and broader training scopes. Emerging technologies and innovative training methods promise to make telehealth training more interactive, personalized, and effective [39].

The integration of advanced technologies (virtual reality, augmented reality) will greatly enrich the training experience. Interactive and immersive training tools will enable healthcare professionals to practice and refine their skills in realistic settings, bridging the gap between theory and practical application. Similarly, intuitive learning aids will simplify the process for patients and caregivers, making it easier for them to understand and use telehealth technologies [40].

Artificial intelligence (AI) is also transforming training by offering personalized learning experiences. AI-driven platforms can adapt to individual performance and learning styles, providing tailored content and feedback. This personalization helps both healthcare professionals and patients overcome specific challenges and enhances the overall effectiveness of the training program [41].

As healthcare continues to evolve toward integrated care models, interdisciplinary training becomes increasingly vital. Programs that include various healthcare disciplines—such as primary care, specialty care, mental health, and social services—promote effective collaboration and improve patient outcomes through coordinated care [15].

Global training initiatives offer additional opportunities for knowledge sharing and standardization. By participating in international collaborations, healthcare professionals can exchange best practices and innovative strategies, contributing to the development of standardized protocols and ensuring consistent quality in telehealth training programs worldwide.

8   Conclusion and Discussion

Telehealth has emerged as a transformative force in healthcare, driven by the necessity to maintain healthcare delivery during the COVID-19 pandemic. By enabling remote consultations and minimizing the need for in-person visits, telehealth has ensured continuity of care, protected healthcare workers and patients, and expanded access to services, particularly in remote and underserved areas. This shift has highlighted telehealth's critical role in addressing chronic shortages of healthcare providers and promoting equitable access to care.

Effective training is essential for optimizing the use of telehealth. Healthcare professionals need to acquire skills to use telehealth technologies proficiently, conduct thorough assessments, make accurate diagnoses, and ensure patient data security. Similarly, patients need training to navigate telehealth platforms confidently, report symptoms accurately, and engage actively in their care. Such training improves care delivery, enhances patient outcomes, and expands healthcare accessibility.

Despite its advantages, telehealth presents challenges, including technology literacy barriers, the need for effective communication in virtual settings, and ensuring data security and privacy. Addressing these challenges through targeted training programs can enhance the effectiveness and equity of telehealth services. By identifying and mitigating these obstacles, healthcare providers can ensure the continued successful implementation and expansion of telehealth.

Investing in comprehensive training will not only improve the proficiency of healthcare professionals and patients in using telehealth but also enhance the overall quality of care. Training programs should be adaptive, incorporating feedback and evolving to meet the changing landscape of healthcare technologies. By prioritizing education and skill development, healthcare systems can ensure that telehealth remains a vital and effective component of healthcare delivery, ultimately providing high-quality, equitable healthcare services to all populations.

References

1. Hincapié MA, et al. Implementation and usefulness of telemedicine during the COVID-19 pandemic: a scoping review. J Prim Care Community Health. 2020;11:215013272098061. https://doi.org/10.1177/2150132720980612.
2. Tajan N, Devès M, Potier R. Tele-psychotherapy during the COVID-19 pandemic: a mini-review. Front Psych. 2023;14 https://doi.org/10.3389/fpsyt.2023.1060961.

3. Wetzlmair L, et al. Teleconsultation in health and social care professions education: a systematic review. Clin Teach. 2022;19(5):e13519. https://doi.org/10.1111/tct.13519.
4. De Simone S, et al. Implementations and strategies of telehealth during COVID-19 outbreak: a systematic review. BMC Health Serv Res. 2022;22(1) https://doi.org/10.1186/s12913-022-08235-4.
5. Yu S, et al. Transformation of chronic disease management: before and after the COVID-19 outbreak. Front Public Health. 2023;11 https://doi.org/10.3389/fpubh.2023.1074364.
6. Zandi D, Kuzmanovic A. Global strategy on digital health 2020–2025. 2021. https://www.who.int/docs/default-source/documents/gs4dhdaa2a9f352b0445bafbc79ca799dce4d.pdf.
7. WHO-ITU global standard for accessibility of telehealth services. Geneva: World Health Organization and International Telecommunication Union, 2022. https://www.who.int/publications/i/item/9789240050464.
8. Tuot DS, Boulware LE. Telehealth applications to enhance CKD knowledge and awareness among patients and providers. Adv Chronic Kidney Dis. 2017;24(1):39–45. https://doi.org/10.1053/j.ackd.2016.11.017.
9. Ramachandran M, et al. The impact of eHealth on relationships and trust in primary care: a review of reviews. BMC Primary Care. 2023;24(1) https://doi.org/10.1186/s12875-023-02176-5.
10. Gonçalves RL, et al. Usability of telehealth systems for noncommunicable diseases in primary Care from the COVID-19 pandemic onward: Systematic review. J Med Internet Res. 2023;25:e44209. https://doi.org/10.2196/44209.
11. Rutledge C, et al. Telehealth and eHealth in nurse practitioner training: current perspectives. Adv Med Educ Pract. 2017;8:399–409. https://doi.org/10.2147/amep.s116071.
12. Pourmand A, et al. Lack of telemedicine training in academic medicine: Are we preparing the next generation? Telemed J E Health. 2021;27(1):62–7. https://doi.org/10.1089/tmj.2019.0287.
13. Johnson AM, et al. A systematic review of the effectiveness of patient education through patient portals. JAMIA Open. 2023;6(1) https://doi.org/10.1093/jamiaopen/ooac085.
14. Miranda R, et al. Towards a framework for implementing remote patient monitoring from an integrated care perspective: a scoping review. Int J Health Policy Manag [Preprint]. https://doi.org/10.34172/ijhpm.2023.7299.
15. Pool MDO, et al. Review of digitalized patient education in cardiology: a future ahead? Cardiology. 2021;146(2):263–71. https://doi.org/10.1159/000512778.
16. Levin-Zamir D, Bertschi I. Media health literacy, eHealth literacy, and the role of the social environment in context. Int J Environ Res Public Health. 2018;15(8):1643. https://doi.org/10.3390/ijerph15081643.
17. Flodgren G, et al. Interactive telemedicine: effects on professional practice and health care outcomes. Cochrane Library. 2015;2016(12) https://doi.org/10.1002/14651858.cd002098.pub2.
18. Odendaal WA, et al. Health workers' perceptions and experiences of using mHealth technologies to deliver primary healthcare services: a qualitative evidence synthesis. Cochrane Library [Preprint]. 2020b; https://doi.org/10.1002/14651858.cd011942.pub2.
19. Risling T, et al. Evaluating patient empowerment in association with eHealth technology: scoping review. J Med Internet Res. 2017;19(9):e329. https://doi.org/10.2196/jmir.7809.
20. Vainauskienė V, Vaitkienė R. Enablers of patient knowledge empowerment for self-management of chronic disease: an integrative review. Int J Environ Res Public Health. 2021;18(5):2247. https://doi.org/10.3390/ijerph18052247.
21. Shaver J. The state of telehealth before and after the COVID-19 pandemic. Prim Care. 2022;49(4):517–30. https://doi.org/10.1016/j.pop.2022.04.002.
22. Brei BK, et al. Telehealth training during the COVID-19 Pandemic: a feasibility study of large group multiplatform telesimulation training. Telemed J E Health. 2021;27(10):1166–73. https://doi.org/10.1089/tmj.2020.0357.
23. González-Fraile E, et al. Remotely delivered information, training and support for informal caregivers of people with dementia. Cochrane Library. 2021;2021(1) https://doi.org/10.1002/14651858.cd006440.pub3.

24. Fitzpatrick PJ. Improving health literacy using the power of digital communications to achieve better health outcomes for patients and practitioners. Front Digit Health. 2023;5 https://doi.org/10.3389/fdgth.2023.1264780.
25. Wijesooriya NR, et al. COVID-19 and telehealth, education, and research adaptations. Paediatr Respir Rev. 2020;35:38–42. https://doi.org/10.1016/j.prrv.2020.06.009.
26. Ewart C, et al. Patient perspectives and experiences of remote consultations in people receiving kidney care: a scoping review. J Ren Care. 2022;48(3):143–53. https://doi.org/10.1111/jorc.12419.
27. Van Kessel R, et al. Mapping factors that affect the uptake of digital therapeutics within health systems: scoping review. J Med Internet Res. 2023;25:e48000. https://doi.org/10.2196/48000.
28. Campanozzi LL, et al. The role of digital literacy in achieving health equity in the third millennium society: a literature review. Front Public Health. 2023;11 https://doi.org/10.3389/fpubh.2023.1109323.
29. Beheshti L, et al. Telehealth in primary health care: a scoping review of the literature; 2022. https://www.ncbi.nlm.nih.gov/pmc/articles/PMC9013222/.
30. Jonnagaddala J, Godinho MA, Liaw S-T. From telehealth to virtual primary care in Australia? A rapid scoping review. Int J Med Inform. 2021;151:104470. https://doi.org/10.1016/j.ijmedinf.2021.104470.
31. Almathami HKY, Win KT, Vlahu-Gjorgievska E. Barriers and facilitators that influence telemedicine-based, real-time, online consultation at patients' homes: systematic literature review. J Med Internet Res. 2020;22(2):e16407. https://doi.org/10.2196/16407.
32. Faheem F, et al. Implementing virtual care in neurology—challenges and pitfalls. J Central Nerv Syst Disease. 2022;14:11795735221109097. https://doi.org/10.1177/11795735221109745.
33. Pang N-Q, et al. Telemedicine acceptance among older adult patients with cancer: Scoping review. J Med Internet Res. 2022;24(3):e28724. https://doi.org/10.2196/28724.
34. Serrano LP, et al. Benefits and challenges of remote patient monitoring as perceived by health care practitioners: a systematic review. Perm J. 2023;27(4):100–11. https://doi.org/10.7812/tpp/23.022.
35. Billis A, Mantziari D, Bamidis P. AD-autonomy: participatory design of an innovative training platform to support the autonomy of Alzheimer disease patients and their carers. Proceedings of the 3rd international conference on medical education informatics, MEI 2018; 2018.
36. Billis A, et al. Co-creation of an innovative vocational training platform to improve autonomy in the context of Alzheimer's disease. ebooks.iospress.nl [Preprint]; 2018. https://doi.org/10.3233/978-1-51499-880-8-309.
37. Karagianni M, et al. Enhancing the adoption of mobile health technologies by persons with mild dementia and their care network though an innovative training program. Proceedings of the 11th international conference on software development and technologies for enhancing accessibility and fighting info-exclusion; 2024. https://dsai.ws/2024/.
38. Mantziari, et al. Participatory design and validation of an innovative training program to maintain autonomy of older adults with Alzheimer's disease. OpenLivingLab Days 2019 Conference Proceedings; 2019.
39. Griffith B, et al. Frontline experiences of delivering remote mental health supports during the COVID-19 pandemic in Scotland: innovations, insights and lessons learned from mental health workers. Psychol Health Med. 2022;28(4):964–79. https://doi.org/10.1080/13548506.2022.2148698.
40. Dafli E, et al. Curricular integration of virtual patients: a unifying perspective of medical teachers and students. BMC Med Educ. 2019;19(1) https://doi.org/10.1186/s12909-019-1849-7.
41. Grunhut J, Marques O, Wyatt ATM. Needs, challenges, and applications of Artificial intelligence in medical education curriculum. JMIR Med Educ. 2022;8(2):e35587. https://doi.org/10.2196/35587.

Symptom Monitoring and Management Digital Platforms: Current Capabilities and Future Research and Clinical Practice Directions

Bridget Nicholson, Elizabeth A. Sloss, and Kathi Mooney

1   Introduction

The illness experience includes a range of symptom occurrences that profoundly impact patients' lives, including their physical and emotional well-being. Thus, symptom evaluation and management are essential components of patient care. Historically, evaluation occurs at clinic visits. This intermittent evaluation leads to episodic symptom care, missing the day-to day fluctuations and resulting in inadequate symptom care, suffering, deterioration, and urgent visits. This is compounded by the traditional approach to patient education for symptom self-management that provides instructions at clinic visits or through scheduled classes offering large amounts of information all at once without tailoring to the patient's current symptom experience. This places the onus on the patient to recall the information or retrieve educational materials and apply them when symptoms appear while at home. Recognizing these inadequacies, advances through digital monitoring technology have enabled new approaches to more systematically evaluate symptoms and tailor management of symptoms as they occur. In addition, technology-based systems are efficient, saving clinician time and are ideal to provide just-in-time automated coaching about self-management strategies. The focus of this chapter is to summarize the state of the science in digital patient symptom monitoring and management, describe monitoring goals, review features of available digital systems, identify issues in integration of systems into healthcare, and project future directions.

B. Nicholson · E. A. Sloss · K. Mooney (✉)
College of Nursing, University of Utah, Salt Lake City, UT, USA
e-mail: bridget.nicholson@nurs.utah.edu; liz.sloss@nurs.utah.edu; kathi.mooney@nurs.utah.edu

2   The Rise of Patient-Reported Outcomes (PROs)

Symptom management aims to keep patient symptom burden low and quality of life high. Patients' symptom experiences impact their health care utilization, quality of life, and functional status. One way to track and improve the symptom experience is by collecting patient-reported outcomes (PROs). PROs come directly from patients and describe their experience of a health condition, including the accompanying symptoms [1]. Early trials that used PRO surveys for symptom assessment revealed that high levels of symptom burden accompanied chronic disease, for example, cancer [2, 3]. Symptom assessments can be utilized at the population level to determine symptom outcomes associated with a disease and/or disease treatments, or they can be utilized at the individual patient level to tailor care to the individual patient experience. Initial studies described the trajectory of symptoms in the population through PRO collection using paper reporting before automated reporting was available. As science advanced, electronic patient reporting (ePRO) was identified as more accurate than paper reporting due to the recall window and systematic collection and documentation of symptom data through electronic or digital mechanisms [4]. As a result, PRO collection moved from pencil-based reporting to electronic kiosks and tablets at clinic visits to now the real-time digital integration of remote patient monitoring systems.

Over the last two decades, the application of both PROs and ePROs have increased significantly. While ePRO collection has been documented primarily within research environments, ePRO reporting systems are rapidly transitioning into real-world practice settings. Successful implementation requires understanding the necessary components of ePRO collection, the barriers and facilitators, as well as the benefit of obtaining key outcome measures.

3   PRO/ePRO Symptom Reporting

Regardless of the collection mechanisms, studies have highlighted the clinical importance of patients' rating of symptoms due to documented variations in the concordance of symptom burden between patient and provider, with clinicians consistently underestimating the severity of symptom distress [5]. Prior to PRO/ePRO collection, clinician visibility into patient reports was incomplete due discrete reporting windows of the symptom experience limited to clinic visits. The use of PROs and ePROs promotes optimal symptom control through frequent systematic tracking and more accurate capture of the symptom trajectory, leading to earlier intervention to reduce symptom burden [6–8]. Research evaluating PRO symptom management platforms has demonstrated lower symptom severity, improved quality of life, and better adherence to treatment regimes, which can result in increased survival length [9, 10].

3.1   ePRO Measures

When considering the collection of ePRO symptom reporting, it is imperative to critically assess the goals and outcome measures for reporting. Depending on the goal to capture population level outcomes or for individual patient care, appropriate measures should be chosen to collect the necessary symptoms to accomplish the overarching purpose. For example, in the cancer research environment, multiple measures have been used to report clinical symptoms, for example, the Edmonton Symptom Assessment Scale (ESAS) [7, 11]; Patient Reported Outcome version of the Common Terminology Criteria for Adverse Events (PRO-CTAE) [12]; and quality of life scales such as Functional Assessment of Cancer Therapy (FACT-G). In addition to cancer, the Patient Reported Outcomes Measurement Information System (PROMIS) scales have been used to evaluate quality of life in cardiology patients [13]. Scales such as the self-assigned New York Heart Association Class of Heart Failure (SA-NYHA) and Kansas City Cardiomyopathy Questionnaire (KCCQ) are PRO symptom-focused assessments that have also been used to evaluate patient symptom burden [14]. While these are examples of validated measures, the choice of scales should reflect the goal of the symptom management program. Choices should be examined by symptoms covered, appropriateness for the disease state, and pragmatic considerations such as scale length and patient reporting burden or complexity of scoring for clinician interpretation. For example, an important consideration for clinicians is whether the chosen measure is granular enough to show specific symptom concerns that require clinical intervention. Global scales or scales with unique scoring approaches may be more suited for population level outcomes. In contrast, pragmatic measures that track on common clinical measurement of symptoms such as 1–10 scales or mild, moderate, and severe scoring may be better suited for clinical care due to patient and clinician familiarity with this type of scaling. How ePRO data is presented to clinicians is an important consideration in gaining clinician use and subsequent action. Patients must also find the reporting easy to do and not unduly burdensome, thus asking patients to compete a battery of individual symptom scales is not practical.

3.2   Frequency of Reporting

Besides the measure selected, a second consideration is the frequency of ePRO reporting and alignment with the anticipated symptom trajectory and collection goals. Initially, ePRO assessment occurred immediately before or at clinic visits to inform clinicians and maximize patient-provider interaction. However, clinic visits are often timed when symptom burden is lower; for example, in cancer, treatment toxicity has lessened before the next treatment cycle. Thus, the actual symptom trajectory is missed. While periodic assessments, weekly or at visits, are standard measurement frequencies, evidence supports more frequent symptom collection, including daily, particularly during active treatment when patients are not in direct contact with providers between visits [15, 16]. While concern exists about the potential burden of frequent patient reporting, patients are willing to report frequently if clinicians are responsive to their reports when poorly controlled symptoms are present. Patients comment that symptom reporting helps them feel connected to their clinical team between visits and adds a sense of security in managing their care at home [17].

3.3   Modality of Reporting of Symptom Rating

Multiple approaches currently exist that can be used to collect patient-generated data, including PROs. In initial symptom studies, patients have reported symptoms before provider visits via email, clinic computer tablets, or kiosks [9, 18]. Other studies utilized interactive voice response (IVR), a phone-based reporting mechanism that does not require the internet since transmission occurs through telephone lines and can be done easily at home [7, 19]. Digital PROs can be collected from multiple mechanisms, such as web-based applications, email, text platforms, or interactive voice recordings to document patient symptom reports. Providing patients multiple ways to access the system and report ePROs increases access and should be considered. Across collection methods, the goal of the patient symptom reporting and assessment remains the same and has been proven effective.

3.4   Equity Considerations and ePRO Platforms

While the use of digital technologies to improve symptom outcomes offers a systematic and efficient approach that has been shown to significantly lower disease and treatment-related symptom burden, digital technology approaches have been criticized for potentially extending inequities that relate to barriers for those with low technology literacy and Internet access. Therefore technology-delivered interventions must address distributive justice concepts of access, reach, and skills needed to engage the technology. While these are not often addressed in research reports, a recent assessment demonstrated that technology-delivered interventions, particularly IVR applications that do not require Internet access, reduced symptom burden for everyone regardless of age, race, and income, and, the improvement was highest for racial minorities and low-income individuals [17]. Further exploration of equitable distribution of access and benefit to digital symptom platforms is warranted.

4   Mobile Health

Thus far we have focused on patient-reported data, however, another growing facet of patient monitoring is remote biometric monitoring. *Mobile health* is a broader category that describes these digital tools that collect patient-generated health data

(PGHD), including ePROs but also passively generated biometric data from sensors or wearables that provide intermittent or continuous monitoring transmitted to centralized telehealth dashboards [20]. PROs, combined with other patient-generated health data monitoring objective physical data holds promise to improve the management of symptoms across the care continuum.

4.1   Sensor-Based Monitoring

Digital sensors include non-invasive commercial and medical-grade sensors to report patient symptoms [21]. Commercial-grade sensors include physical activity trackers, such as Garmin®. Medical-grade sensors, which some governments regulate such as the U.S. Food and Drug Administration (FDA) in the USA, monitor patient-generated data including but not limited to vital signs, respiratory rate, oxygenation, heart rate and rhythm, heart rate variability, sleep, positioning (for fall detection), and step count [21]. Medical-grade sensors typically involve a user platform or tablet with which the provider can visualize patient data and respond to patient changes. Many commercial-grade sensors and medical-grade sensors can provide direct visualization to the patient for personal health tracking.

The explosion of sensor technology to record patient biometrics has led to applications in certain disease states, such as detecting heart failure symptoms for patients at home [22]. Similarly, for cancer, passively collected measures such as step count, skin temperature monitoring, and evaluation for dehydration while patients are at home may lead to earlier identification of impending acute episodes. Combined data collection of ePRO and sensor biometric data may overcome the disparity in severity reporting of symptoms between clinicians and patients [23] and identify signs of increasing symptoms in a more timely manner [24].

Objective data measures are appealing for integration into care due to long periods between clinical visits, rapid changes in symptoms, variability in patient ePRO reporting behavior and the ability to detect symptom changes before the patient senses them. Studies to establish risk prediction for symptom deterioration are rapidly advancing and have been aided by the use of AI, machine learning methods. One example in cancer is the biometric measurement utilized to understand the relationship between declining step count and symptom burden [25]. Decreased step count has been linked to symptom burden and downstream outcomes such as lower performance status, hospitalization risk, and survival [26]. Step count as a biometric marker may provide direct insight into the patient's increasing symptom burden and anticipate downstream markers of declining treatment tolerance and changes in performance status. Combined sensor and ePRO monitoring for determining early dehydration risk in head and neck cancer patients demonstrated feasibility and acceptability for both patients and clinicians [27]. In addition, investigators found that decreased weight, blood pressure, and increased pulse, combined with ePRO reporting, predicted early dehydration [28]. In the future, systems such as these will become an integral part of care so that symptoms changes are detected much earlier and acute escalations are prevented.

Another mechanism for early detection of symptoms is monitoring febrile neutropenia with skin sensors to predict temperature changes and is particularly useful for the early detection of neutropenic fever [29]. While concerns exist about the reliability and specificity of fever detection [29], some reports have indicated the detection of fever is possible hours prior to patients sensing fever symptoms [30]. While additional studies are needed prior to integration in real-world clinical settings, in the future, early detection systems will transform symptom care.

Integrated medical-grade sensor platforms to monitor symptom changes in acute and subacute patients are common in care delivery for health systems seeking to move care from acute care facilities to care at home, such as hospital-at-home or virtual wards programs. Hospital at home programs promise to improve patient quality of life by allowing patients to remain at home through the use of technology alongside rigorous clinical care. Study findings show that use of the combination of biometric remote monitoring paired with home-based clinical care can allow patients to be safely treated at home rather than through traditional hospitalization [31, 32]. In the United Kingdom, delivery of inpatient level care at home coined "virtual wards" underwent rapid growth during the COVID-19 pandemic providing remote monitoring without face-to-face clinical care [32]. The integration of sensor-based programs to rapidly respond to patients' symptom changes will continue to evolve as technology becomes increasingly available, creating new models of care after continued testing in subpopulations to ensure effective and tailored use.

Multiple research and clinical applications of sensor-based evaluation of symptoms are currently under study. These applications hold great promise for increasing responsiveness to patient symptom burden. Many use case applications are currently in feasibility and acceptability testing. Propelling this work forward will necessitate large-scale clinical trials, with attention to user-centered design and rigorous data analysis to help understand the optimal clinical applications and contribution to value-based care models. Incorporating artificial intelligence methods into these studies so risk profiles for earlier detection are established will further advance the field.

4.2   Telehealth

Telehealth is defined as the "use of electronic information and telecommunications technologies to support long-distance clinical healthcare patient and professional health-related education" [33]. However, telehealth is often pragmatically more narrowly considered the synchronous exchange of medical information between providers and patients in a remote virtual visit. It encompasses the digital monitoring of patient symptoms and the technologies and interactions necessary for remote healthcare provider responses [33]. Mobile health monitoring can occur with or without the capacity for a telehealth virtual visit.

Telehealth underwent explosive growth during the COVID-19 pandemic. Unfortunately, telehealth utilization has decreased overall, for example, in the USA, Medicare reported that 25% of patients eligible for telehealth visits utilized the service in 2023, down from 48% at the height of the COVID-19 pandemic [34].

Telehealth (including virtual visits and phone calls) can continue to be a mechanism to monitor symptoms in routine, chronic, and acute reporting but need continued clinician incentives and an appropriate level of reimbursement to be viable. Many programs have integrated telehealth to provide follow-up for reported patient symptoms, across disease types. One novel program has delivered entirely virtual provider visits for patients undergoing radiation therapy for their cancer diagnoses with similar clinical efficacy [35]. A recent systematic review of synchronous teleconsultation among patients with Type 2 diabetes mellitus resulted in a greater hemoglobin A1c decrease when compared to usual care [36]. Virtual telehealth visits can continue to provide symptom management and be integrated with ePRO and sensor-based monitoring platforms providing a comprehensive and efficient approach to supportive care that is patient-centric and accessible.

Mobile applications have been developed and are primarily used on patient smartphones to report symptoms [37]. The advantages of these mobile platforms include the ability to respond to patient symptoms securely and the integration of the platform into the electronic health record (EHR) to facilitate communication and response by clinicians. Mobile platforms may require downloading the application, which can be burdensome or create barriers for patients with less technical skills. Direct texting platforms that deliver ePRO survey text directly to patients are increasingly being used as a response to decrease technology burden on patients. However, texting platforms have security concerns that must be diligently addressed. Ultimately, transitioning to using patient-facing EHR portals decreases the security risk for patients and providers. Though patient portal engagement in the cancer population is increasing, efforts to facilitate patient use and decrease the burden should persist. When choosing a successful platform to report data, balancing patient confidentiality and ease of patient and provider integration are concerns. Consideration of these factors are key to maintain high patient engagement levels across populations. Since ePRO and sensor monitoring are relatively new in health care, both patients and clinicians need to embrace this technology innovation into their daily routines, seeing it as a normal part of health care communication and delivery. Additional research that focuses on best practices for engagement and adoption will be important to successful integration in routine clinical care [also refer to chapter on Telemonitoring and Teleconsultation in Cancer Care].

5 ePRO Platforms That Combine ePRO Assessment with Automated Patient Self-Management

In addition to facilitating the sharing of patient-reported data to clinicians, PRO/ePRO systems can also offer automated just-in-time self-management coaching for patients. Self-management refers to an individual's ability to manage symptoms, and self-management support often includes educational and supportive interventions that facilitate knowledge and skill acquisition and boost patients' confidence in managing their health problems [38, 39]. Automated delivery through ePRO platforms improves on current approaches by delivering the right self-management information based on the symptom report at the time the patient needs to take action with self-management. Ideally this delivery is seamless and does not require extra steps for the patient like clicking on a link and pulling up the correct information. Research shows that digital self-management support tools effectively improve the quality of life among patients with cancer [38].

Similar to ePRO platforms, digital self-management support tools are available across platforms and delivered through various modalities, including an interactive voice response (IVR) system, mobile application, and website [7, 40–42]. However, not all ePRO platforms include a self-management support component. A review of the literature that was published in 2019 found that only 17 of 41 (41%) ePRO systems provided the patient with information about their cancer treatment and side effects, and fewer (12 of 41, or 9%) provided patients with automated advice or guidance based on their reported symptoms [43]. Evidence suggests that ePRO systems with self-management support components result in improved patient outcomes, including lower symptom burden [7] and faster return to normal activity following surgery [44].

The content and method of self-management information delivery to patients varies across ePRO systems. For example, OncoKompas is a web-based, behavioral symptom management application developed in the Netherlands that automatically provides patients with cancer tailored information specific to reported symptoms through reasoning pathways [39, 45]. eSyM is another oncology electronic symptom management platform developed by a United States team that provides links to over 70 open-source symptom management tip sheets for symptoms that patients report [42]. All tip sheets contain four components: (1) self-management strategies that patients can do on their own, (2) over-the-counter medications, (3) strategies that can be implemented with the help of the patient's care team, and (4) when the patient should call their care team [42].

Self-management support tools have been shown to be feasible and acceptable and are generally well-liked by patients [40, 41]. In addition to satisfaction with tailored symptom support, patients report feelings of empowerment and reduced isolation [17, 40]. However, evidence on the use of self-management support tools on clinical outcomes is mixed [45, 46]. While studies show very positive impact on symptom burden and quality of life, a few studies have found no difference between intervention and control groups [46, 47]. This may be due to the effectiveness of the self-management content as opposed to the automated delivery and requires further study. In addition, effectiveness of self-management tools has been linked to self-efficacy [39], suggesting that subsets of populations may experience different benefits. For example, evaluation of the Oncokompas platform found that those with lower self-efficacy but higher personal control and health literacy obtained higher benefit [46]. In the future, automated delivery of self-management coaching may become more sophisticated through AI, machine learning techniques to tailor content to the learning style and preferences of individual patients.

6   Clinician Use of ePRO for Symptom Management

Since many ePRO platforms are multicomponent and include assessment, self-management coaching, and clinician alerts, it is difficult to determine if all components contribute to symptom improvement. One study utilizing the U.S. developed Symptom Care at Home platform, evaluated the efficacy of ePRO system components and found that while self-management support alone showed no statistically significant difference between component groups, self-management support combined with alert notification and clinician follow-up resulted in the greatest reduction in symptom burden [48]. In this example, ePRO collection combined with automated self-management coaching and clinician follow-up may enhance the personalized and tailored response to better meet a patient's individualized needs. The combination might also offer a two-pronged, synergistic approach where clinicians decrease moderate to severe symptoms and self-management coaching assists the patient to maintain symptoms at mild levels or eliminates them entirely [7].

Reporting of ePRO to clinicians at in-person visits has focused primarily on providing clinicians with additional information regarding symptoms occurring around the time of the visit. Increasingly, platforms offer more distributive escalation to clinical teams, particularly for high-level symptoms. Alerts are generated when symptom severity reaches a preset threshold, prompting clinician response. Alert triggers range from simple symptom levels (e.g., severe pain) to complex algorithms, including artificial intelligence (AI) or machine learning (ML)-based, that take into account previous patient-reported symptom data and detect pattern changes over time.

Clinicians assigned to respond to symptom alerts vary by discipline and level of education. Studies have utilized centralized nurse-led synchronous telehealth to respond, and this real-time follow-up has demonstrated significant symptom improvement [7, 10, 49]. Patients report high satisfaction when clinicians respond to their symptoms. Other platforms send symptom results to the patient's clinical team with integration of reports into the clinical workflow. Concerns exist that current levels of staffing and patient volumes receiving in-clinic visits may limit the ability for a timely response to home-based electronic patient reports and thereby decrease the effectiveness of this strategy. Besides the development of ePRO and remote sensor monitoring systems, their integration into clinical care requires implementation science studies to enhance adoption.

7   Integration into Clinical Care

There is broad consensus that implementing ePROs into routine care is feasible [50, 51]. The collection of ePRO has been validated across multiple studies at various sites and geographic locations, but there has been limited large-scale implementation into clinical practice. One example of real-world integration is the Cancer Care

Canada system. Cancer Care Canada has been collecting the ePRO since 2007, utilizing both the Edmonton Symptom Assessment Revised (ESAS-r) and, more recently, collecting performance status measures using the Eastern Cooperative Oncology Group (ECOG) [11]. The collection of ESAS-r across thousands of Canadian patients provide significant population level insights into patient burden and management techniques [11]. From this work, recommendations for criteria for selecting ePRO measures for monitoring symptoms have been developed [52]. Additionally, the National Cancer Institute recommends collecting specific, common oncology symptoms via an electronic platform [53].

Despite the confirmed consensus on benefit and feasibility of ePRO systems, the implementation and outcomes related to ePRO symptom management systems in real-world clinical settings have been mixed. There is some evidence that ePRO symptom management system implementation positively impacts clinical outcomes, for example, lower rates of treatment discontinuation [54] and fewer visits for problematic symptoms [55] among patients with cancer. Other studies find, however, that there were no changes in clinical outcomes pre- and post-implementation [47, 56]. Continued implementation and outcome evaluations should occur to ascertain the optimal integration and utilization of ePRO digital tools into routine care.

7.1   Barriers to Implementation

Barriers to ePRO implementation exist at all levels, from patient- and clinician-facing to health system organizations. Common patient-facing barriers to implementation include patient engagement, lack of reminders or prompts for missed reports, and the integration with the patient-facing electronic portal [51, 56, 57]. Though patients generally have moderate reporting adherence when using an ePRO system, strategies specific to patient uptake and engagement include having a technology navigator or clinician explain the ePRO system for symptom management to the patient and using patient nudges (reminders) in establishing reporting routines [39]. Best practices for patient engagement and long-term use need to be established.

Clinician-facing barriers include increased workload or work burden, lack of ePRO integration into clinical workflow and clinician valuing additional approaches to achieve symptom reduction [51, 56]. In the initial study of the digital system, Symptom Care at Home, we reported no benefit in decreasing symptom burden due to a lack of clinician response to moderate or severe symptoms, emphasizing the importance of both clinician incentives to respond to patient reports and the need to better integrate ePRO symptom management system components into the workflow [58]. Lack of integration with the electronic health record (EHR) is a significant barrier at both individual and organizational levels. In 2014, in the USA, only 40% of ePRO systems were integrated with an EHR [59], though the integration of ePRO systems into the EHR is improving due to enhanced interoperability standards such as HL7 and Fast Healthcare Interoperability Resources (FHIR) in countries where this standard is adopted. A recent international scoping survey found that clinicians who work in facilities with PRO infrastructure, or have standing operating procedures regarding the collection of PROs, were less likely to perceive barriers to implementation [60].

7.2   Facilitators to Implementation

Lack of integration is a significant barrier to ePRO implementation, and integration with an organization's EHR is an important facilitator. Along with having an integrated system, appropriate workflow development and ease of use are key contributors to successful implementation [39, 56]. To promote clinical use, ePRO systems should present symptom data to clinicians in a clinically actionable way and be fully integrated into their workflow [39]. Other facilitators include organizational and leadership support, adequate resources for implementation, feedback to clinicians on results or outcomes of ePRO use, and reinforcement of ePRO data collection as a tool for symptom management [39, 51, 56]. At a broader health system level, national guidelines that recommend or policies that provide incentives for ePRO integration through reimbursement could compel broader adoption of ePRO systems. For example, the U.S. Centers for Medicare and Medicaid Services (CMS) will require PRO monitoring in the updated Enhancing Oncology Model (EOM) for reimbursement [57].

7.3   Implementation Recommendations

Recommendations for implementing ePRO systems into routine care can generally be assigned to three stages: (1) pre-implementation, (2) implementation, and (3) post-implementation. During pre-implementation, it is important to identify, engage, seek feedback from and iterate with key end-users including patients, clinicians, and organizational leadership. Next steps include selecting the ePRO tool and/or measures, identifying the technical specifications for integration, analyzing existing workflow then developing integrated workflows, and building end-user engagement [50, 56, 61]. Outcome measures for implementation evaluation should be identified at this stage and followed post-implementation.

7.4   Implementation and Post-Implementation

The implementation stage should include ongoing training, support for, and engagement of all key interest groups. Recommendations include employing an iterative process with repeated evaluation and modification to processes and workflows [50]. This process continues into post-implementation, with ongoing evaluation of implementation outcomes and modifications to workflows as necessary.

8   Future Research and Clinical Practice Directions

Though we have seen rapid expansion of PRO collection and use over the last two decades, opportunities related to PROs and ePRO systems will continue to expand. Future opportunities in ePRO research and clinical practice span increased health promotion applications and broader chronic disease management. The broader implementation of ePRO systems stands to improve patient quality of life through stricter disease and symptom control, and improved responsiveness of the health care system. Care must be taken to correctly measure and respond to patient associated symptom burden to ensure real improvement in the lived experience of patients with chronic disease.

8.1   Expansion Beyond Cancer Treatment Populations

To date, PRO and ePRO systems for cancer have primarily focused on symptom management for patients actively receiving cancer treatment. Yet, advances in cancer treatment have resulted in increasing numbers of individuals living with cancer as a chronic condition that includes ongoing symptom burden. The development and implementation of ePRO systems for cancer survivorship is new and can continue to grow to support the increasing numbers of cancer survivors. Furthermore, with the increasing distribution of orally administered chemotherapeutic and immunotherapy agents as part of oncology treatment plans, remote patient monitoring becomes more important because of increased time between clinic visits and fewer in-person encounters with the clinical care team. This is an example for cancer but other chronic disease management should similarly examine applications for each phase and component of the disease spectrum.

ePRO symptom management systems are being used to alleviate symptom burden among patients with kidney disease, chronic obstructive pulmonary disease (COPD), and heart failure [62, 63]. In another instance, the impact of real-time monitoring using ePROs to prevent adverse events during care transitions is being evaluated [64]. More research is needed to establish clinical efficacy of ePRO use particularly when used in combination with sensor or other integrated patient-generated health data.

It is also important to consider patients for whom coming to the bricks and mortar of a health system is burdensome. Specialty care disease management is usually concentrated in population centers leaving rural residents to travel great distances to receive this care. Development of health care delivery systems that bridge this disparity is long overdue. Technology-based systems provide the bridge to overcome access barriers to specialty services, even at a distance, including specialized symptom care.

8.2   Leveraging AI

As integrating ePRO systems with self-management support continues to grow, there is an opportunity to build upon current system capabilities by leveraging

AI. These emerging analytic capabilities can be incorporated into both backend and patient-facing components of ePRO systems and self-management support tools. For example, machine learning has been and can continue to be used to predict personalized symptom trajectories, allowing for tailored monitoring and early detection so interventions can be applied earlier to prevent symptom escalations [65]. Additionally, chatbots that use generative AI rather than preset algorithms can be developed to assess and respond to patients' individualized symptom needs in real time.

8.3   Dissemination of ePRO Systems

To broaden the dissemination of ePRO systems worldwide, more attention is needed on the development of effective implementation strategies. In particular, governmental policies supporting PRO collection and incentivizing proactive symptom management among patient populations would support widespread adoption and sustainment of effective ePRO systems. Additionally, implementation questions remain: What are effective strategies to implement ePRO systems into routine care delivery while maintaining the fidelity of symptom management interventions? How can we reduce health disparities through improved access to and use of ePRO systems? How can we encourage patients and clinicians to remain engaged in daily symptom reporting and responding? As the field of PRO and ePRO systems advances along the translational continuum, these and other questions regarding equitable and optimal implementation of ePRO systems need to be addressed.

9   Conclusion

Historically symptom burden during disease treatment has been seen as unpleasant but of secondary importance to the primary goal to treat and where possible, cure disease. The emergence of technology innovations that facilitate sophisticated symptom monitoring and management approaches, provides the opportunity to change that perspective on symptom care from treating symptom escalations as needed through emergency department visits and rehospitalizations to ongoing monitoring of a patient's health status and intervening at the earliest indication of symptom deterioration facilitating high quality of life and physical and psychosocial well-being no matter the disease state.

Over the past 20 years, digital ePRO systems have been developed, evaluated, and found to be efficacious. Futher work is now needed to develop systems that not only monitor patient symptoms reports, but are comprehensive, providing timely and tailored reponses as symptoms emerge. Advances in remote sensor monitoring will provide additional approaches to ongoing assessment that lead to a paradigm shift to symptom prevention prior to patients even experiencing the detrimental effects of symptoms These technology-aided systems will revolutionize care delivery, permitting high-level symptom care that reaches patients no matter where they live while at the same time, being efficient and widely deployable. Thus advancing the development and clinical adoption of digital symptom monitoring and management systems into everyday clinical care processes is of upmost importance.

References

1. Cracchiolo JR, Arafat W, Atreja A, Bruckner L, Emamekhoo H, Heinrichs T, et al. Getting ready for real-world use of electronic patient-reported outcomes (ePROs) for patients with cancer: a National Comprehensive Cancer Network ePRO workgroup paper. Cancer. 2023;129(16):2441–9.
2. Fortner B, Baldwin S, Schwartzberg L, Houts AC. Validation of the cancer care monitor items for physical symptoms and treatment side effects using expert oncology nurse evaluation. J Pain Symptom Manag. 2006;31(3):207–14.
3. Henry DH, Viswanathan HN, Elkin EP, Traina S, Wade S, Cella D. Symptoms and treatment burden associated with cancer treatment: results from a cross-sectional national survey in the U.S. Support Care Cancer. 2008;16(7):791–801.
4. Dale O, Hagen KB. Despite technical problems personal digital assistants outperform pen and paper when collecting patient diary data. J Clin Epidemiol. 2007;60(1):8–17.
5. Falchook AD, Green R, Knowles ME, Amdur RJ, Mendenhall W, Hayes DN, et al. Comparison of patient- and practitioner-reported toxic effects associated with Chemoradiotherapy for head and neck cancer. JAMA Otolaryngol—Head Neck Surg. 2016;142(6):517–23.
6. Berry DL. Patient-reported symptoms and quality of life integrated into clinical cancer care. Semin Oncol Nurs. 2011;27(3):203–10.
7. Mooney KH, Beck SL, Wong B, Dunson W, Wujcik D, Whisenant M, et al. Automated home monitoring and management of patient-reported symptoms during chemotherapy: results of the symptom care at home RCT. Cancer Med. 2017;6(3):537–46.
8. Ruland CM, Holte HH, Roislien J, Heaven C, Hamilton GA, Kristiansen J, et al. Effects of a computer-supported interactive tailored patient assessment tool on patient care, symptom distress, and patients' need for symptom management support: a randomized clinical trial. J Am Med Inform Assoc. 2010;17(4):403–10.
9. Basch E, Deal AM, Dueck AC, Scher HI, Kris MG, Hudis C, et al. Overall survival results of a trial assessing patient-reported outcomes for symptom monitoring during routine cancer treatment. JAMA. 2017;318(2):197.
10. Basch E, Deal AM, Kris MG, Scher HI, Hudis CA, Sabbatini P, et al. Symptom monitoring with patient-reported outcomes during routine cancer treatment: a randomized controlled trial. J Clin Oncol. 2016;34(6):557–65.
11. Barbera L, Lee F, Sutradhar R. Use of patient-reported outcomes in regional cancer centres over time: a retrospective study. CMAJ Open. 2019;7(1):E101–8.
12. Basch E, Reeve BB, Mitchell SA, Clauser SB, Minasian LM, Dueck AC, et al. Development of the National Cancer Institute's patient-reported outcomes version of the common terminology criteria for adverse events (PRO-CTCAE). J Natl Cancer Inst. 2014;106(9):dju244.
13. Masterson Creber R, Spadaccio C, Dimagli A, Myers A, Taylor B, Fremes S. Patient-reported outcomes in cardiovascular trials. Can J Cardiol. 2021;37(9):1340–52.
14. Rothmund M, Pilz MJ, Egeter N, Lidington E, Piccinin C, Arraras JI, et al. Patient-reported outcome measures for emotional functioning in cancer patients: content comparison of the EORTC CAT Core, FACT-G, HADS, SF-36, PRO-CTCAE, and PROMIS instruments. Psychooncology. 2023;32(4):628–39.
15. Daly B, Nicholas K, Flynn J, Silva N, Panageas K, Mao JJ, et al. Analysis of a remote monitoring program for symptoms among adults with cancer receiving antineoplastic therapy. JAMA Netw Open. 2022;5(3):e221078.

16. Innominato PF, Komarzynski S, Dallmann R, Wreglesworth NI, Bouchahda M, Karaboué A, et al. Impact of assessment frequency of patient-reported outcomes: an observational study using an eHealth platform in cancer patients. Support Care Cancer. 2021;29(11):6167–70.

17. Mooney K, Beck SL, Wilson C, Coombs L, Whisenant M, Moraitis AM, et al. Assessing patient perspectives and the health equity of a digital cancer symptom remote monitoring and management system. JCO Clin Cancer Inform. 2024;8:e2300243.

18. Berry DL, Blumenstein BA, Halpenny B, Wolpin S, Fann JR, Austin-Seymour M, et al. Enhancing patient-provider communication with the electronic self-report assessment for cancer: a randomized trial. J Clin Oncol. 2011;29(8):1029–35.

19. Piette JD, Rosland AM, Marinec NS, Striplin D, Bernstein SJ, Silveira MJ. Engagement with automated patient monitoring and self-management support calls: experience with a thousand chronically ill patients. Med Care. 2013;51(3):216–23.

20. Dias D, Cunha PS, J. Wearable health devices—vital sign monitoring, systems and technologies. Sensors. 2018;18(8):2414.

21. Majumder S, Mondal T, Deen M. Wearable sensors for remote health monitoring. Sensors. 2017;17(1):130.

22. Stevenson LW, Ross HJ, Rathman LD, Boehmer JP. Remote monitoring for heart failure management at home. J Am Coll Cardiol. 2023;81(23):2272–91.

23. Xiao C, Polomano R, Bruner DW. Comparison between patient-reported and clinician-observed symptoms in oncology. Cancer Nurs. 2013;36(6):E1–16.

24. Taylor AE, Olver IN, Sivanthan T, Chi M, Purnell C. Observer error in grading performance status in cancer patients. Support Care Cancer Off J Multinatl Assoc Support Care Cancer. 1999;7(5):332–5.

25. Nicholson BL. Step count and symptom burden during cancer treatment. 2024 Jun 27; Lille, France.

26. Gresham G, Hendifar AE, Spiegel B, Neeman E, Tuli R, Rimel BJ, et al. Wearable activity monitors to assess performance status and predict clinical outcomes in advanced cancer patients. NPJ Digit Med. 2018;1:27.

27. Peterson SK, Shinn EH, Basen-Engquist K, Demark-Wahnefried W, Prokhorov AV, Baru C, et al. Identifying early dehydration risk with home-based sensors during radiation treatment: a feasibility study on patients with head and neck cancer. JNCI Monogr. 2013;2013(47):162–8.

28. Peterson SK, Shinn EH, Garden AS, Patrick K, Shete S, Shen C, et al. Identifying dehydration risk in head and neck cancer patients undergoing radiation therapy using remote, sensor-based monitoring: a randomized controlled trial. J Clin Oncol. 2016;34(3_suppl):152.

29. Verma N, Haji-Abolhassani I, Ganesh S, Vera-Aguilera J, Paludo J, Heitz R, et al. A novel wearable device for continuous temperature monitoring & fever detection. IEEE J Transl Eng Health Med. 2021;9:2700407.

30. Dambrosio N, Porter M, Bauer E, Levitan N, Liedtke D, De Lima M, et al. Identifying neutropenic fever earlier: an application of a skin patch for continuous temperature monitoring. Blood. 2018;132(Suppl 1):4713.

31. Nicholson B, Sloss EA, Fausett A, Davis C, Dumas K, Littledike M, et al. Rural access to the cancer hospital at home care model. NEJM Catal [Internet]. 2024;5(3) http://catalyst.nejm.org/doi/10.1056/CAT.23.0336

32. Shi C, Dumville J, Rubinstein F, Norman G, Ullah A, Bashir S, et al. Inpatient-level care at home delivered by virtual wards and hospital at home: a systematic review and meta-analysis of complex interventions and their components. BMC Med. 2024;22(1):145.

33. Official Website of The Office of the National Coordinator for Health Information Technology (ONC) [Internet]. 2024. https://www.healthit.gov/faq/what-telehealth-how-telehealth-different-telemedicine.

34. Data.CMS.gov[Internet].2024.https://data.cms.gov/summary-statistics-on-use-and-payments/medicare-service-type-reports/medicare-telehealth-trends.

35. Cuaron JJ, McBride S, Chino F, Parikh D, Kollmeier M, Pastrana G, et al. Patient safety and satisfaction with fully remote management of radiation oncology care. JAMA Netw Open. 2024;7(6):e2416570.

36. Zhang J, Ji X, Xie J, Lin K, Yao M, Chi C. Effectiveness of synchronous teleconsultation for patients with type 2 diabetes mellitus: a systematic review and meta-analysis. BMJ Open Diabetes Res Care. 2023;11(1):e003180.

37. Fjell M, Langius-Eklöf A, Nilsson M, Wengström Y, Sundberg K. Reduced symptom burden with the support of an interactive app during neoadjuvant chemotherapy for breast cancer—a randomized controlled trial. Breast. 2020;51:85–93.

38. Adriaans DJ, Dierick-van Daele AT, van Bakel MJHM, Nieuwenhuijzen GA, Teijink JA, Heesakkers FF, et al. Digital self-management support tools in the care plan of patients with cancer: review of randomized controlled trials. J Med Internet Res. 2021;23(6):e20861.

39. van den Hurk CJG, Mols F, Eicher M, Chan RJ, Becker A, Geleijnse G, et al. A narrative review on the collection and use of electronic patient-reported outcomes in cancer survivorship care with emphasis on symptom monitoring. Curr Oncol. 2022;29(6):4370–85.

40. Richards HS, Portal A, Absolom K, Blazeby JM, Velikova G, Avery KNL. Patient experiences of an electronic PRO tailored feedback system for symptom management following upper gastrointestinal cancer surgery. Qual Life Res. 2021;30(11):3229–39.

41. Avery KNL, Richards HS, Portal A, Reed T, Harding R, Carter R, et al. Developing a real-time electronic symptom monitoring system for patients after discharge following cancer-related surgery. BMC Cancer. 2019;19(1):463.

42. Schrag D, Osarogiagbon RU, Wong SL, Hazard H, Bian JJ, Dizon DS, et al. Development of self-management tip sheets for medical oncology and surgical patients electronically reporting symptoms in the home-care recovery setting. J Clin Oncol. 2020;38(29_suppl):299.

43. Warrington L, Absolom K, Conner M, Kellar I, Clayton B, Ayres M, et al. Electronic systems for patients to report and manage side effects of cancer treatment: systematic review. J Med Internet Res. 2019;21(1):e10875.

44. van der Meij E, Anema JR, Leclercq WKG, Bongers MY, Consten ECJ, Koops SES, et al. Personalised perioperative care by e-health after intermediate-grade abdominal surgery: a multicentre, single-blind, randomised, placebo-controlled trial. Lancet. 2018;392(10141):51–9.

45. van der Hout A, Holtmaat K, Jansen F, Lissenberg-Witte B, Van Uden-Kraan CF, Nieuwenhuijzen GAP, et al. The eHealth self-management application "Oncokompas" that supports cancer survivors to improve health-related quality of life and reduce symptoms: which groups benefit most? Acta Oncol. 2021;60(4):403–11.

46. Dirven L, Taphoorn MJB. Evaluating the lack of impact of the e-health application Oncokompas on outcomes in incurably ill cancer patients. Lancet Reg Health—Eur [Internet]. 2022;18. https://www.thelancet.com/journals/lanepe/article/PIIS2666-7762(22)00089-8/fulltext

47. Schuit AS, Holtmaat K, Lissenberg-Witte BI, Eerenstein SEJ, Zijlstra JM, Eeltink C, et al. Efficacy of the eHealth application Oncokompas, facilitating incurably ill cancer patients to self-manage their palliative care needs: a randomized controlled trial. Lancet Reg Health—Eur [Internet]. 2022;18:100390. https://www.thelancet.com/journals/lanepe/article/PIIS2666-7762(22)00083-7/fulltext

48. Mooney K, Gullatte M, Iacob E, Echeverria C, Brown K, Donaldson G. A randomized control trial to determine necessary intervention elements to achieve optimal symptom outcomes for a remote symptom management system. J Clin Oncol. 2022;40(16_suppl):12008.

49. Mooney K, Gullatte M, Iacob E, Alekhina N, Nicholson B, Sloss EA, Lloyd J, Moraitis AM, Donaldson G. Essential Elements of an Electronic Patient-Reported Cancer Symptom Monitoring and Management System. JAMA Network Open. 2024;7(9):e2433153. https://doi.org/10.1001/jamanetworkopen.2024.33153

50. Kwok C, Degen C, Moradi N, Stacey D. Nurse-led telehealth interventions for symptom management in patients with cancer receiving systemic or radiation therapy: a systematic review and meta-analysis. Support Care Cancer. 2022;30(9):7119–32.

51. Wintner LM, Sztankay M, Riedl D, Rumpold G, Nickels A, Licht T, et al. How to implement routine electronic patient-reported outcome monitoring in oncology rehabilitation. Int J Clin Pract. 2021;75(4):e13694.

52. Patt D, Wilfong L, Hudson KE, Patel A, Books H, Pearson B, et al. Implementation of electronic patient-reported outcomes for symptom monitoring in a large multisite community

oncology practice: dancing the Texas two-step through a pandemic. JCO Clin Cancer Inform. 2021;5:615–21.

53. The Cancer Care Ontario Patient Reported Outcome Advisory Committee, Montgomery N, Howell D, Ismail Z, Bartlett SJ, Brundage M, et al. Selecting, implementing and evaluating patient-reported outcome measures for routine clinical use in cancer: the Cancer Care Ontario approach. J Patient-Rep Outcomes. 2020;4(1):101.

54. Reeve BB, Mitchell SA, Dueck AC, Basch E, Cella D, Reilly CM, et al. Recommended patient-reported core set of symptoms to measure in adult cancer treatment trials. JNCI J Natl Cancer Inst. 2014;106(7):dju129.

55. Dickson NR, Beauchamp KD, Perry TS, Roush A, Goldschmidt D, Edwards ML, et al. Real-world use and clinical impact of an electronic patient-reported outcome tool in patients with solid tumors treated with immuno-oncology therapy. J Patient-Rep Outcomes. 2024;8(1):23.

56. Girgis A, Bamgboje-Ayodele A, Rincones O, Vinod SK, Avery S, Descallar J, et al. Stepping into the real world: a mixed-methods evaluation of the implementation of electronic patient reported outcomes in routine lung cancer care. J Patient-Rep Outcomes. 2022;6(1):70.

57. Generalova O, Roy M, Hall E, Shah SA, Cunanan K, Fardeen T, et al. Implementation of a cloud-based electronic patient-reported outcome (ePRO) platform in patients with advanced cancer. J Patient-Rep Outcomes. 2021;5(1):91.

58. Basch E, Rocque G, Mody G, Mullangi S, Patt D. Tenets for implementing electronic patient-reported outcomes for remote symptom monitoring during cancer treatment. JCO Clin Cancer Inform. 2023;7:e2200187.

59. Mooney KH, Beck SL, Friedman RH, Farzanfar R, Wong B. Automated monitoring of symptoms during ambulatory chemotherapy and oncology providers' use of the information: a randomized controlled clinical trial. Support Care Cancer Off J Multinatl Assoc Support Care Cancer. 2014;22(9):2343–50.

60. Jensen RE, Snyder CF, Abernethy AP, Basch E, Potosky AL, Roberts AC, et al. Review of electronic patient-reported outcomes systems used in cancer clinical care. J Oncol Pract. 2014;10(4):e215–22.

61. Eng L, Chan RJ, Chan A, Charalambous A, Darling HS, Grech L, et al. Perceived barriers toward patient-reported outcome implementation in cancer care: an international scoping survey. JCO Oncol Pract. 2024;20(6):816–26.

62. Group COS of A (COSA) PROW, Koczwara B, Bonnamy J, Briggs P, Brown B, Butow PN, et al. Patient-reported outcomes and personalised cancer care. Med J Aust. 2021;214(9):406–408.e1.

63. Tang E, Yantsis A, Ho M, Hussain J, Dano S, Aiyegbusi OL, et al. Patient-reported outcome measures for patients with CKD: the case for patient-reported outcomes measurement information system (PROMIS) tools. Am J Kidney Dis. 2024;83(4):508–18.

64. Erturkmen GBL, Juul NK, Redondo IE, Gil AO, Berastegui DV, de Manuel E, et al. Design, implementation and usability analysis of patient empowerment in ADLIFE project via patient reported outcome measures and shared decision making. BMC Med Inform Decis Mak. 2024;24(1):185.

65. Real-time symptom monitoring using ePROs to prevent adverse events during care transitions. Digital Healthcare Research [Internet]. [cited 2024 Jul 23]. https://digital.ahrq.gov/ahrq-funded-projects/real-time-symptom-monitoring-using-epros-prevent-adverse-events-during-care-transitions.

66. Bennett AV, Jensen RE, Basch E. Electronic patient-reported outcome systems in oncology clinical practice. CA Cancer J Clin. 2012;62(5):336–47.

Twenty-First Century Cancer Care: Follow the Data

Mark Lawler

1 Introduction: Nothing Makes Sense Except in the Light of Data

This chapter will address the critical importance of data (in all of its diverse forms)—in accelerating our understanding of cancer, its impact and its mitigation through the use, and more importantly the sharing of, multi-modal data, data tools and code;—in highlighting initiatives and approaches to measuring and codifying cancer inequalities and their origins;—in mitigating the impact of these inequalities on cancer patients and cancer systems;—and in deploying the intelligence that we garner from a variety of different data sources to inform and implement effective cancer policy.

We have entered a data-driven era (increasingly known as the digital health era) that is much more about the data, their collection, their evaluation, their interpretation and ultimately their deployment to enhance human health and well-being. From a cancer perspective, digital oncology approaches are enabling us to maximise the use, value and impact of retrospective information from the many pre-existing data collections that are often siloed and/or non-compatible, while it is also informing prospective data collection and their use. Establishing a more collaborative ethos that recognises and promotes the value of a cross-disciplinary culture, together with an approach that supports the collation, refinement and deployment of multi-modal data intelligence, have helped deliver a series of valuable new insights into the critical drivers involved in cancer development and progression and their potential mitigation.

M. Lawler (✉)
Patrick G Johnston Centre for Cancer Research, Queen's University Belfast, Belfast, UK

European Cancer Organisation, Brussels, Belgium
e-mail: mark.lawler@qub.ac.uk

While this chapter may to a certain degree emphasise a more European focus and ascertain what has been achieved across the European continent, the international perspective is also highlighted, as is the recognition that the intelligence as a community that we have gathered and used, the impact that we have achieved and the lessons that we have learned, can tangibly and effectively inform our responses to many of the global challenges of cancer.

2 Changing the Mindset: A Bottom-Up Approach to Data Sharing and Its Deployment

Back in 2011, a feature article appeared in the Wall Street Journal which highlighted a refreshingly new approach to performing scientific research that was gaining significant momentum and support at that time, and which reflected a change in ethos across the scientific and medical communities. The prescient article was entitled *"The New Einsteins Will Be Scientists Who Share,"* with an accompanying strapline *From cancer to cosmology, researchers could race ahead by working together— online and in the open.* The article described how an unprecedented change in the way in which scientists interacted with each other had started to develop, driven by a more outward looking culture that sought to replace the multiple siloed approaches that were the norm at the time by individual researchers to achieve scientific evidence and impact, with a much more collaborative and cross-disciplinary research ethos that valued a team-based approach. This "reformation" was particularly evident within and across the genomics and data sciences communities, where an innovative bottom-up approach underpinned the creation of an initiative that became known as the Global Alliance for Genomics and Health (GA4GH https://www.ga4gh.org), an exciting new venture which united researchers from around the world within a common aim and ambition to work more collaboratively together, including through cross-disciplinary linkages so that disciplines previously remote from each other now embraced a common collaborative ethos. Changing the mindset and adopting this collective approach facilitated the creation of a supercharged cooperative, with the ambition to grasp both the currently available and future opportunities to address some of the most significant challenges in human health that would benefit from a data-driven strategy.

The GA4GH Cancer Task Team, which I had the pleasure to co-lead, with my colleague Charles Sawyers from the Memorial Sloan Kettering Cancer Centre in New York, was particularly active and productive, breaking down the many silos that existed at the time. This more collaborative-style effort provided a distinct pathway to empower the cancer community to share data, code, and expertise for common benefit and the advancement of cancer research, while also providing insights for enhanced cancer care [1]. One of our early successes was the creation of a *"Framework for the Sharing of Health Related and Genomic Data,"* a framework which provided a common set of rules and processes that we would abide by to ensure responsible, ethical and effective sharing of data for the common good [2].

3   Cancer Data and Team Science: Driving a Culture Change

From a cancer perspective, a series of high impact papers have been published [1–3], culminating in the founding principle of a "Cancer Knowledge Network", which was articulated in a key "call to arms" paper published in the *New England Journal of Medicine*, with a determination and ambition to move from the previously more closed "selfish silo" mentality and ethos to a much more open collaborative culture [4]. A series of data analysis tools was created to support, enable and empower the cancer data research community, including a "Cancer Meta Knowledgebase", an innovative data "translator" (as we coined it), which captured together in a single location for the first time the knowledge on potential/actual mutations linked to a particular cancer. These data were aggregated into a single knowledgebase and, emphasising the collaborative culture principles of GA4GH, which was shared online for anyone to access freely, thus ensuring a more open "team science" approach that we felt would resonate strongly and more effectively with the global cancer research community [5].

3.1   Realising the Importance of Trust in the Use of Data: Embedding the Patient/Public Perspective

Critical to the use of data to better understand disease and enhance patient care is the importance of ensuring absolute public trust in the use of those data. As part of our evolving approach, we reached out across the cancer patient, cancer researcher and cancer professionals communities to bring together a so-called coalition of the willing and developed a consensus landscape statement on the trustworthy and effective use of data, which resonated well with all communities. In an accompanying paper in *The Lancet Oncology* [6], we recognised and articulated the central role of the public and patients as both "data donors" and equal partners. We established a blueprint that articulated the key approaches that ensure the safe, effective and trustworthy use of data.

In the UK, the focus on cancer data and its deployment gave rise to DATA-CAN, the UK's Health Data Research Hub for Cancer [7]. DATA-CAN is part of Health Data Research UK (HDR UK), the UK's health data science institute (https://www.hdruk.ac.uk). Emphasising the importance of working together for mutual benefit, DATA-CAN's key philosophy is one of Fair Value—whereby all stakeholders, whether they be patients, health services, academic researchers or industry all get fair value from the use of patient data—the principles of fair value are ones that we frequently articulate and uphold. Patients are embedded within DATA-CAN—they were co-applicants in the original funding bid, they sit as equal partners on all steering, management and project committees, and they are present for all discussions, including with those that take place with industry [7].

DATA-CAN's Patient and Public Involvement and Engagement (PPIE) activities have resulted in it widely being acknowledged as an exemplar of how to achieve effective, truly collaborative PPIE that respects the views of patients and the public [7]. This type of philosophy is best captured in the words of DATA-CAN's PPIE group member and breast cancer survivor Jacqui Gath—*"Patients want their data to be used to improve care and enhance research. In fact, they're often surprised it's not used already."* Jacqui's words are frequently echoed in the views of other patients, and as such need to be heard more clearly in the sometimes-challenging debate on data privacy and the secondary use of data for research. Data privacy and trust in the use of data must be balanced with the need to deploy data to help enhance human health and well-being [8]. During the COVID-19 pandemic, it was necessary to relax data privacy rules and simplify data access procedures, so as to effectively conduct more effective and timely research and innovation. Otherwise, we could not have readily accessed the vital data required to understand how COVID-19 worked and spread, so that we could have the relevant data to both inform development of COVID-19 diagnostic tests and vaccines, but also to test their accuracy (in terms of the diagnostic tests) and their efficacy (in terms of the vaccines). Cancer has regrettably killed many more people than COVID-19 and thus deserves due consideration to help balance both the debate and its consequences on data privacy and secondary data use.

4   How Data Intelligence Identified the Disastrous Impact of COVID-19 on Cancer Services and Cancer Patients

While the initial focus within DATA-CAN was to provide a more nuanced data-informed understanding of cancer, particularly in the UK, and deploy this data to enhance cancer diagnosis and cancer treatment, the onset of the COVID-19 pandemic and the introduction of national lockdowns caused us to pivot to address their collective impact on cancer services and cancer patients. In response to the pandemic and its potential impact on cancer services and cancer patients [9], a multi-institution study was established to collect cancer data from hospital trusts across the UK in near real-time to evaluate the impact of COVID-19 and national lockdowns on both the cancer diagnostic and treatment pathways. The results uncovered for the first time the disastrous impact of the COVID-19 pandemic on cancer patients and cancer services in the UK [10]. The data indicated that 7 out of 10 people with suspicion of cancer either did not attend cancer clinics or were not seen by cancer specialists; results for the cancer treatment pathway were also disturbing, with 4 out of 10 patients not receiving their chemotherapy at the right time [11]. These results were shared immediately (given their gravity) with the four Chief Medical Officers of the UK nations and contributed to a recalibration of the response to the COVID-19 pandemic from a cancer perspective. This body of work emphasised the significant negative impact on delays in 2-week wait times on cancer survival [12–14], highlighted the potential impact of Faecal Immunochemical Testing (FIT) to mitigate the impact of delays in the 2-week wait pathway in colorectal cancer [15] and emphasised the profound impact on endoscopies, with a 91% drop in endoscopies during the pandemic [16].

The UK data that had been generated were presented to WHO Europe and to the Board of the European Cancer Organisation (ECO), the largest multi-professional cancer organisation in Europe. On the basis of the data intelligence presented and its impact, ECO immediately established a Special Focussed Topic Network on COVID-19 and Cancer (https://www.europeancancer.org/topic-networks/impact-of-covid-19-on-cancer.html). As part of the Network's activities, a pan-European study was initiated to study the impact of the COVID-19 pandemic on cancer patients and cancer services Europe-wide. Key findings of the impact of the COVID-19 pandemic and national lockdowns included—100 Million (M) cancer screening tests were not performed;—1 M cancer diagnoses were missed;—there was a 50% reduction in both chemotherapy and surgical treatment; 4 out of 10 cancer health professionals were recognised as being burnt out, with 3 out of 10 showing signs of clinical depression [17, 18]. This intelligence led to the establishment of a data-informed Pan European Time To Act Campaign (https://www.european-cancer.org/timetoact), launched in the European Parliament by Health and Food Safety Commissioner Stella Kyriakides and subsequently launched in 12 individual countries in Europe. The Time to Act Campaign has been translated into 32 different languages, amplifying its message and the impact of COVID-19 on cancer across Europe (https://www.europeancancer.org/timetoact/impact/campaign.html) A Time To Act Data Navigator has been created, broadening the message and highlighting the data intelligence that informed the Time To Act Campaign and allowing the impact of COVID-19 on cancer to be captured and visualised in different countries, significantly informing cancer research and policy in those countries and Europe-wide https://www.europeancancer.org/timetoact/impact/building-back.html.

5   Addressing Inequalities in Cancer: The Critical Role of Data Intelligence

Capturing data on cancer inequalities is increasingly key to understanding the challenges that both patients and healthcare professionals face, providing the critical evidence to help inform the development of transparent and tangible solutions to address the cancer inequalities that are identified. World Cancer Day 2024 marked the tenth Anniversary of the European Cancer Patient's Bill of Rights, a patient-centred initiative that was launched through a partnership of patient advocates and healthcare professionals in the European Parliament or World Cancer Day 2014 [19]. One of the key drivers that led to the creation of the Bill of Rights was the most comprehensive analysis that had been undertaken at the time of cancer inequalities experienced by patients and healthcare systems across Europe [20]. This study provided the crucial data intelligence required to enable the co-creation of a series of rights that addressed the cancer care inequalities that had been revealed by this comprehensive data analysis.

The European Cancer Patient's Bill of Rights was widely seen as an enabling catalyst to help effect meaningful change and was deployed as a charter for action for those affected by cancer in Europe. It received the prestigious European Health

Award at the European Health Forum Gastein in 2018, an award which recognises health initiatives with Europe-wide impact. Further data analyses and a series of modelling approaches of the impact of cancer inequalities and what would need to be done to mitigate these inequalities informed the creation of a 70:35 Vision, an ambitious but achievable vision for 70% long term survival for cancer patients across Europe by 2035 [21, 22].

As part of this 70:35 Vision and underpinned by data intelligence that had been gathered, working across the European Cancer Organisation (ECO), we created the European Code of Cancer Practice [23], a series of ten patient-centred rights that define what cancer patients must expect from their health system, in order to receive optimal care, informed by research (Fig. 1). The Code of Practice, which has been translated into over 30 different languages to date and highlighted in a series of national launches supported by national Ministers of Health or their counterparts, has resonated significantly across the continent of Europe.

Key aspirations of the European Code of Cancer Practice are:

- To empower cancer patients to be active participants rather than passive recipients in their own care.
- To address the inequalities that many patients are experiencing every single day of their lives.
- To ensure that cancer patients receive quality treatment to achieve the best possible outcomes, no matter where they live.
- To achieve the aim of an average of 70% long term survival for cancer patients by 2035 (The 70/35 Vision) with progress on cancer control, patient experience and quality-of-life.

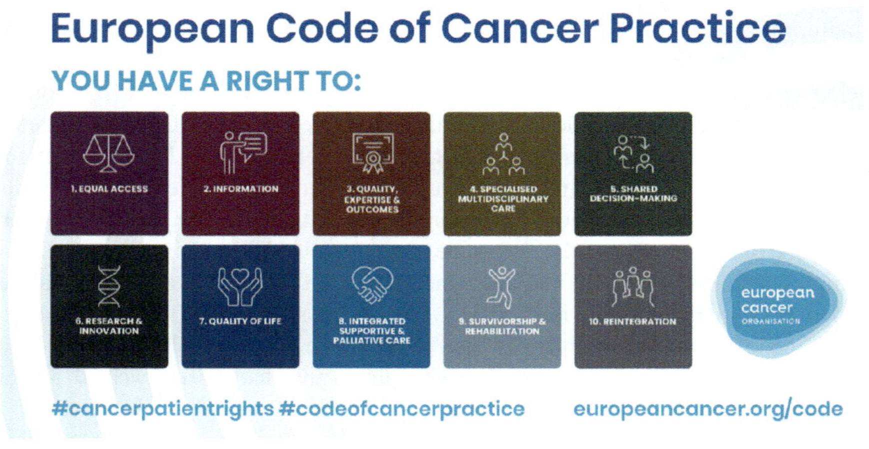

Fig. 1 The European Code of Cancer Practice—what patients should expect from their health system

- To embed rights that patients should expect from their health system into European cancer policy.

The European Code of Cancer Practice sets out a series of ten key overarching rights, and in particular signposts what patients should expect from their health system, in order for them to achieve the best possible outcomes. It is an empowerment tool to ensure the best available care is delivered for European citizens and patients. Each of the ten overarching rights is linked to three questions that a patient/parent/guardian may choose to ask their healthcare professionals. Within the Code of Cancer Practice, there is a particular focus on survivorship, reflected in the last four rights of the code—Quality-of-Life; Integrated, Supportive and Palliative Care; Survivorship and Rehabilitation; Re-integration. There is a clear need to focus on the challenges faced by the 20 million Europeans who are living beyond their cancer [24].

Recognising that rural and coastal regions represent areas of even greater cancer inequalities, the European Code of Cancer Practice has now been adapted to address the cancer inequalities that people living in these regions/communities face [25].

6 The European Cancer Pulse: Providing the Evidence Base for Cancer Inequalities in Europe

Recognising the importance of capturing and deploying data to enhance our understanding of cancer inequalities and to narrow the inequalities gap in Europe, the European Cancer Organisation has created the European Cancer Pulse, a data collection initiative that provides an interactive tool to navigate and map the cancer data inequalities that exist across the WHO Europe region [26]. It includes over 250 data indicators and greater than 13,000 data measurements across 50 European countries, capturing a wide variety of data sources [27]. It has informed the development of a series of country data reports, which highlight both inequality domains where countries are doing well and those that require often urgent recalibration of effort to address significant cancer inequalities and their sequelae. The Pulse specifically calls out over 20 categories where there is significant evidence of cancer inequalities, both within and between countries. Certain thematic domains require access to more data sources to capture the inequalities including surgery, work force, quality-of-life and patient recorded outcome measures. This unique data tool provides invaluable intelligence to national cancer agencies in order to modify/change/enhance their cancer policies and strategies.

7 It's All About the Data: No Matter Where You Live

The principles that underpinned the creation of the European Cancer Patient's Bill of Rights, the 70:35 Vision, the European Code of Cancer Practice and the European Cancer Pulse should inform all of our collective efforts that seek to inform, improve or enhance cancer healthcare delivery. Initiatives such as Concord [28], Eurocare [29], and the International Cancer Benchmarking Partnership (ICBP) [30] provide comparative information that facilitate a greater understanding of the challenges that health systems face, but also help identify the opportunities for improvement that will ensue from sharing data and best practice. Deploying this type of intelligence to inform our decision-making is critically important to ensure the best possible outcomes for our patients.

8   Making the Economic Case for Cancer Policy Change

The data required to inform changes in cancer policy can come from unusual sources. A key patient-informed campaign, led by Bowel Cancer UK in collaboration with a number of academic institutions and patient advocates, sought to provide the evidence base that would end the surprising practice in England (not in place in any other of the UK nations) whereby colorectal cancer patients who were receiving cetuximab treatment were not permitted to go on treatment breaks, despite lack of evidence that these treatment breaks were having any negative impact on patient outcomes, and in the face of potential indicators of slightly better quality-of-life and tumour re-sensitisation with an intermittent cetuximab treatment strategy. Despite this data intelligence and a series of patient testimonials, the crucial evidence that underpinned a change in policy by NHS England was the in depth health economic analysis which was performed, which among other things indicated that a change in policy to an intermittent treatment approach could save £1.2 billion for the NHS [31]. The impact of this particular piece of work was such that it was recognised by the Health Data Research UK's Impact of the Year Award in 2022.

9   How Consistent Cancer Policy Informed by Data, Leads to Better Cancer Outcomes

Crucial to ensuring that the innovations that are developed through high quality cancer research and optimal cancer care lead to better outcomes for cancer patients is the presence and implementation of a national cancer control strategy for each country or jurisdiction. But the policy that underpins national cancer control must be consistent. ICBP is an international partnership of clinicians, researchers, data experts and policy makers which involves 21 different international jurisdictions (Canada, Australia and New Zealand have federal health systems, hence there will be several to many jurisdictions in individual countries). ICBP explores the differences that it observes (mostly through data collected and analysed from cancer registries) in cancer survival and outcomes between these jurisdictions, and evaluates which are the factors that may be contributing to these differences. These data underpin the cancer intelligence and evidence that informs policy and ultimately may lead to clinical practice change, in order to ensure better patient outcomes.

A comprehensive study undertaken by the ICBP highlighted how an observed consistency of cancer policy improved cancer outcomes in six of seven cancers that were analysed [32]. This led to the development of a cancer policy scorecard, which ranked each jurisdiction/country for their consistency of cancer policy. Denmark was ranked highest, closely followed by New South Wales (Australia) and Ontario (Canada); countries including Norway and Ireland were, as it were mid-table, while the UK nations (England, Scotland, Wales and Northern Ireland) and New Zealand were found at the bottom of this particular league table. Despite this evidence, which supports the need for a National Cancer Plan, England has abandoned its cancer strategy and moved to a major conditions strategy [33], This goes against international best practice, with Europe having both a Beating Cancer Plan [34] and a Cancer Mission [35], while the US has, last year, launched its first National Cancer Plan [36]. The ICBP data were presented to the Health and Social Care select Committee's Inquiry on the Future of Cancer, providing strong evidence to reverse the abandonment of the national cancer control strategy [37]. A group of UK cancer experts have captured the evidence to support a UK-wide National Cancer Plan [38] which they launched in the House of Commons in November 2023.

10   Conclusions

A by-product of the COVID-19 pandemic and society's response to it, has meant that as a global community we are now more familiar with health data and its use to draw particular conclusions and agree specific actions to enhance human health and well-being. We must ensure that data intelligence is always part of our armamentarium against cancer. Historically, decisions in relation to approaches and policies on cancer tended to be based more on opinion, rather than hard data. This was partially because of the paucity of good data sources and lack of relevant intelligence to inform policy, but also the product of a particular mindset. Categorically this is no longer the case. A cancer health system informed by evidence not opinion will ensure that we make the correct decisions that will have the greatest impact for both patients and citizens. Data have, and will continue to save lives.

Acknowledgements ML is supported in this work by a grant from the Higher Education Authority North South Research Programme and a grant from Health Data Research UK.

References

1. Lawler M, Siu LL, Rehm HR, Chanock SJ, Alterovitz G, Burn J, Calvo F, Lacombe D, Teh BT, North KN, Sawyers CL. All the world's a stage. Facilitating discovery science and improved cancer care through the global alliance for genomics and health. Cancer Discov. 2015;5:1133–6. https://doi.org/10.1158/2159-8290.cd-15-0821
2. Siu LL, Lawler M, Haussler D, Knoppers BM, Lewin J, Vis DJ, Liao RG, Andre F, Banks I, Barrett JC, Caldas C, Camargo AA, Fitzgerald RC, Mao M, Mattison JE, Pao W, Sellers WR, Sullivan P, Teh BT, Ward RL, ZenKlusen JC, Sawyers CL, Voest EE. Facilitating a culture of

responsible and effective sharing of cancer genome data. Nat Med. 2016;22:464–71. https://doi.org/10.1038/nm.4089.

3. Vis DJ, Lewin J, Liao RG, Mao M, Andre F, Ward RL, Calvo F, Teh BT, Camargo AA, Knoppers BM, Sawyers CL, Wessels LFA, Lawler M, Siu LL, Voest E, Clinical Working Group of the Global Alliance for Genomics and Health. Towards a global cancer knowledge network: dissecting the current international cancer genomic sequencing landscape. Ann Oncol. 2017;28:1145–51. https://doi.org/10.1093/annonc/mdx037.

4. Lawler M, Haussler D, Siu LL, Haendel MA, McMurry JA, Knoppers BM, Chanock SJ, Calvo F, The BT, Walia G, Banks I, Yu PP, Staudt LM, Sawyers CL. Clinical cancer genome task team of the Global Alliance for Genomics and Health(GA4GH) sharing clinical and genomic data on cancer—the need for global solutions. N Engl J Med. 2017;376:2006–9. https://doi.org/10.1056/NEJMp1612254.

5. Wagner AH, Walsh B, Mayfield G, Tamborero D, Sonkin D, Krysiak K, Deu-Pons J, Duren RP, Gao J, McMurry J, Patterson S, Del Vecchio FC, Pitel BA, Sezerman OU, Ellrott K, Warner JL, Rieke DT, Aittokallio T, Cerami E, Ritter DI, Schriml LM, Freimuth RR, Haendel M, Raca G, Madhavan S, Baudis M, Beckmann JS, Dienstmann R, Chakravarty D, Li XS, Mockus S, Elemento O, Schultz N, Lopez-Bigas N, Lawler M, Goecks J, Griffith M, Griffith OL, Margolin AA, Variant Interpretation for Cancer Consortium. A harmonized meta-knowledgebase of clinical interpretations of somatic genomic variants in cancer. Nat Genet. 2020;52:448–57. https://doi.org/10.1038/s41588-020-0603-8.

6. Lawler M, Morris AD, Sullivan R, Birney E, Middleton A, Makaroff L, Knoppers BM, Horgan D, Eggermont A. A roadmap for restoring trust in big data. Lancet Oncol. 2018;19:1014–5. https://doi.org/10.1016/S1470-2045(18)30425-X.

7. Wheatstone P, Gath J, Carrigan C, Hall G, Cook Y, DATA-CAN, Sujenthiran A, Peach J, Davie C, Lawler M. DATA-CAN: a co-created cancer data knowledge network to deliver better outcomes and higher societal value. BMJ Partnerships Practice. 2021; https://blogs.bmj.com/bmj/2021/08/11/data-can-a-co-created-cancer-data-knowledge-network-to-deliver-better-outcomes-and-higher-societal-value/.

8. Lawler M, Maughan T. From Rosalind Franklin to Barack Obama: data sharing challenges and solutions in genomics and personalised medicine. New Bioeth. 2017;23:64–73. https://doi.org/10.1080/20502877.2017.1314883.

9. Vrdoljak E, Sullivan R, Lawler M. Cancer and coronavirus disease 2019; how do we manage cancer optimally through a public health crisis? Eur J Cancer. 2020;132:98–9. https://doi.org/10.1016/j.ejca.2020.04.001.

10. Lai AG, Pasea L, Banerjee A, Hall G, Denaxas S, Chang WH, Katsoulis M, Williams B, Pillay D, Noursadeghi M, Linch D, Hughes D, Forster D, Turnbull C, Fitzpatrick NK, Boyd K, Foster GR, Enver T, DATA-CAN, Cooper M, Jones M, Pritchard-Jones K, Sullivan R, Davie C, Lawler M, Hemingway H. Estimating excess mortality in people with cancer and multimorbidity in the COVID-19 emergency medRxiv 2020. https://doi.org/10.1101/2020.05.27.20083287.

11. Lai AG, Pasea L, Banerjee A, Hall G, Denaxas S, Chang WH, Katsoulis M, Williams B, Pillay D, Noursadeghi M, Linch D, Hughes D, Forster MD, Turnbull C, Fitzpatrick NK, Boyd K, Foster GR, Enver T, Nafilyan V, Humberstone B, Neal RD, Cooper M, Jones M, Pritchard-Jones K, Sullivan R, Davie C, Lawler M, Hemingway H. Estimated impact of the COVID-19 pandemic on cancer services and excess 1-year mortality in people with cancer and multimorbidity: near real-time data on cancer care, cancer deaths and a population-based cohort study. BMJ Open. 2020;10(11):e043828. https://doi.org/10.1136/bmjopen-2020-043828.

12. Sud A, Torr B, Loveday C, Jones M, Broggio J, Scott S, Gronthoud F, , Nicol DL, Garrett A, Jhanji S, Boyce SA, Williams M, Lyratzopoulos G, Barry C, Riboli E, Kipps E, Larkin Navani N, Swanton C, McFerran E, Muller DC, Lawler M, Houlston R, Turnbull C. Effect of delays in the 2-week-wait cancer referral pathway during the COVID-19 pandemic on cancer survival in the UK: a modelling study Lancet Oncol 2020 21:1035–1044. https://doi.org/10.1016/S1470-2045(20)30392-2.

13. Greene G, Griffiths R, Han J, Akbari A, Jones M, Lyons J, Lyons RA, Rolles M, Torabi F, Warlow J, Morris ERA, Lawler M, Huws DW. Impact of the SARS-CoV-2 pandemic on female breast, colorectal and non-small cell lung cancer incidence, stage and healthcare pathway to diagnosis during 2020 in Wales, UK, using a national cancer clinical record system. Br J Cancer. 2022;127(3):558–68. https://doi.org/10.1038/s41416-022-01830-6.

14. Greene GJ, Thomson CS, Donnelly D, Chung D, Bhatti L, Gavin AT, Lawler M, Huws DW, Rolles MJ, Bennée F, Morrison DS. Whole-population trends in pathology-confirmed cancer incidence in Northern Ireland, Scotland and Wales during the SARS-CoV-2 pandemic: a retrospective observational study. Cancer Epidemiol. 2023;84:102367. https://doi.org/10.1016/j.canep.2023.102367. Epub 2023 Apr 21.

15. Loveday C, Sud A, Jones M, Broggio J, Scott S, Torr B, Garrett A, Nicol DL, Jhanji S, Boyce SA, Williams M, Lyratzopoulos G, Barry C, Riboli E, Kipps E, McFerran E, Muller DC, Lawler M, Abulafi M, Houlston R, Turnbull C. Prioritisation by FIT to mitigate the impact of delays in the 2-week wait colorectal cancer referral pathway during the COVID-19 pandemic: a UK modelling study. Gut. 2020;70(6):1053–60. https://doi.org/10.1136/gutjnl-2020-321650.

16. Ho KMA, Banerjee A, Lawler M, Rutter MD, Lovat LB. Predicting endoscopic activity recovery in England after COVID-19: a national analysis. Lancet Gastroenterol Hepatol. 2021;6:381–90. https://doi.org/10.1016/S2468-1253(21)00058-3.

17. Lawler M, Crul M. Data must underpin our response to the COVID-19 pandemic's disastrous impact on cancer. BMJ. 2022;376:o282. https://doi.org/10.1136/bmj.o282.

18. Banerjee A, Sudlow C, Lawler M. Indirect effects of the pandemic: highlighting the need for data-driven policy and preparedness. J R Soc Med. 2022;10:1410768221095245. https://doi.org/10.1177/01410768221095245.

19. Lawler M, Le Chevalier T, Banks I, Conte P, De Lorenzo F, Meunier F, Pinedo HM, Selby P, Murphy MJ, Johnston PG, European Cancer Concord (ECC). A bill of rights for patients with cancer in Europe. Lancet Oncol. 2014;15:258–60. https://doi.org/10.1016/S1470-2045(13)70552-7.

20. Lawler M, Le Chevalier T, Murphy MJ Jr, Banks I, Conte P, De Lorenzo F, Meunier F, Pinedo HM, Selby P, Armand JP, Barbacid M, Barzach M, Bergh J, Bode G, Cameron DA, de Braud F, de Gramont A, Diehl V, Diler S, Erdem S, Fitzpatrick JM, Geissler J, Hollywood D, Højgaard L, Horgan D, Jassem J, Johnson PW, Kapitein P, Kelly J, Kloezen S, La Vecchia C, Löwenberg B, Oliver K, Sullivan R, Tabernero J, Van de Velde CJ, Wilking N, Wilson R, Zielinski C, Zur Hausen H, Johnston PG. A catalyst for change: The European cancer patient's bill of rights. Oncologist. 2014;19:217–24. https://doi.org/10.1634/theoncologist.2013-0452.

21. Lawler M, Selby P, Banks I, Law K, Albreht T, Armand JP, Barbacid M, Barzach M, Bergh J, Cameron D, Conte P, de Braud F, de Gramont A, De Lorenzo F, Diehl V, Diler S, Erdem S, Geissler J, Gore-Booth J, Henning G, Højgaard L, Horgan D, Jassem J, Johnson P, Kaasa S, Kapitein P, Karjalainen S, Kelly J, Kienesberger A, La Vecchia C, Lacombe D, Lindahl T, Löwenberg B, Luzzatto L, Malby R, Mastris K, Meunier F, Murphy M, Naredi P, Nurse P, Oliver K, Pearce J, Pelouchov J, Piccart M, Pinedo B, Spurrier-Bernard G, Sullivan R, Tabernero J, Van de Velde C, van Herk B, Vedsted P, Waldmann A, Weller D, Wilking N, Wilson R, Yared W, Zielinski C, Zur Hausen H, Le Chevalier T, Johnston P. The European cancer patient's bill of rights, update and implementation 2016. ESMO Open. 2017;1:e000127. https://doi.org/10.1136/esmoopen-2016-000127.

22. Lawler M, Davies L, Oberst S, Oliver K, Eggermont A, Schmutz A, La Vecchia C, Allemani C, Lievens Y, Naredi P, Cufer T, Aggarwal A, Aapro M, Apostolidis K, Baird AM, Cardoso F, Charalambous A, Coleman MP, Costa A, Crul M, Dégi CL, Di Nicolantonio F, Erdem S, Geanta M, Geissler J, Jassem J, Jagielska B, Jonsson B, Kelly D, Kelm O, Kolarova T, Kutluk T, Lewison G, Meunier F, Pelouchova J, Philip T, Price R, Rau B, Rubio IT, Selby P, Južnič Sotlar M, Spurrier-Bernard G, van Hoeve JC, Vrdoljak E, Westerhuis W, Wojciechowska U, Sullivan R. European Groundshot-addressing Europe's cancer research challenges: a lancet oncology commission. Lancet Oncol. 2023;24(1):e11–56. https://doi.org/10.1016/S1470-2045(22)00540-X. Epub 2022 Nov 16.

23. Lawler M, Oliver K, Stefan Gijssels S, Aapro M, Abolina A, Albreht A, Erdem S, Geissler J, Jassem J, Karjalainen S, La Vecchia C, Lievens Y, Meunier F, Morrisey M, Naredi P, Oberst S, Poortmans P, Price R, Sullivan R, Velikova G, Vrdoljak E, Wilking N, Yared W, Selby P. The European code of cancer practice. J Cancer Policy. 2021;28:100282. https://doi.org/10.1016/j.jcpo.2021.100282.

24. Lawler M, De Lorenzo F, Lagergren P, Mennini FS, Narbutas S, Scocca G, Meunier F, European Academy of Cancer Sciences. Challenges and solutions to embed cancer survivorship research and innovation within the EU Cancer Mission. Mol Oncol. 2021;15:1750–8. https://doi.org/10.1002/1878-0261.13022.

25. Nelson D, Selby P, Kane R, Harding-Bell A, Kenny A, McPeake K, Cooke S, Hogue T, Oliver K, Gussy M, Lawler M. Implementing the European code of cancer practice in rural settings. J Cancer Policy. 2024;39:100465. https://doi.org/10.1016/j.jcpo.2023.100465. Online ahead of print.

26. Couespel N, Venegoni E, Lawler M. The European cancer pulse: tracking inequalities in cancer control for citizen benefit. Lancet Oncol. 2023;24(5):441–2. https://doi.org/10.1016/S1470-2045(23)00140-7.

27. European Cancer Organisation. Tracking inequalities in cancer: The European Cancer Pulse. 2024. https://www.europeancancer.org/pulse.

28. EUROCARE Survival and prevalence of cancer patients in Europe. 2023. https://www.iss.it/eurocare-il-progetto.

29. CONCORD Programme. 2024. https://csg.lshtm.ac.uk/research/themes/concord-programme/.

30. International Cancer Benchmarking Partnership 2024. https://www.cancerresearchuk.org/health-professional/data-and-statistics/international-cancer-benchmarking-partnership-icbp.

31. Henderson RH, French D, McFerran E, Adams R, Wasan H, Glynne-Jones R, Fisher D, Richman S, Dunne PD, Wilde L, Maughan TS, Sullivan R, Lawler M. Spend less to achieve more: economic analysis of intermittent versus continuous cetuximab in KRAS wild-type patients with metastatic colorectal cancer. J Cancer Policy. 2022;33:100342. https://doi.org/10.1016/j.jcpo.2022.100342. Online ahead of print.

32. Nolte E, Morris M, Landon S, McKee M, Seguin M, Butler J, Lawler M. Exploring the link between cancer policies and cancer survival: a comparison of international cancer benchmarking partnership countries. Lancet Oncol. 2022;23(11):e502–14. https://doi.org/10.1016/S1470-2045(22)00450-8.

33. Policy paper. Major conditions strategy: case for change and our strategic framework. 21 Aug 2023. https://www.gov.uk/government/publications/major-conditions-strategy-case-for-change-and-our-strategic-framework/major-conditions-strategy-case-for-change-and-our-strategic-framework%2D%2D.

34. Europe's Beating Cancer Plan Communication from the commission to the European Parliament and the Council. February 2022. https://health.ec.europa.eu/system/files/2022-02/eu_cancer-plan_en_0.pdf.

35. EU Mission: Cancer. https://research-and-innovation.ec.europa.eu/funding/funding-opportunities/funding-programmes-and-open-calls/horizon-europe/eu-missions-horizon-europe/eu-mission-cancer_en.

36. About the National Cancer Plan. 9 July 2024. https://nationalcancerplan.cancer.gov/about.

37. Future cancer—oral evidence. 9 January 2024. https://committees.parliament.uk/event/20227https://committees.parliament.uk/event/20227.

38. Aggarwal A, Choudhury A, Fearnhead N, Kearns P, Kirby A, Lawler M, Quinlan S, Palmieri C, Roques T, Simcock R, Walter FM, Price P, Sullivan R. The future of cancer care in the UK-time for a radical and sustainable National Cancer Plan. Lancet Oncol. 2024;25(1):e6–17. https://doi.org/10.1016/S1470-2045(23)00511-9.

Challenges and Future Directions

Andreas Charalambous

1 Introduction

The healthcare industry evolution from Healthcare 1.0 to 4.0 has paved the way for the introduction of many innovations within the healthcare context. Perhaps one of the main innovations came from the development and integration of technological solutions as means to enhance services across the disease continuum provided in the healthcare domain. In recent years, different technological solutions have been introduced to enhance the provided care, optimize treatment options, improve medical diagnoses, support health decision making, increase patient's self-management, and remotely monitor the health status of the patient to name a few.

The progress of technological solutions in the realm of healthcare can also be viewed in the evolution of patient health records. Patient's health records manual storing from the physician (Healthcare 1.0) has been replaced in Healthcare 2.0 by holding the patient's health history in electronic form. In Healthcare 3.0, the wearable devices were introduced as an innovative way to retrieve health data for medical diagnosis purposes and real-time health monitoring. When Healthcare 4.0 came, the focus was shifted to ensuring the privacy and integrity of health data [1]. Advanced medical wearable devices were developed and complemented with artificial intelligence (AI) and machine learning algorithms to track, for example, blood pressure, glucose level, temperature, electrocardiogram (ECG), electroencephalogram (EEG), and perform medical diagnoses as well as supporting health decision making. Internet of Medical Things (IoMT) technologies allowed seamless connectivity between patients and doctors using communication technologies like Bluetooth, Wi-Fi, Zigbee, COAP, MQTT, and many more. They opened ideas to new domains like

A. Charalambous (✉)
Faculty of Health Science, Department of Nursing Science, Cyprus University of Technology, Limassol, Cyprus
e-mail: Andreas.charalambous@cut.ac.cy

© The Author(s), under exclusive license to Springer Nature Switzerland AG 2025
A. Charalambous (ed.), *Critical Perspectives on Technological Innovations in Healthcare*, https://doi.org/10.1007/978-3-031-87158-0_13

telehealthcare where the patient is continuously monitored using data collected by wearable sensors, and the electronic health record (EHR) is updated frequently with this data in a central database. This form of EHR also allowed the accessibility of the data not only between service providers but also between countries to facilitate the mobility of patients and the continuation of their treatment [2].

Despite the many technological breakthroughs in the healthcare domain, the evolution has not been recorded on a global scale. Conventional healthcare systems have been generating various challenges for the evolution to be fully manifested. Challenges that have been identified include network latency, fragmented and erroneous health data, gaps in workflows due to incompatible and vendor-specific healthcare solutions, lack of privacy and integrity of health data, lack of complete and comprehensive health history of patients, and lack of a trusted, secure health data-sharing platform to process data gathered from different healthcare systems. Furthermore, regulatory and interoperability challenges have also been identified as main contributors to the efficient and effective integration and sustainability of technology within healthcare.

2 Challenges

2.1 Regulatory Framework: Safeguarding the Future of Technologies in Healthcare

AI provides endless possibilities that are not merely limited to analyze and act on big data at speed and at levels of accuracy that exceed those of humans. Machine learning can also be built into AI algorithms, enabling them to learn from their mistakes, evolve and improve their performance (also refer to chapter "How SARS-CoV-2 Changed the Landscape of Healthcare: Opportunities for Technological Innovation"). Although the benefits of healthcare AI are great and new possibilities and areas of infiltration are identified on a constant basis, patients still need protection from defective diagnosis, unacceptable use of personal data, and the elimination of bias built into algorithms. With the rapid development and integration of technologies in healthcare, the need for a regulatory framework has become now more than ever more necessary.

Regulating technologies such as healthcare AI are a challenging task due to the dynamic nature of this technology that is complex to regulate. The difficulties in this filed are reflected on the fact that their regulation is still in its infancy and regulators are playing catch-up. While both the EU and US have taken tentative steps in this area—signaling the need for regulation and issuing proposals—there are still no concrete laws in place.

The European Commission, published in 2020 a "White Paper on Artificial Intelligence—A European approach to excellence and trust." The paper deals with policy and regulatory options toward an ecosystem for excellence and trust. The European Commission's (EC) white paper evolved to the proposed Artificial Intelligence Act, the first comprehensive regulation on AI by a major regulator anywhere, published in April 2021 [3] and subsequently updated with a final draft in April 2024 [4], aims to fill the regulatory void, creating the first legal framework on AI—turning Europe into a global hub for trustworthy AI. The AI Act classifies AI according to its risk:

- Unacceptable risk is prohibited (e.g., social scoring systems and manipulative AI).
- Most of the text addresses high-risk AI systems, which are regulated.
- A smaller section handles limited risk AI systems, subject to lighter transparency obligations: developers and deployers must ensure that end-users are aware that they are interacting with AI (i.e., chatbots and deepfakes).
- Minimal risk is unregulated (including the majority of AI applications currently available on the EU single market, such as AI enabled video games and spam filters—at least in 2021; this is changing with generative AI) [5].

The implementation of the AI Act will become the responsibility of the AI Office which will be established, sitting within the Commission, to monitor the effective implementation and compliance of general-purpose AI (GPAI) model providers. Downstream providers can lodge a complaint regarding the upstream providers infringement to the AI Office. The AI Office may conduct evaluations of the GPAI model to:

- assess compliance where the information gathered under its powers to request information is insufficient.
- investigate systemic risks, particularly following a qualified report from the scientific panel of independent experts [5].

In the USA, there have been similar efforts toward this path, resulting in the FDA's Artificial Intelligence/Machine Learning (AI-ML)-Based Software as a Medical Device (SaMD) Action Plan, which was published in January 2021 [6]. It is envisioned that the plan will enable the FDA to provide a reasonable assurance of safety and effectiveness while embracing the iterative improvement power of AI and machine learning-based software as a medical device. Toward achieving this, the AI/ML-Based Software as a Medical Device Action Plan focuses on five areas of action including:

- Further developing the proposed regulatory framework, including through issuance of draft guidance on a predetermined change control plan (for software's learning over time);
- Supporting the development of good machine learning practices to evaluate and improve machine learning algorithms;
- Fostering a patient-centered approach, including device transparency to users;
- Developing methods to evaluate and improve machine learning algorithms; and
- Advancing real-world performance monitoring pilots [7].

Despite the efforts on regulating technologies in healthcare, the proposed regulatory frameworks are not without limitations. One of the most important issues to highlight is that these regulations do not apply to certain AI applications (e.g., software intended to support people in maintaining a healthy lifestyle, software that provides clinical support or recommendations to healthcare professionals) [8]. The reason for such limitation is attributed to the fact that the individual is expected to be qualified to make his or her own rational decisions based on the recommendations provided by the AI application [9]. A review of the varying strategies for regulatory frameworks across the world for the use of AI in healthcare shows that regulations currently mostly adopt a soft-law approach. Soft-law approaches can include professional guidelines, voluntary standards, and codes of conduct that are adopted by governments and the industry [8]. Such soft-law approach for regulating AI in healthcare, place substantial expectations for the relevant stakeholders to consider during the development of AI's technological innovations; however, they are not directly enforced by governments which can be considered as a significant limitation [10].

2.2 Interoperability and Devices Heterogeneity

The healthcare setting is becoming increasingly complex, governed by novel diagnostic and therapeutic regimes, new procedures, and the existence of multiple professional groups, each with its own set of characteristics, requirements, and working methods. In this complex environment, the introduction of health information systems (e.g., software, devices) was required to ensure the long-term stability of the healthcare system. However, the systems currently in use are proprietary, may differ from one health institution to the next, and were developed for local access, resulting in heterogeneity in the existing ecosystems [11]. Similarly, each manufacturer has its proprietary protocol, which means, for example, that devices and sensors made by different manufacturers cannot necessarily communicate with each other. Device management requires directories of devices' functionality, protocols, terminologies, and standards compliance [12]. Because of segregated data and legal regulations, many of these technologies cannot operate together, leaving healthcare providers and personnel to undertake the manual job, which comes at a high cost. Therefore, these conditions generate interoperability issues which hinder the deployment and operability of the health information systems to their full capacity. A recent systematic review by Pournik et al. [13] showed that interoperability challenges can be varying in the field of Internet of Medical Things (IoMT) and include the following categories: of device heterogeneity, system heterogeneity, data standardization, security and safety, system and architecture standard, system and workflow integration, and regulatory and compliance requirements.

Interoperability is a significant challenge in creating medical devices that easily connect with other devices and sensors to health providers' electronic medical record systems. Interoperability refers to the ability of different medical devices, systems, and software applications to communicate, exchange data, and work together effectively [14]. Interoperability allows the huge amount of data generated and collected by medical devices and systems such as wearable sensors, remote monitoring devices, electronic health records, and healthcare management systems to be shared, integrated, and utilized across different devices and platforms, enabling healthcare providers to make informed decisions, improve care coordination, and ultimately achieve a more efficient and patient-centered care [13]. However, it takes time to corroborate such a massive amount of data with the different terminologies and standards on every system and might even yield inaccurate results.

Interoperability is a complex concept which affects different elements of the health information system thus, the necessary actions to address the problems of interoperability need to be addressed at different areas of these systems. Another aspect that needs to be considered is that interoperability also has the local characteristics and reality incorporated. Therefore, some of the aspects of any proposed solutions for addressing the barriers to interoperability need to be center-specific. The path to interoperability is one that goes through policy as many of the aspects that generate interoperability barriers require policy amendments. In the USA for example, as a means to promote interoperability, the twenty-first Century Cures Act (21CCA; 21CCA 2016) mandated the sharing of certain data elements, placed restrictions on information blocking, and promoted the use of application programming interfaces (APIs; e.g., Fast Healthcare Interoperability Resources [FHIR]) [15]. The 21CCA also established the Trusted Exchange Framework Common Agreement (TEFCA) that provides an infrastructure model and governing approach for health information exchange (HIE) networks [16]. Another aspect to be considered within the context of interoperability is the development and adoption of universal standards for the collection and validation of data. As a mean to create a health system that enables continuous improvements, we need systems that collect the data that are most important for patient care, for accomplishing critical analyses, for enhancing the level of evidence, and for addressing public health challenges [17, 18]. There needs to be an effort to develop universal standards for the collection and validation of the most clinically important data. These standards can ensure that only valid information is being correctly captured and delivered. Moreover, from a technological perspective, the diverse software, transfer engines, and information technology systems need to be able to correctly interpret these standards, and process standard nomenclatures and notations without corruption [19].

3 Future Directions

As the evolution of technology is moving at a fast pace constantly changing the landscape of healthcare, it is difficult to predict of how the future might look like as a result of the heavy infiltration of technologies across all healthcare domains. However, what is expected is that current technologies will be further developed, seamless integrated and more fine-tuned for example by the collection of large quality data from multiple resources (e.g., Real-World Data and Real-World Evidence) contributing to the earlier and accurate diagnosis, more personalized treatment regimes, and disease prevention to name a few.

Treatment decisions, for example, can be augmented by clinical decision support (CDS) systems and enriched with advanced analytics. AI-based systems offer the unique opportunity to augment clinician performance by creating order and transforming vast amounts of mostly unstructured data into clinically actionable information to support optimal care [20]. In the future, these systems will become more efficient in presenting the necessary information (removing for example "noisy" data) so that appropriate actions can be timely taken. For example, AI has been used to improve the speed of prediction and diagnosis of sepsis [21]. Integrated with the care delivery workflow, these technologies could identify patterns, form linkages between disparate data sources, and suggest treatment options for clinicians to review. In this context, it is expected that these breakthroughs will also evolve the capabilities of telemonitoring and teleconsultation as well as increasing the empowerment of the person through increased self-management. With the collection of more accurate patient data from multiple sources, decision-making processes at the home setting can be simplified, while the patient and informal caregiver can also attain information that can allow them to take actions (with or without healthcare oversight) toward the better management of the disease. While at the moment self-management at the home setting includes rather simple tasks, these developments of the technology (e.g., machine learning) and the more complete data will allow for more complex procedures to be undertaken independently at the home setting.

AI, particularly deep learning algorithms, has demonstrated remarkable capabilities in extracting valuable insights from medical images [22]. Deep learning models, trained on large datasets, are capable of recognizing complex patterns and features that may not be readily discernible to the human eye [23]. These algorithms can even provide a new perspective about what image features should be valued to support decisions. One of the key advantages of AI in medical imaging is its ability to enhance the accuracy and efficiency of disease diagnosis [24]. Through this process, AI can assist healthcare professionals in detecting abnormalities, identifying specific structures, and predicting disease outcomes [25].

Another tool that has been cautiously introduced in medical image-to-image translation are generative adversarial networks (GANs). Preceding studies showed that GANs are far from being equal as some are ill-suited for medical imaging applications while others are much better off [26]. The advantages and performance that have been successively achieved with their development have allowed GANs to become a successful technology that in the future will be more widely adopted within the imaging domain [25].

One of the major concerns generated by the rapid development of technology in healthcare is maintaining the focus on the person. Focusing too much on the technological aspects of the intervention (i.e., designing and delivering) poses as a potential threat to the person-centeredness and person-center care [27]. Fully engaging individuals in their health and well-being through digital health, responding to public demand for participation in the growing digital health ecosystem, and balancing demand for consistent, transparent protections for health data within and outside of the health care system is a priority in achieving a fully realized future for digital health. There needs to be acknowledged that health data are intensely personal, and unintentional exposure of that data has the potential to upset an individual's life. Capturing the full potential of digital health will require broad confidence in health systems and commercial ventures to protect the individual from negative outcomes [28].

The rapid development and application of digital health is also accompanied by the need for vigilance on equity and equality issues that include availability and access to the benefits of digital health, racial bias in AI, and misuse of personal information in discriminatory practices. For digital health to improve health and well-being, a data-centric and patient-centric approach to developing and deploying these tools is essential, and data must reflect the diverse communities and populations across the USA.

4 Conclusion

Envisioning and achieving a seamless, healthier future through digital innovation will require a deeper investment in evidence-based research, more clinical and field studies, and commitment from diverse stakeholders especially policy makers. Nevertheless, the potential impact of digital innovation which extends beyond the healthcare realm is enormous. Technological solutions have allowed for validated information (i.e., data from different sources), curated across the health data continuum and easily shared, enabling an insight at the point of care (i.e., also detecting shifts in health status as they manifest), easing provider burden and augmenting clinical reasoning skills. An "Internet of Things" in health care serves the public's need for accurate health advice, and a digital health ecosystem that provides high-quality, personalized, equitable care to all who need it is achievable and worthy of our best individual and collective efforts.

As healthcare technology becomes more advanced and available, the way that healthcare professionals and organizations interact with patients is rapidly shifting from the traditional in-person model of interaction. While these interactions will always be central to the healthcare industry, the rapid onset of COVID-19 caused a digital health revolution practically overnight. Now we are emerging into a new era, where technology walks hand in hand with traditional approaches—elevating the overall quality of care. In this new reality of healthcare, there needs to be efforts to maintain the center where it has always been, on the person. The introduction of technology should not be left to alter the nature of the interactions with the patients, which now more than even should be person-center. Technology should be developed with co-design approaches that provide the opportunity to potential end-users (i.e., patients) shape the features of the newly developed technology, placing emphasis not only on personalization but also customization [27].

The integration of technological solutions with healthcare system poses particular challenges like practical implementation feasibility, scalability, cost, network, power and resource requirements, seamless interoperability, and invasion of privacy of the patients, for example, devices attached to a person's body or constant monitoring could be invasive. These are problems that scholars, researchers, and other stakeholders need to turn the attention so that sustainable solutions can be devised without the technology losing its potential along the way (e.g., as a result of regulatory frameworks).

Future research needs to target developing more robust and reliable systems that can scale well, be energy efficient, and be easily integrated into the clinical pathways of healthcare systems. These systems need to take into consideration the realities and the capabilities of the host organization so that the end product can last over time. They should address privacy, security, scalability, seamless connectivity, interoperability, accuracy, and precision that can be achieved in forecasting and treating time-critical applications like asthma, strokes, seizures, or heart attacks. Another aspect that needs to be pursued in this context is to fully realize the vision of a learning health system. In the digital age, regardless of the specific barrier to the creation and support of individual and population health (e.g., staff burnout, financial restrains, and equity), digital health can and should act as a "force multiplier" of the interventions to combat these challenges.

The future is already here, it is just not very evenly distributed [29]

References

1. Krishnamoorthy S, Dua A, Gupta S. Role of emerging technologies in future IoT-driven Healthcare 4.0 technologies: a survey, current challenges and future directions. J Ambient Intell Human Comput. 2023;14:361–407. https://doi.org/10.1007/s12652-021-03302-w.
2. Shaver J. The state of telehealth before and after the COVID-19 pandemic. Prim Care. 2022;49(4):517–30. https://doi.org/10.1016/j.pop.2022.04.002. Epub 2022 Apr 25.
3. European Commission. The AI Act. https://artificialintelligenceact.eu/wp-content/uploads/2021/08/The-AI-Act.pdf. Accessed 13 Jul 2024.
4. European Commission. The AI Act. CORRIGENDUM https://www.europarl.europa.eu/doceo/document/TA-9-2024-0138-FNL-COR01_EN.pdf. Accessed 24 Jul 2024.
5. European Commission. The AI Act. Executive summary https://artificialintelligenceact.eu/high-level-summary/. Accessed 23 Jul 2024.
6. U.S. Food and Drug Administration. Intelligence/machine learning (AI/ML)-based software as a medical device (SaMD) action plan. https://www.fda.gov/news-events/press-announcements/fda-releases-artificial-intelligencemachine-learning-action-plan. Accessed 21 Jul 2024.
7. U.S. Food and Drug Administration. Intelligence/machine learning (AI/ML)-based software as a medical device (SaMD) action plan. Media Release. https://www.fda.gov/media/145022/download. Accessed 21 Jul 2024.
8. Palaniappan K, Lin EYT, Vogel S. Global regulatory frameworks for the use of artificial intelligence (AI) in the healthcare services sector. Healthcare. 2024;12(5):562. https://doi.org/10.3390/healthcare12050562.
9. Tsang L, Kracov DA, Mulryne J, Strom L, Perkins N, Dickinson R, Wallace VM, Jones B. The impact of artificial intelligence on medical innovation in the European Union and United States. Intellect Prop Technol Law J. 2017;29:3.
10. Taeihagh A. Governance of artificial intelligence. Polic Soc. 2021;40:137–57.
11. Dixon BE, Rahurkar S, Apathy NC. Interoperability and health information exchange for public health. In: Public health informatics and information systems. Cham: Springer; 2020. p. 307–24.

12. Torab-Miandoab A, Samad-Soltani T, Jodati A, Rezaei-Hachesu P. Interoperability of heterogeneous health information systems: a systematic literature review. BMC Med Inform Decis Mak. 2023;23(1):18. https://doi.org/10.1186/s12911-023-02115-5.
13. Pournik O, Mukherjee T, Ghalichi L, Arvanitis TN. How interoperability challenges are addressed in healthcare IoT projects. Stud Health Technol Inform. 2023;309:121–5. https://doi.org/10.3233/SHTI230754.
14. Yasmeen G, Javed N, Ahmed T. Interoperability: a challenge for IoMT. ECS Trans. 2022;107(1):4459.
15. Walker DM, Tarver WL, Jonnalagadda P, Ranbom L, Ford EW, Rahurkar S. Perspectives on challenges and opportunities for interoperability: findings from key informant interviews with stakeholders in Ohio. JMIR Med Inform. 2023;11:e43848. https://doi.org/10.2196/43848.
16. Pronovost P, Johns MM, Palmer S. Procuring interoperability: achieving high-quality, connected, and person-centered care. Washington, DC: National Academy of Medicine; 2018.
17. Parsons A, Unaka NI, Stewart C, Foster J, Perez V, Jones NY, Kahn R, Beck AF, Riley C. Seven practices for pursuing equity through learning health systems: notes from the field. Learn Health Syst. 2021;5(3):e10279. https://doi.org/10.1002/lrh2.10279.
18. Ros F, et al. Addressing the COVID-19 pandemic and future public health challenges through global collaboration and a data-driven systems approach. Learn Health Syst. 2020;5(1):e10253. https://doi.org/10.1002/lrh2.10253.
19. Szarfman A, Levine JG, Tonning JM, Weichold F, Bloom JC, Soreth JM, Geanacopoulos M, Callahan L, Spotnitz M, Ryan Q, Pease-Fye M, Brownstein JS, Ed Hammond W, Reich C, Altman RB. Recommendations for achieving interoperable and shareable medical data in the USA. Commun Med (Lond). 2022;2:86. https://doi.org/10.1038/s43856-022-00148-x.
20. Charalambous A, Dodlek N. Big data, machine learning, and artificial intelligence to advance cancer care: opportunities and challenges. Semin Oncol Nurs. 2023;39(3):151429. https://doi.org/10.1016/j.soncn.2023.151429. Epub 2023 Apr 20.
21. Goh KH, Wang L, Yeow AYK, Poh H, Li K, Yeow JJL, Tan GYH. Artificial intelligence in sepsis early prediction and diagnosis using unstructured data in healthcare. Nat Commun. 2021;12:711. https://doi.org/10.1038/s41467-021-20910-4.
22. Ghaffar NN, Kaplanoglu E, Nasab A. Evaluation of artificial intelligence techniques in disease diagnosis and prediction. Discov Artif Intell. 2023;3:5. https://doi.org/10.1007/s44163-023-00049-5.
23. Kumar Y, Koul A, Singla R, Ijaz MF. Artificial intelligence in disease diagnosis: a systematic literature review, synthesizing framework and future research agenda. J Ambient Intell Humaniz Comput. 2023;14:8459–86. https://doi.org/10.1007/s12652-021-03612-z.
24. Lazic I, Agullo F, Ausso S, Alves B, Barelle C, Berral JL, Bizopoulos P, Bunduc O, Chouvarda I, Dominguez D, et al. The holistic perspective of the INCISIVE project—artificial intelligence in screening mammography. Appl Sci. 2022;12(17):8755.
25. Pinto-Coelho L. How artificial intelligence is shaping medical imaging technology: a survey of innovations and applications. Bioengineering (Basel). 2023;10(12):1435. https://doi.org/10.3390/bioengineering10121435.
26. Kazeminia S, Baur C, Kuijper A, van Ginneken B, Navab N, Albarqouni S, Mukhopadhyay A. GANs for medical image analysis. Artif Intell Med. 2020;109:101938. https://doi.org/10.1016/j.artmed.2020.101938.
27. Charalambous A. Personalising the technological experience. In: Charalambous A, editor. Developing and utilizing digital technology in healthcare for assessment and monitoring. Cham: Springer; 2020. https://doi.org/10.1007/978-3-030-60697-8_2.
28. Abernethy A, Adams L, Barrett M, Bechtel C, Brennan P, Butte A, Faulkner J, Fontaine E, Friedhoff S, Halamka J, Howell M, Johnson K, Lee P, Long P, McGraw D, Miller R, Perlin J, Rucker D, Sandy L, Savage L, Stump L, Tang P, Topol E, Tuckson R, Valdes K. The promise of digital health: then, now, and the future. NAM perspectives. Discussion Paper. Washington, DC: National Academy of Medicine; 2022. https://doi.org/10.31478/202206e.
29. The science in science fiction. NPR; 2018. www.npr.org/2018/10/22/1067220/the-science-in-science-fiction?t=1655297648031.